Development and Evolution
of Brain Size

Behavioral Implications

Development and Evolution of Brain Size

Behavioral Implications

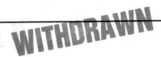

Edited by

MARTIN E. HAHN

Department of Biology
William Paterson College
Wayne, New Jersey

CRAIG JENSEN

Behavior Adjustment Program
Agnews State Hospital
San Jose, California

BRUCE C. DUDEK

Department of Psychology
State University of New York at Binghamton
Binghamton, New York

ACADEMIC PRESS

A Subsidiary of Harcourt Brace Jovanovich, Publishers

New York   London   Toronto   Sydney   San Francisco

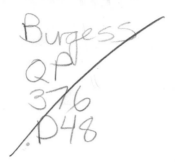

ACADEMIC PRESS, INC.
111 Fifth Avenue, New York, New York 10003

United Kingdom Edition published by
ACADEMIC PRESS, INC. (LONDON) LTD.
24/28 Oval Road, London NW1 7DX

Library of Congress Cataloging in Publication Data
Main entry under title:

Development and evolution of brain size.

Includes bibliographies and index.
1. Brain. 2. Neuropsychology. 3. Brain--Evolu-
tion. I. Hahn, Martin E. II. Jensen, Craig.
III. Dudek, Bruce C. IV. Title: Brain size.
QP376.D48   612'.82   79–23145
ISBN 0–12–314650–X

PRINTED IN THE UNITED STATES OF AMERICA

79 80 81 82   9 8 7 6 5 4 3 2 1

To John L. Fuller,
our mentor

Contents

Chapter I

Introduction: Toward Understanding the Brain–Behavior Relationship

CRAIG JENSEN, MARTIN E. HAHN, AND BRUCE C. DUDEK

Chapter II

Evolutionary Theory and the Evolution of the Human Brain

ERNST W. CASPARI

The Evolution of Diversity in Brain Size

HARRY J. JERISON

Brain Size, Allometry, and Reorganization: Toward a Synthesis

RALPH L. HOLLOWAY

Cerebral Indices and Behavioral Differences

WILLIAM I. RIDDELL

Correlated Brain and Intelligence Development in Humans

HERMAN T. EPSTEIN

Chapter VII

Genetic Techniques as Tools for Analysis of Brain–Behavior Relationships

THOMAS H. RODERICK

Chapter VIII

Correlates of Mouse Brain Weight: A Search for Component Morphological Traits

CYNTHIA WIMER

Chapter IX

Brain Weight, Brain Chemical Content, and Their Early Manipulation

STEPHEN ZAMENHOF AND EDITH VAN MARTHENS

Chapter XIV

Responsiveness of Brain Size to Individual Experience: Behavioral and Evolutionary Implications

MARK R. ROSENZWEIG

Chapter XV

Experience-Induced Changes in Brain Fine Structure: Their Behavioral Implications

WILLIAM T. GREENOUGH AND JANICE M. JURASKA

Chapter XVI

Effects of Early Undernutrition on Brain and Behavior of Developing Mice

Z. MICHAEL NAGY

List of Contributors

Numbers in parentheses indicate the pages on which the authors' contributions begin.

PETER J. BERMAN* (221), Department of Psychology, State University of New York at Binghamton, Binghamton, New York 13901

ERNST W. CASPARI (9), Department of Biology, University of Rochester, Rochester, New York 14627

BRUCE C. DUDEK† (1, 221, 371), Department of Psychology, State University of New York at Binghamton, Binghamton, New York 13901

HERMAN T. EPSTEIN (111), Biology Department, Brandeis University, Waltham, Massachusetts 02154

JOHN L. FULLER (187), Department of Psychology; State University of New York at Binghamton, Binghamton, New York 13901

WILLIAM T. GREENOUGH (295), Department of Psychology and Neural and Behavioral Biology Program, University of Illinois at Urbana-Champaign, Champaign, Illinois 61820

MARTIN E. HAHN (1, 239, 371), Department of Biology, William Paterson College, Wayne, New Jersey 07470

NORMAN D. HENDERSON (347), Department of Psychology, Oberlin College, Oberlin, Ohio 44074

*Present address: St. George's University, School of Medicine, Grenada, West Indies.
†Present address: Department of Psychology, State University of New York at Albany, Albany, New York 12222.

RALPH L. HOLLOWAY (59), Department of Anthropology, Columbia University, New York, New York 10027

CRAIG JENSEN (1, 205, 371), Behavior Adjustment Program, Agnews State Hospital, San Jose, California 95134

HARRY J. JERISON (29), Departments of Psychiatry and Biobehavioral Sciences, University of California, Los Angeles, School of Medicine, Los Angeles, California 90024

JANICE M. JURASKA (295), Department of Psychology and Neural and Behavioral Biology Program, University of Illinois at Urbana-Champaign, Champaign, Illinois 61820

Z. MICHAEL NAGY (321), Department of Psychology, Bowling Green State University, Bowling Green, Ohio 43403

WILLIAM I. RIDDELL (89), State University of New York at Brockport, Brockport, New York

THOMAS H. RODERICK (133), The Jackson Laboratory, Bar Harbor, Maine 04609

MARK R. ROSENZWEIG (263), Department of Psychology, University of California, Berkeley, Berkeley, California 94720

EDITH VAN MARTHENS (163), Mental Retardation Research Center and Brain Research Institute, University of California, Los Angeles, School of Medicine, Los Angeles, California 90024

CYNTHIA WIMER (147), Division of Neurosciences, City of Hope National Medical Center, Duarte, California 91010

STEPHEN ZAMENHOF (163), Mental Retardation Research Center and Brain Research Institute, University of California, Los Angeles, School of Medicine, Los Angeles, California 90024

Preface

The relationship between brain and behavior is a fascinating and extremely complex topic that has long interested man. Its formal study is interdisciplinary and multidisciplinary, encompassing such diverse techniques as electron microscopy and avoidance-learning paradigms. The results of the study appeal to a broad range of interests from evolutionary biology to clinical psychology, with numerous disciplinary stops in between.

The idea for our volume on this topic was rooted in the association among the editors and our mutual association with John L. Fuller. Each of us studied with Fuller and became involved in his research on genetic selection for brain size and its behavioral ramifications. As we became involved in the selection program, we were struck with some different notions: the importance of brain size for learning, the biochemical correlates of selection, and the impact of selection on developing behaviors. We were also struck with a common question—what is the importance of brain size per se? Lacking a satisfying answer, we decided to bring together a number of investigators in related areas to interact and share data and ideas.

The result was a plan for a book and a symposium entitled "Development and Evolution of Brain Size: Behavioral Implications." The symposium was held at William Paterson College in April 1978 and was highly successful in initiating contact and exchange of ideas among all.

Following the symposium, each participant wrote or rewrote his or her contribution to the book, taking into account the other presentations, as well as the formal and informal discussions. The volume that resulted integrates divergent areas and synthesizes thought on several aspects of the brain–behavior relationship. In particular, we believe that the reader will come away with a far greater understanding of the relationship between evolution and development as it impacts on brain size and behavior.

Acknowledgments

We thank the Academic Development Office and the School of Science at William Paterson College for support in the preparation of the manuscript for this book. We wish to thank our manuscript typist Ms. Maria Lavooy for her excellent and dedicated work, our indexer Ms. B.B. Huck, and, of course, the very professional work of the editorial and production staffs of Academic Press.

The symposium that preceeded the book was supported by the Academic Development Office and the Biopsychology Honors Program of William Paterson College. Five individuals deserve particular mention for their roles in making the symposium run smoothly: Dean Cliff Adelman, Jim Crawford, Jackie Lavooy, Pam Huck, and Dr. James Walters. We would also like to thank all the students of the Biopsychology Honors Program who gave freely of their time.

Chapter I

Introduction:
Toward Understanding the
Brain–Behavior Relationship

CRAIG JENSEN
MARTIN E. HAHN
BRUCE C. DUDEK

Most of the important questions regarding the relationship between brain size and behavior were asked prior to this century (for further details on the history of this problem, see Chapter XIV, this volume). Among them were

Do bigger brains allow more complex behaviors?
Is absolute brain size (weight or volume) an appropriate measure or should the "apropriate" measure somehow consider body size?
How and why have bigger brains evolved in hominids and other groups?
Does overall brain size predict values of brain substructures?
Can experience modify the substructure size or overall brain size?

While all of these and more questions have been posed previously, the experimental techniques required to answer these questions have only recently been developed.

It is now recognized that brain size is a dimension upon which organisms can be ordered meaningfully between as well as within species. Recent work has shown that overall brain size is influenced by many factors, including genes, hormones, nutrition, allometry, environmental enrichment, and maternal behavior. It is also recognized that brain size is related to behavior. Species with larger average brains, in relation to average body size, show greater ability to process and utilize complex

1

DEVELOPMENT AND EVOLUTION
OF BRAIN SIZE

information. With recent within-species demonstrations that brain size is related to learning performance and rate of behavioral development, the implications of variation in brain size for behavioral variation is also becoming apparent on a within-species level. Finally, it has been shown that the brain is a malleable organ, showing remarkable responsiveness to genetic and environmental influences.

Because these developments have taken place only recently, because of the tremendous volume of work in this area, and because the developments come from such diverse sources as evolutionary theory, anthropology, the neurosciences, and behavior genetics, there has necessarily been little intergration of separate areas. In order to obtain an integrated picture of the general relationship between brain size and behavior, it is necessary to consider such topics as brain evolution, brain development and plasticity, variation in brain size (both overall and substructure), genetic and environmental manipulation of brain parameters, behavioral capabilities (both between and within species), and behavioral development.

To provide an opportunity for the integration of diverse areas and to make investigators in these areas more aware of parallel developments in related fields, a symposium on the *Development and Evolution of Brain Size: Behavioral Implications* was held at William Paterson College in Wayne, New Jersey. In organizing the conference we were interested in the general question of the relationship between brain size and behavior. Of necessity, we delimited the area and settled on three questions for careful examination.

1. What is the importance of brain size for behavior?
2. What are the effects of genetic selection for brain size on brain substructures and behavior?
3. Do genetic and environmental manipulations of brain size have similar consequences?

Some readers may consider these questions to be heavily interrelated and some may not. While the questions seemed related to us, our reading suggested that the major names associated with research on each question were different and we hoped that by bringing these investigators together in a symposium we could help forge an integration of these seemingly divergent areas and points of view.

What Is the Importance of Brain Size for Behavior?

In order to bring contemporary points of view to bear on the first question, "What is the importance of brain size for behavior?" we invited the participation of Ernst Caspari, Harry Jerison, Ralph Holloway, William Riddell, and Herman Epstein.

Caspari set a general tone for all the papers by discussing the general relationship among evolution, brain size, and behavior. His prior writing on this topic (e.g., Caspari, 1963, 1967) indicates his expertise in the area, particularly on the topic of the mechanisms of evolution and their relationship to behavior.

Jerison was an obvious choice to discuss the importance of brain size. His germinal volume, *Evolution of the Brain and Intelligence* (1973) provided a fascinating theoretical approach to the relationship between brain size and behavior through the concept of the number of extra cortical neurons above that needed for basic functioning. While Jerison's previous work had dealt primarily with brain size and behavior on a between species basis, on this occasion he discusses that relationship on a within-species basis.

In contrast to Jerison, Holloway has consistently argued that brain size per se is unimportant unless it can be shown to predict sizes of brain substructures (Holloway, 1974). Holloway emphasizes the importance of relative growth and the timing of events in organizing the brain for the understanding of the brain–behavior relationship.

The brain–behavior relationship from the behavioral side has been studied extensively by Riddell. In his previous work (e.g., Riddell, Corl, & Gravetter, 1976) he carefully investigated the classic comparative problem of making behavioral comparisons on animals of different taxonomic groups. After instituting controls to minimize species "special abilities," he has correlated general ability or intelligence with Jerison's index of cerebral development, *Nc* (number of extra cortical neurons).

Another approach to the question of the behavioral implications of brains size is that taken by Epstein. In two intriguing papers (Epstein, 1974a, 1974b), he studied increases in brain size occurring during ontogeny and correlated them with patterns of mental development. He found that brain growth in humans occurs in spurts and plateaus rather than at a uniform rate, and that mental development as defined by Piaget is correlated with the growth spurts.

What Are the Effects of Genetic Selection for Brain Size on Brain Substructures and Behavior?

If evolutionary pressures have produced differences in brain size (with concomitant behavioral changes) across species, evidence for the adaptive value of bigger brains should be available within species. While there are a variety of possible ways to study the brain–behavior relationship within a species, we chose to concentrate on approaches that employed selection for brain weight. This approach may mimic the effects of selection pressure across species and provides a convenient way of examining the brain substructure and behavioral manifestations of selection for brain size. In order to examine this area in detail, we invited the contributions of Thomas Roderick, Cynthia Wimer, Stephan Zamenhof, Edith van Marthens, John Fuller, Craig Jensen, Bruce Dudek, Peter Berman, and Martin Hahn.

It would be fair to say that Roderick is the father of the work on genetic selection for brain size. His early collaborations at Berkeley gave impetus to the idea of genetic selection for a brain character (Roderick, Wimer, & Wimer, 1976). The brain weight selections done by Roderick and the Wimers have resulted in interesting substructure and behavioral changes in their selected lines. Roderick speaks to the general issue of genetic methods in this area and, via hindsight, comments on the virtues and vices of selection for a brain parameter as a means of unraveling the brain–behavior relationship.

While Roderick and colleagues demonstrated behavioral correlations with brain weight, Cynthia Wimer, who was involved in the original selections, pursued the question of the substructure results of brain weight selection. Earlier work summarized in Roderick, Wimer, and Wimer (1976) had suggested that the volume of certain brain areas correlated highly with overall brain volume. Wimer discusses the possibility of common or separate genetic control of the growth of substructure areas.

While neuroanatomy can be studied directly by size measurement, it can also be studied indirectly by neurochemical techniques. Zamenhof and van Marthens had previously investigated the development of the brain by examining DNA and protein contents. Their work on the Roderick–Wimer lines (Zamenhof & van Marthens 1976) demonstrated that the differences in brain weight between high and low lines were due to cell number rather than cell size or density. They also found developmental differences in cell proliferation between the selected lines. Here they refine and extend those results by presenting the results of further investigations in this area.

Fuller continued the selection approach of Roderick but introduced several modifications. Fuller's investigations began with a different gene pool and a different selection criterion than Roderick, and Fuller was more interested in rates of development in lines of mice selected for brain weight than in their adult behavior. Fuller demonstrated that brain growth occurs at different rates, and that behavioral development is strongly influenced by selection for brain weight (Fuller & Geils, 1972;

Fuller & Herman, 1974). Fuller recalls the history and results of his selection experiment and summarizes their importance.

Investigations of brain–behavior relations would have greater generality if they included in their subject pool mice of several selection projects. Jensen has intensively studied the learning behavior of lines of mice from the Roderick–Wimer and Fuller selections (Jensen, 1977). In general, he found no reliable relationship between brain size and learning ability. In this volume he offers an explanation of those results and extends his search for brain–behavior relationships to mice that were not selected for brain size.

Neuroanatomical and neurochemical investigations similar to those by Zamenhof and van Marthens and by Wimer have begun on the Fuller BWS lines. Dudek and Berman studied the genetic regulation of neurochemical development in the Fuller BWS lines and report the results of that study. Results similar to those found in the Roderick–Wimer lines add substantiation to the technique of genetic selection for brain size as a way of unraveling the brain–behavior complex.

In a developing animal, genotype and environment interact in a complex fashion to produce behavior. Hahn has previously investigated this process with respect to agonistic behavior in the Fuller BWS mice (Hahn, Haber & Fuller, 1973). Here he describes his most recent work in which he used fostering procedures to examine the effects of genes and environment on developing behaviors, or the degree to which selection has indirectly altered behavior through pleiotropic effects on parental or similar behaviors.

Do Genetic and Environmental Manipulations of Brain Size Have Similar Behavior Consequences?

It is clear that both genes and environments contribute to variation in brain size and behavior. We were interested in the similar and dissimilar effects of these two variables, and invited the contributions of Mark Rosenzweig, William Greenough and Janice Juraska, Michael Nagy, and Norman Henderson.

The relations between brains, chemistry, environment, and behavior have long been an interest of Rosenzweig. Perhaps the most significant finding to emerge from his group is that enriched environments produced animals with bigger brains, altered neurochemistry, and enhanced learning ability (e.g., Rosenzweig & Bennett, 1976). Rosenzweig describes his most recent work on the complex question of how enriched environments alter various brain measures.

Greenough and Juraska have been involved in fascinating work on the neuroanatomical effects of enriched environments (e.g., Greenough, Volkmar & Fleischmann, 1976). They have shown that enrichment is associated with increased dendritic branching and changes at the synapse such as increases in post synaptic thickening. They summarize their past results and discuss extentions of that work. Their work help establish a basis for comparison of genetically induced and environmentally induced changes in neuroanatomy.

While adult brains and behaviors are significantly altered by environmental manipulations, the brains and behaviors of very young animals are certainly more plastic. Nagy has done important work on the characteristics of infant learning and memory (Nagy, Misanin, Newman, Olson, & Hinderliter, 1972). He reports on his most recent work that involves altering the rate of development of learning, memory and retention processes.

Under certain circumstances, very brief exposures to enriched environments alter the genetic determination of a brain character (Henderson, 1976). This interesting effect fits into the general topic of Gene × Environment interaction, about which our final participant has thought and written extensively. He discusses Gene × Environment interactions particularly as they affect research designed to find within-species genetic relationships between brain size and behavior.

Emphases and Omissions

In any attempt to integrate diverse areas of research, some are emphasized, some are neglected, and some fall in between. In assembling this volume, we were confronted with an overwhelming literature that concerned the classic question of the relationship between brain size and behavior. The choice of which areas and points of view to emphasize and which to neglect was a function of our perception of the potential for integrating areas, as well as our training and interests. Our experiences in working with John L. Fuller had created a deep interest in genetic selection for brain weight and had demonstrated that selection experiments alone could not address the question of the importance of brain size in a more general sense. If the results from selection studies were integrated with the theory and results from the study of the evolution of brain size and intelligence and with studies dealing with environmental effects on brain development and behavior, we believed that the results would benefit research and theory in each of these areas. Another potential benefit of bringing diverse theories and research approaches together in a single volume is that new ideas for research, not covered in the volume, would emerge for the readers. We hope that this volume will accomplish these objectives.

References

Caspari, E. Selective forces in the evolution of man. *American Naturalist*, 1963, *97*, 5–14.
Caspari, E. Introduction to Part 1 and remarks on evolutionary aspects of behavior. In J. Hirsch (Ed.), *Behavior-genetic analysis*. New York: McGraw-Hill, 1967.
Epstein, H. T. Phrenoblysis: Special brain and mind growth periods. I. Human brain and skull development. *Developmental Psychobiology*, 1974, *7*, 207–216.(a)
Epstein, H. T. Phrenoblysis: Special brain and mind growth periods. II. Human mental development. *Developmental Psychobiology*, 1974, *7*, 217–224.(b)
Fuller, J. L., & Geils, H. D. Brain growth in mice selected for high and low brain weight. *Developmental Psychobiology*, 1972, *5*, 307–318.
Fuller, J. L., & Herman, B. H. Effect of genotype and practice upon behavioral development in mice. *Developmental Psychobiology*, 1974, *7*, 21–30.
Greenough, W. T., Volkmar, F. R., & Fleischmann, T. B. Environmental effects on brain connectivity and behavior. In D. I. Mosotofsky (Ed.), *Behavior control and modification of physiological activity*. Englewood Cliffs, N. J.: Prentice-Hall, 1976.
Hahn, M. E., Haber, S. B., & Fuller, J. L. Differential agonistic behavior of mice selected for brain weight. *Physiology and Behavior*, 1973, *10*, 759–762.
Henderson, N. D. Short exposures to enriched environments can increase genetic variability of behavior in mice. *Developmental Psychobiology*, 1976, *9*, 549–553.
Holloway, R. L. On the meaning of brain size. Book review of Jerison's 1973, *Evolution of brain and intelligence*. *Science*, 1974, *184*, 677–679.
Jensen, C. Generality of learning differences in brain-weight-selected mice. *Journal of Comparative and Physiological Psychology*, 1977, *91*, 629–641.
Jerison, H. J. *Evolution of the brain and intelligence*. New York: Academic Press, 1973.
Nagy, Z. M., Misanin, J. R., Newman, J. A., Olsen, P. L., & Hinderliter, C. F. Ontogeny of memory in the neonatal mouse. *Journal of Comparative and Physiological Psychology*, 1972, *81*, 380–393.
Riddell, W. I., Corl, K. G., & Gravetter, F. J. Cross-order comparisons using indexes of cerebral development. *Bulletin of the Psychonomic Society*, 1976, *8*, 578–580.
Roderick, T. H., Wimer, R. E., & Wimer, C. C. Genetic manipulations of neuroanatomical traits. In L. Petrinovich & J. L. McGaugh (Eds.), *Knowing, thinking and believing*. New York: Plenum Publishing, 1976.
Rosenzweig, M. R., & Bennett, E. L. Enriched environments: Facts, factors and fantasies. In L. Petrinovich & J. L. McGaugh (Eds.), *Knowing, thinking and believing*. New York: Plenum Publishing, 1976.
Zamenhof, S., & van Marthens, E. Neonatal and adult brain parameters in mice selected for adult brain weight. *Developmental Psychobiology*, 1976, *9*, 587–593.

Chapter II

Evolutionary Theory and the Evolution of the Human Brain

ERNST W. CASPARI

The XI International Conference of Genetics at the Hague, 1963, was the first one in which a symposium on behavior genetics was presented. The symposium had been organized by J. H. F. van Abeelen, I was appointed chairman, and John Fuller gave the first invited lecture, entitled "From genes to behavioral traits." After the lecture there was a vivid discussion, during which the biochemist S. Granick raised the question of why behavior geneticists are concerned mostly with responses in psychological tests instead of with studying the genetics of size of the brain, which he assumed to be related to intelligence. I do not remember John Fuller's answer, except that I was disappointed that he did not refer to a slide showing Storer's preliminary results on differences of brain size between mouse strains, which he had presented in his talk.

This anecdote seems to me a suitable introduction to the present volume because Granick asked the question that we want to consider here: In what way do genes influence the development and structure of the brain? This question is of particular interest to biologists and psychologists, since in the evolution of the human species conspicuous changes in brain size and structure must have occurred. Implied in Granick's question is the assumption that an increase in the size of the brain would be expressed as favorable changes in behavior, and particularly in an increase in intelligence; this topic will also be dealt with in

9

DEVELOPMENT AND EVOLUTION
OF BRAIN SIZE

this volume. Finally, implied in the question is the widespread assumption that intelligence is advantageous for the species, and therefore
an increase of intelligence in the population is highly desirable. Whether
this is really the case cannot be argued in the present intellectual climate,
because in our present culture high intelligence is probably the most
highly valued human quality.

In this chapter I shall be concerned primarily with the theory of evolution. This is a more difficult undertaking than it would have been
10 years ago. At that time, there was agreement among population
geneticists concerning the main mechanisms of evolution, mutation,
selection, genetic adaptation, and speciation, and there were only dis-
agreements concerning the basis of genetic variability within populations. This situation has changed within the last decade. New theories
and viewpoints have developed primarily under the influence of molecular biology and of ecological theory. It is impossible to summarize
all these developments in the space at my disposal. I shall, therefore,
select some aspects of the present theory, which I think may have some
bearing on the evolution of the brain. But I want to emphasize that there
is much less unanimity among population biologists on the genetic basis
of evolution now than there has been in the past, and that many possibilities have opened up which were not considered in the past. Thus,
population biology will not give us the firm foundation for our discussions, which it would have done formerly.

In the second part of my presentation I will make some remarks on
the evolution of the human brain. In 1963 I proposed an hypothesis
suggesting some selective conditions responsible for the growth of the
human brain during the course of evolution. Since that time, more
material concerning human evolution has accumulated, and our picture
of human evolution has changed to a certain degree. It is, therefore,
necessary to reconsider the old hypothesis under the new evidence. .

Some Present Problems in Evolution

Neutralist and Selectionist Theories
of Genetic Polymorphism

When I was a student around 1930, evolutionary theories were not
in fashion. The classical work of Darwinists trying to clarify the phylogenetic relationships of different groups of organisms was falling into
disrepute. Most geneticists were more or less agnostic with respect to
evolution, or assumed that mutations were responsible for evolution,

and that evolution was, therefore, proceeding in sudden jumps and not gradually, as Darwin had assumed. Most biologists were unaware that the mathematical theory of evolution by selection, worked out by Fisher, Haldane and Wright, existed already, and many of those who knew of the work did not have the mathematical background to appreciate it. The demonstration by Chetverikov (1926 and later) that genetic polymorphism is widespread in natural populations of *Drosophila* remained unknown in the West. And the experimental approach to evolution, introduced by L'Héritier and Teissier in 1934, was ignored by most biologists. Evolutionary work became greatly stimulated only beginning in the late 1930s and 1940s when Dobzhansky (1937), Mayr (1942) and Simpson (1944) reviewed the evidence from genetics, systematics and paleontology and showed that they fit well together into a coherent theory that has become known as the Neodarwinian theory. All three scientists initiated vigorous research programs, which at that time consisted mostly in the collection of data which generally substantiated the theory.

One controversy that arose in the 1940s concerned the nature of genetic variation within populations, a problem that had puzzled Darwin and Galton much earlier. The theory favored by Muller, Crow and many others assumed that populations are mostly homozygous, that most mutations are harmful and eliminated by selection, and that only the rare favorable mutations form the basis of evolution. Dobzhansky, Wallace and their students, on the other hand, proposed that two or more alleles of the same gene can be maintained in a population by heterosis, and thus a plentiful raw material of genetic variation is present in every sexually reproducing species. The controversy was decided by direct studies of the amount of genetic variation within natural populations. The method uses specific enzymes and proteins, each determined by a single gene locus, and tests them for genetic polymorphism by means of electrophoresis. The results of Lewontin and Hubby (1966) and Harris (1966) were incompatible with the theory that most genes in natural populations are homozygous: On the average about 30% of all loci tested turned out to be polymorphic in a population, and every individual showed on the average about 12% heterozygosity for polymorphic genes. This result has been borne out by a large number of further investigations on different animals and plants. The frequency of polymorphic loci is sometimes even higher than found by Lewontin and Hubby.

The neutralist theory was introduced as an alternative to the balance theory in order to explain the high degree of polymorphism in natural populations (Kirmura, 1969; King & Jukes, 1969). The theory assumes that most of the polymorphic forms of an enzyme are neutral in adaptive value, and can thus be kept in populations by chance. The mathematical theory of adaptively neutral and near neutral genes has been worked out by Kimura and Ohta (summarized in 1971), and there is no doubt that the theory can account for a large amount of polymorphism within large populations. Furthermore, the balance theory has been criticized on the grounds that a large number of genes held in a population by heterozygote superiority would strongly reduce the fitness of the population, because the inferior homozygotes would continue to segregate. The amount of polymorphism actually found should result in a higher loss of fitness due to inbreeding than is experimentally observed. The suggestion has, therefore, been made that frequency dependent selection and different adaptive values in different ecological niches may account for a large amount of polymorphism. But a recent paper by Lewontin, Ginsberg, & Tuljapurkar, (1978) demonstrates that it is highly unlikely that the large number of alleles found at one locus (27 different alleles among 146 genes for xanthine dehydrogenase tested) can be held in equilibrium by heterosis, and the same is suspected for frequency dependent selection. Even though niche selection has not been ruled out as a mechanism for the maintenance of genetic polymorphism, this observation has weakened the theory of selection as the cause of polymorphism. On the other hand, the large number of alleles found at one locus also presents difficulties for the neutralist theory. For the maintenance of such a large amount of polymorphism by chance, the breeding populations must be excessively large and the mutation rates considerably higher than those observed. To prevent a wrong impression, it still appears that a high proportion of all structural loci in populations are monomorphic.

One factor which seemed to favor the neutralist theory is the finding of a molecular evolutionary clock for protein evolution. If the amino acid sequences of homologous proteins of different species are compared, it is found that they differ in certain amino acids, and that the number of amino acid substitutions parallels the taxonomic distance between the species, closely related species showing fewer substitutions than remotely related ones. If the number of amino acid substitutions is plotted against the time when the species compared are assumed to have diverged in evolution, according to the paleontological record, a straight line is obtained (Margoliash & Fitch, 1968). This has been most thoroughly shown for cytochrome c, but other proteins show the same straight line relationship.

The lines for different proteins differ in slope. In other words, some proteins evolve faster than others, probably because more or less amino acid substitutions are forbidden by the function of the protein. Kimura and Ohta (1974) have shown that if random replacement is the only cause of protein divergence, one would expect divergence rate to be equal to the rate of neutral mutations; under selection, the rate of divergence would depend on mutation rates, selection coefficients and effective population size and thus give a more complex relationship.

More recent investigations have shown that the rate of change of particular proteins is not as constant as had been assumed when only few amino acid sequences had been analyzed. More specifically, the rate of protein divergence may differ in different taxonomic groups for homologous proteins (Fitch & Langley, 1976). This finding may be assumed to invalidate the argument in favor of neutralism from the molecular clock, but is easily accounted for by the occurrence of adaptively favorable mutations.

Thus, it appears that the neutralist–selectionist controversy is not resolved, though many students of evolution tend at present to lean more towards neutralism. It should be pointed out that the controversy is an exact repetition of the controversy between R. A. Fisher and Sewall Wright about the relative role of random drift versus selection in evolution that took place in the 1930s. This is not accidental: Some of the most prominent neutralists, Crow and Kimura, have worked with Wright, while among the defenders of selectionism are many collaborators of Dobzhansky, and several British evolutionists, who have been influenced by Fisher and E. B. Ford. From the point of our discussion it should be kept in mind that the facts to be explained by either theory are polymorphism in natural populations and biochemical divergence in evolution. In genetic adaptation and speciation, selection is assumed to play a prominent role also under the neutralist theory.

The role of selection under the neutralist theory is twofold. First of all, it reduces the rate of change in the structure of proteins below the rate of mutations by random base substitutions. It explains, thus, that a protein with a well understood function such as cytochrome c evolves more slowly than the fibrinopeptides, whose function does not depend on their structure and whose changes are therefore regarded as indicating the rate of evolution in the absence of selection. In this respect, selection has a stabilizing role. But it is also admitted that changes or differences in environment can lead to adaptive selective events that would lead to directional and diversifying selection. The latter aspect would also apply if a selectionist theory of polymorphism is assumed. The only difference consists in the assumption by selectionists that within a population selective forces establish dynamic equilibria at many gene loci, while according to the neutralist point of view, chance plays a large role in establishing particular alleles in populations.

Evolution of Regulatory Genes and Polygenic Inheritance

The evolutionary processes affecting the structure of proteins that were discussed in the last section are reflections of changes in the DNA of their structural genes. The structure of DNA has been studied directly in the last decade, and even though these methods have not been as specific as those used for the analysis of proteins, they have given much unexpected information that shows that the organization of eukaryote DNA is more complex than that of bacteria and viruses. The methods employed use primarily the kinetics of reassociation of single-stranded, heat-denatured DNA under different conditions. Also, the frequency of mismatched nucleotide pairs can be estimated from the thermal stability of reassociated DNA.

With the aid of these techniques it can be shown that eukaryote DNA consists of two main fractions: unique or single copy DNA and repetitive DNA. The single copy DNA makes up a relatively large part of the total DNA, most frequently 50–75%, depending on species, and contains the structural DNA which is transcribed into the mRNA which is in turn translated into protein. But only a small proportion, perhaps 10–20%, of the single copy DNA is made up of structural DNA; the remainder consists of DNA of unknown function. A considerable proportion of single copy DNA is transcribed and its RNA is found in the nucleus in the hnRNA fraction. But only a small proportion of the single copy DNA gives rise to cytoplasmic polysomal mRNA in particular cells (e.g., 2.7% in the sea urchin gastrula).

Repetitive DNA can be further subdivided into several fractions: short repeats, long repeats and very short sequences, frequently called satellite DNA. The latter consists of tandem clusters, 2–10 nucleotide pairs long, which may be repeated 10^3–10^6 times. Many organisms have low or undetectable amounts of satellite DNA, in others it accounts for more than 50% of the total DNA. The facts that: (*a*) it is found accumulated in the centromeric heterochromatin; (*b*) that closely related species have strikingly different amounts and sequences of satellite DNA; and (*c*) that it is not transcribed, have led to the conclusion that it probably carries no genetic information.

The short repeats are some 100 nucleotide pairs in length and are singly interspersed between single copy DNA sequences; in *Drosophila* and some other insects this repetitive DNA is present in longer stretches. Structural gene sequences are frequently adjacent or near to short repetitive sequences. The short repeats occur in families, more or less closely related in structure, each comprising about one hundred to several thousand repeats. Short repeats can be transcribed, and transcripts of short repeats are found in the hnRNA fraction. The concentration of RNA derived from particular families varies during development. Many properties of short repeats have been interpreted to mean that they are involved in the regulation of the activity of structural genes (Britten & Davidson, 1976).

The long repetitive sections seem to be a heterogeneous group. They consist of DNA sequences repeated 100 to over 1000 times in tandem at the same place in the genome. Among them are repeated gene sequences such as the ribosomal DNA, t-RNA–DNAs, the genes determining the histones and possibly some other ubiquitous proteins. But these genes account only for a fraction of the long repeats, and the function of the remainder is unknown.

The main conclusion from these studies is that the DNA of higher organisms consists of a number of different types of sequences that can be distinguished by their behavior in reassociation experiments. Only about one-tenth of these sequences are made up of the structural genes that determine the structure of proteins. The function of the remainder of the DNA is largely unknown. It is suspected that some of them are regulatory elements for the control of structural genes and batteries of structural genes, and since the mechanism of their control in development is believed to be complex, a certain proportion of the remaining DNA may be involved in this function. There are certainly some spacer DNAs which separate different structural genes, some non-translated DNA within genes, and there is still enough DNA left not to exclude the existence of "junk" DNA, (i.e., DNA without informational function). Still, the fact remains that there are measurable quantities of DNA in the genome of higher organisms whose functions we cannot indicate with any precision. As far as evolutionary theory is concerned, all theories have been based on models dealing with structural genes, making the implicit assumption that other sequences in the DNA are either functionally negligible or behave like structural genes.

Some species comparisons are available for the single copy DNA of related species. Kohne (1970) has studied the DNA sequences of some mammals, particularly primates, and Angerer, Davidson, & Britten, (1976) compared four species of sea urchins, three belonging to the same genus and the fourth to a different order. The rates of change of nucleotide substitutions found in the two sets of experiments are similar, about .1% per million years or about 3–$4 \cdot 10^6$ nucleotide pairs (Kohne, Chiscon, & Hoyer, 1972). These values agree well with the rates for fast evolving proteins such as the fibrinopeptides, which do not determine a selected phenotype. This rate is thus regarded as the basal rate of incorporation of nucleotide substitutions (Britten & Davidson, 1976), which is attained in the absence of selection. As Ohta and Kimura (1971) pointed out, selection reduces the rate of change below the basal level. Angerer *et al.* (1976) have found that in sea urchins, the subset represented by structural genes diverges at a lower rate than the total single copy DNA, indicating the action of selection.

The study of the evolution of repetitive DNA is technically more difficult, and it has been studied only recently since techniques involving recombinant DNA have made it possible to isolate single sequences of a family of short repeats. In this way repeat frequency of individual sequences could be compared for related species, for instance in sea urchin species (Moore, Scheller, Davidson, & Britten, 1978) and in birds (Eden, Hendrick & Gottlieb, 1978). It was found that different families of sequences differ in the frequency of repeats in closely related species, while in remotely related species many families of repeats cannot be identified with each other. In their nucleotide constitutions the repeats tend to be conserved in evolution and change more slowly than unique sequences. The quantitative changes in family size, on the other hand, progress with great speed, about $4 \cdot 10^{-8}$ fractions of the repeated sequence being added per year, for one full sequence every 50 years. Thus, the short repeats seem to be relatively constant in nucleotide sequence but change rapidly in number per family. The possibility that sequences will be reduced, lost, and transposed has also been suggested (Britten & Davidson, 1976).

Long, repetitive sequences are highly conserved in evolution, indicating either selection for constancy or recent appearance. The number of repeats per sequence can change, possibly by unequal crossing over. Histones belong to the most highly conserved proteins: In histones H3 and H4, the difference between one plant, pea seedlings, and one animal (calf), is only two amino acids. The histone genes are long tandem repeats, and it is hard to see how evolution can act to keep the different elements of the repeat free of base substitutions, such as led to divergence between the repeated hemoglobin genes α, β, γ and δ. Comparison of histone RNAs in two sea urchin species has shown that they vary considerably in their nucleotide composition. Thus, variation is apparently restricted to third position bases of the codon, and possible intercalary DNA segments (Grunstein, Schedl, & Kedes, 1976). Similar observations apply to the ribosomal RNA genes. In comparisons of the frogs *Xenopus laevis* and *X. mulleri* it was found that the ribosomal DNA sequences were conserved while the spacer sequences of the same genes were very different (Brown, Wensink, & Jordan, 1972). This indicates that natural selection determines the maintenance of the highly conserved long, repetitive DNA sequences, even though we cannot define the mechanisms of natural selection involved. It is known that in *Drosophila* rDNA can vary quantitatively by unequal crossing over, and in the mouse rDNA can change its position in the genome.

It is thus clear that repetitive DNAs behave differently in evolution than single copy DNA. If some of them control regulatory developmental processes, they may be expressed phenotypically by quantitative rather than alternative characters, such as relative growth rates, relative timing of developmental events, and tissue specificity. It had early been proposed by Mather (1943) that the genes responsible for quantitative variation constitute a different class of genes, the polygenes. They act in groups of genes, segregate like structural genes since they are located on the chromosomes, but cannot be individually identified and are located in the heterochromatin. Mather's theory did not find much acceptance among geneticists. First of all, there was no evidence that genes for quantitative characters are concentrated in heterochromatic regions. Experiments by Thoday (1961) showed that a high proportion of the difference between two strains developed by selection for a quantitative character could be due to a few well defined and localized pairs of alleles. But more important was the widespread assumption that most quantitative effects are pleiotropic effects of orthodox Mendelian genes. It is indeed a common experience that Mendelian mutant genes have secondary effects on quantitative characters such as fitness, viability, fertility, speed of development, size, and many behavioral characters (Caspari, 1952). It was thus concluded that the polygenes were nothing but collections of phenotypically minor alleles of structural genes that were, for practical reasons, investigated by the methods of quantitative genetics: selection experiments, diallel crosses and others. These techniques used in polygenic analysis will be discussed in this volume in the contributions by Fuller, Roderick and Henderson. Since many behavioral characters have a polygenic basis, the question of whether polygenic characters are completely controlled by orthodox structural genes or by other types of genes that have a higher rate of variation, and whose variation may affect the pattern of action of different structural genes, is pertinent to our topic. Such a possibility has been suggested by Britten and Davidson (1976), and Mather's ideas have also been revived in Carson's (1975) evolutionary theory (see following). Lewontin (1974, pp. 66–68) reviews experimental evidence that fitness characters and other quantitative characters acquire spontaneously considerable quantitative variation starting out from homozygous chromosomes, and suggests that this variation is derived from recombination rather than from the much less effective mutation process. In addition, transposable elements, first discovered by McClintock in maize, are known to control the activity and the timing of activation of structural genes and to change their position in the genome (McClintock, 1965).

All these well-established observations can be easily understood if it is assumed that there are genetic elements in the chromosomes that control the action of structural genes in development, and that evolve by mechanisms additional to nucleotide substitution, such as changes in frequency, sequence, and position. Repetitive DNA may include some of these elements.

Macroevolution: Speciation and Extinction

The Neodarwinian theory is mainly concerned with the genetic adaptation of populations by natural selection. This is true for both neutralist and selectionist theories that differ in the accounts of the origin of genetic variation, the raw material upon which selection acts. The result of selection is the formation of populations adapted to local conditions, and possibly subspecies—processes subsumed under the term microevolution. There has been little interest in macroevolution, the formation and extinction of species. Both were assumed to be extensions of microevolution. The appearance of genetic isolation between populations would gradually lead to further genetic divergence, and extinction of reproductive lines and populations is a frequent event within species.

But there persisted a suspicion expressed, for example, by Goldschmidt (1940 and later), that microevolution is in principle a different process from macroevolution and involves a more thoroughgoing reorganization of the genome. This was already indicated in the early development of Neodarwinism: Simpson (1944) proposed the existence of "quantum" evolution, in contrast to gradual evolution. Mayr's (1963) founder effect, in which a single or few individuals give rise to a new species if they find themselves isolated from the main body of the population, assumes that the unique assortment of genes isolated by chance in the founder serves as a starting point for selection different from that offered by a population in genetic equilibrium. Mayr regards the species as the real unit of evolution and suggests that the origin of a new species involves a "genetic revolution."

Reorganization of the genotype of a species has been put into more concrete terms by Carson (1975). Carson assumes that a species may have, besides the Mendelian genes and polygenes, systems of coadapted gene complexes that he calls "closed gene systems." These coadapted genes are held together by epistatic interactions in *cis* position, that is, the genes are linked and interact only when they are located on the same chromosome. Therefore, recombinants between coadapted genes are strongly reduced in fitness and are not found under usual conditions of selection. They might, however, survive and multiply when selection is relaxed. If, after some time, selection becomes stringent again and the population is drastically reduced in size, it is possible that recombinants for these previously closed gene systems would survive and give rise, under selective pressure, to a line presenting a new genetic organization. It is obvious that Carson's model combines aspects of Mayr's genetic revolution and of Goldschmidt's old idea of the "happy monster."

Theories purporting that macroevolution is in principle a different process from microevolution imply that speciation is not a gradual process but proceeds suddenly and in spurts. Darwin had observed that the fossil record did not bear out the gradualism postulated by his theory, but he attributed this to gaps in the record. In the meantime, much more material has been collected, but the gaps have not disappeared. This has led some paleontologists to assume that the gaps are real and represent periods at which evolution proceeds at great speed. Gould and Eldredge (1977) designate this type of saltatory evolution as "punctuated equilibria." The theory of sudden speciation is widely accepted among paleontologists, but most geneticists are skeptical and feel that the data are more in agreement with gradual evolution (e.g., Avise & Ayala, 1975).

Paleontologists have also become concerned with the problem of the extinction of species. This problem was previously neglected because it seemed to offer no theoretical problems. Species not sufficiently fit, or not sufficiently versatile to adapt to changing environmental conditions, were doomed to extinction. This attitude toward extinction had a definite moralistic flavor—it was regarded as a penalty paid by a species for lack of fitness.

Evolutionists have recently suggested that extinction, rather than being looked upon as a penalty, may be regarded as a chance phenomenon. This idea was first expressed by Van Valen (1973). He plotted, for different taxonomic groups, the logarithm of surviving taxons against geologic time, and obtained for each of the groups a straight line that differed in slope from the others. He concluded that extinction proceeds at a rate that can be described as a random process, and that the probability of extinction varies among the different taxonomic groups.

In considering the geological record, it should always be kept in mind that taxa can only be distinguished morphologically; genetic and biochemical differences remain unknown. Morphology is the outcome of developmental processes, and it is not certain that developmental processes evolve at the same rate as Mendelian genes and enzymes. If, as Britten and Davidson (1976) suggest, repeated sequences control the action of structural genes in development, and these sequences are affected by quantitative changes, a molecular basis is obtained for morphological variation that differs in rate from the variation by nucleotide substitution that forms the basis for enzyme variation. That biochemical and morphological evolution may not proceed at the same rate has been suggested by Wilson, Sarich, & Maxson, (1974). However, all these ideas will remain speculative until a better understanding of the function of the repetitive DNA sequences has been obtained.

Ecological Theory and Selection

In the last decade, ecological theory has made great strides, thanks to the mathematical models developed by MacArthur, Wilson, Levins, May and others. Previously, ecology was mostly a descriptive discipline, but it has developed into a rapidly growing, quantitative science. Journals like THE AMERICAN NATURALIST and EVOLUTION are at present filled with papers that develop mathematical models for different ecological situations. This work has had a deep impact on evolutionary theory primarily because ecological conditions constitute the environment through which selection acts. It is impossible to review here all the interactions between ecological and evolutionary theory. I only want to point to one aspect.

Ecological interactions are obviously very important for the purpose of this volume, which focuses on the evolution of brain size and the behavioral consequences of increased brain size. In particular, we assume that in some ways brain size is correlated with increased plasticity or modifiability of behavior. But the ecological conditions under which modifiability of behavior increases Darwinian fitness have only recently been discussed. It is well understood that in present human populations intellectual superiority, though necessary for social success, is not necessarily correlated with increased Darwinian fitness, nor is there good reason to believe that higher learning ability increases reproductive fitness in other organisms. Arnold (1978) has developed a model comparing the advantage of a particular type of avoidance learning for a predator compared to a nonmodifiable predator preying on a model and its mimic. It turns out that the ability to learn under these conditions is of Darwinian advantage only in certain specifiable ecological conditions.

Since all behavioral characters derive their fitness value from their importance in adapting an organism to its environment, including conspecific animals, quantitative ecological models of this type are needed to interpret our knowledge of the evolution of behavior, which up to now has been based on comparative descriptive data.

Human Evolution and the Evolution of the Human Brain

In this chapter I want to address myself to certain evolutionary questions that either have been controversial in the recent past or that have a special interest in the context of this volume.

Morphological and Biochemical Evolutionary Rates

There now exists a reasonably large amount of fossil material pertaining to hominid evolution. From the Lower Pleistocene and Upper Pliocene, numerous remains belonging to the genera *Homo* and *Australopithecus* have been found. The dating is not always very exact, but the oldest are probably over 3.8 million years old. There are few hominid remains during the earlier Pliocene. But from the Miocene remains of an ape *Ramapithecus* have been found that according to its jaws and dentition may belong to the Hominid, and not to the Pongid, line. The conclusion has thus been drawn that these two lines diverged at least 12 million years ago.

This conclusion has been challenged by Wilson and Sarich (1969), who on immunological and biochemical evidence claim that man and chimpanzee cannot have diverged more than 5 million years ago, that is, during the Upper Pliocene. Immunological methods have been used in phylogenetic studies ever since Nuttall (1904) compared a large number of vertebrate and invertebrate species with each other by measuring the volumes of precipitate produced in serum-antibody reactions. The reactions corresponded in general to the phylogenetic scheme derived by morphological methods, but inconsistencies also occurred. An antihuman antibody, for instance, produced more precipitate with chimpanzee than with human antigen, a result that has been explained by the assumption that the antibody-chimpanzee antigen precipitate may have bound more water. This finding shows, however, how careful one has to be in the interpretation of immunological data.

In the meantime, the sensitivity of the immunological reactions has been improved, and Wilson and Sarich worked with a sensitive and reliable method, quantitative micro complement fixation. This method is assumed to be able to detect single amino acid substitutions in a protein, and to measure the number of protein substitutions. The latter assumption is, however, open to question. It has been shown that single amino acid substitutions can be detected by micro complement fixation. But no systematic studies have been reported that show that all amino acid substitutions can be demonstrated; the possibility that only changes in certain positions on the protein chain are detected cannot be excluded.

On the basis of results achieved with this method, and accepting the original concept of the molecular clock, Wilson and Sarich conclude that man and chimpanzee diverged 5 million years ago. There are, however, some puzzling observations in these data: the gorilla has two amino acid substitutions in its hemoglobin, whereas man and chimpanzee have identical proteins. Some comparable discrepancies from expectation are discussed by Sarich (1970). In this paper, the stochastic nature of amino acid substitutions is used to account for the unexpected immunological behavior of Tupaia serum albumen, which appears closer to man and higher monkeys than to Prosimians. A similar explanation might be invoked for the close biochemical similarity of man and chimpanzee.

The discrepancy between the paleontological and the biochemical evidence can be resolved in several ways. It may be argued that the conclusion from the fossils is wrong and that *Ramapithecus* does not belong in the Hominid line, but constitutes a convergent line. This assumption is strengthened by the finding that Upper Pliocene Australopithecines are more "primitive", i.e. less similar to modern man, in some dental characters than *Ramapithecus*. (Johanson & White 1979). On the other hand, the molecular clock may not be as constant for short time periods as was originally assumed from a comparison of taxonomically widely separated species. As discussed under the heading "Neutralist and Selectionist Theories of Genetic Polymorphism", there is evidence that the molecular clock may not be identical for different taxa. Finally, there is the possibility that morphology and protein structure may not diverge at the same rate. This is particularly true if, as suggested in our section "Macroevolution: Speciation and Extinction," evolution may not be gradual but proceeds in spurts. Wilson *et al.* (1974) have pointed out that chromosome number and morphological characters evolve 20 times faster in mammals than in frogs, but the rate of divergence of serum albumens is the same. King and Wilson (1975), pointing to the strong biochemical similarity between humans and chimpanzees, suggest that the large morphological differences between these two genera may be due to chromosomal rearrangements rather than to point mutations. Their opinion is similar to that discussed under the heading, Macroevolution: Speciation and Extinction," except that "genetic reorganization" is not necessarily identical with "chromosomal rearrangements."

Selective Factors Affecting the Increase in Size of the Human Brain

In an earlier paper (Caspari, 1963) it has been pointed out that the increase in the size of the human cranial capacity, and implicitly of the human brain, proceeded very fast at the *Homo erectus* stage. It was assumed at the time that *Australopithecus* evolved into *H. erectus* at the border of Lower and Middle Pleistocene and *H. erectus* in turn evolved into *Homo sapiens*. This process involved mainly an increase in the size of the brain; in other anatomical structures *Australopithecus* was already essentially human. This picture has changed through more recent fossil finds. There is now good evidence that the genus *Homo* is older than previously assumed, and that in the Lower Pleistocene there lived at least three species of Hominids all but one of which became extinct before the Middle Pleistocene. The Upper Pliocene Hominids are described as a different species of *Australopithecus* (Johanson & White 1979).

The cranial capacity of these Pliocene Australopithecines is not certain but is assumed to be similar to that of later Australopithecines. Two different populations of Pliocene Australopithecines have been studied which are separated by at least 1 million years. Johanson & White emphasize their strong morphological similarity and speak of an evolutionary "stasis". The Lower Pleistocene *Homo* skulls had a cranial capacity slightly larger than *A. africanus* but both species showed no conspicuous change in cranial capacity during the Lower Pleistocene. Thus the genus *Homo* lived for a considerable period with little change in cranial size, though with some variation, and evolved a larger cranium within a relatively short time. The essential aspect of this picture is that during the Lower Pleistocene little change occurred for 1–2 million years, whereas at the *Homo erectus* stage cranial capacity almost doubled in the course of about 800,000 years; for the last 200,000 years, cranial capacity has stayed constant or has somewhat decreased. Although this is a fast rate of evolutionary change it is not an unusual rate; it becomes more striking if the long generation time of Hominids and Pongids is taken into consideration. The fast change in cranial capacity is in agreement with the idea that macroevolution does not always proceed gradually, but may occur in spurts.

It was further suggested in the earlier paper that the reason for this change in cranial capacity was strong selective pressure created by the environment constituted by man's own cultural activities. This was described in terms of a positive feedback relationship between man's cultural activities and the organization of the human brain. It was known that tool making, a cultural activity, preceded in time the conspicuous growth of cranial capacity; it was plausible, therefore, to assume that the existence of cultural activities such as tool making increased the adaptive value of mental abilities such as learning, communication and cooperation, and that selective pressure in this way favored the increase in brain size. The increase in brain size in turn made possible increased and more varied cultural activities, which in turn affected the brain until a limit in cranial size was reached, probably quite early, since the cranial capacity of late *Homo erectus* approaches that of modern man. It is supportive of this hypothesis that during the *H. erectus* stage advances in cultural activities can be observed: The stone tools became more sophisticated, and fire was invented.

These considerations are based on the naive assumption that a large brain is correlated with higher intelligence, and that in human evolution genes favoring higher intelligence have been selected for. Under present conditions, higher intelligence does not necessarily confer higher Darwinian fitness on individuals, nor, as far as we know, in animals. The proposed hypothesis suggests how increased Darwinian fitness may have, for a short time, resulted from higher intelligence. There is still the difficulty that group selection rather then individual selection would have been the most likely result of this type of selection pressure, and group selection presents some theoretical difficulties. Although there is no necessity to reject the hypothesis that selection for brain size at the *H. erectus* level took place because it permitted the development of higher intelligence, alternative possibilities may be considered.

One alternative which at first sight may appear farfetched may be presented here: this alternative is based on pleiotropic gene action. As has been pointed out earlier (Caspari 1952), most genes are pleiotropic, and if one character is selected for, other characters in the population will also change. And it is possible that under changed environmental conditions it is these correlated characters, which originally became established as a byproduct of natural selection, that will prove adaptive.

It is a well known fact, first pointed out by Friedenthal (1910), that in a comparison of different mammalian species a correlation is found between relative brain weight and maximum life expectancy. This has been confirmed by Sacher (1959 and later) and others. It suggests that there are genes that affect brain size and life expectancy in the same direction, and that selection for long life span might thus result in an increase in brain size. This hypothesis could be easily tested on the mouse strains of large and small brain size on which Roderick, Wimer, and Wimer will report in this volume. It remains then to establish ecological conditions in which a higher life expectancy results in higher Darwinian fitness. This is not true in monogamous societies where the last part of the life span is reproductively wasted, but it may occur in polygamous societies where a few powerful males are married to the majority of the females.

Considerations of this type may lead to an agnostic position concerning selective conditions in the past. It will serve to remind us that the conditions providing for superior fitness of a particular character or genotype are often hard to define.

Conclusions

We have seen that for the theory of evolution this is a period of uncertainty. Neither the selectionist nor the neurtralist theory can account for all the facts known about genetic polymorphism within species. The information on the evolution of DNA seems to suggest that, besides the evolution of structural genes and of other unique sequences that evolve faster than structural genes and are presumed not to be subject to stabilizing selection, there is another type of genetic material: repeated sequences. These repeated sequences evolve primarily by an increase and reduction in the number of repeats, which proceeds much faster than base substitution. Repeated sequences are assumed to function in the control of the action of structural genes. In this function, they resemble the controlling elements first described by McClintock in maize and also demonstrated in *Drosophila* and other organisms. These controlling elements also show a type of change that occurs more frequently than base substitution: transposition to another part of the genome. Since the methods used in DNA research in the past did not permit identification of the position of repeated sequences in the genome, identification of controlling elements with repeats will be possible only in the future.

Both techniques indicate, however, the existence of genetic materials that can undergo changes in quantity and position at relatively fast speeds. Phenotypically, the effects of these genetic elements may be assumed to be quantitative and to represent part of what is usually known as polygenic systems. Since it is known that populations react on selective forces by changes in polygenic systems, the possibility of faster rates of change in controlling systems may be of great importance in natural selection. Particularly in such unspecific developmental processes, such as relative growth rates and allometric growth, which underlie the morphological changes we see in fossils, controlling elements may play a significant role.

The evolutionary process with which we are dealing is the process of encephalization in mammals and its relation to learning ability and intelligence. Riddell demonstrates a correlation in interspecies comparisons, and intraspecies comparisons will be presented by several other participants. Here it is only necessary to point out that Darwinian theory predicts that inter- and intraspecific variation have fundamentally the same basis insofar as that during the course of speciation intraspecific variation is transformed by isolation and selection into the differences between two species.

Even if a correlation between relative brain size and plasticity of behavior can be established, it cannot be concluded that the observed effect, encephalization, is a consequence of selection for the behavioral character. We have mentioned an alternative; it should be pointed out that in addition to encephalization, lateralization and other structural changes of the brain have occurred at some period of evolution, and that the latter processes may have been very important in the determination of the particular human behavioral capacities. It is always attractive to speculate on the evolution of man and on the selective forces that have shaped him. But this question appears to me transscientific in the sense of Weinberg (1977). It is scientifically a meaningful question that can, however, never be answered because we will never be able to fully reconstruct the genetic structure, population size, and ecological conditions for populations living in the past.

Acknowledgments

I am very grateful to Robert C. Angerer, Uzi Nur, Robert K. Selander, and G. Lawrence Vankin for reading the manuscript and for many informative, stimulating, and critical discussions.

References

Angerer, R. C., Davidson, E. H., & Britten, R. J. Single copy DNA and structural gene sequence relationships among four sea urchin species. *Chromosoma*, 1976, 56, 213–226.
Arnold, S. J. The evolution of a special class of modifiable behaviors in relation to environmental pattern. *American Naturalist*, 1978, 112, 415–427.

Avise, J. C., & Ayala, F. J. Genetic change and rates of cladogenesis. *Genetics*, 1975, *81*, 757–773.

Britten, R. J., & Davidson, E. H. DNA sequence arrangement and preliminary evidence on its evolution. *Federation Proceedings*, 1976, *35*, 2151–2157.

Brown, D. D., Wensink, P. C., & Jordan, E. A comparison of the ribosomal DNAs of *Xenopus laevis* and *Xenopus mulleri*: The evolution of tandem genes. *Journal of Molecular Biology*, 1972, *63*, 57–73.

Carson, H. L. The genetics of speciation at the diploid level. *American Naturalist*, 1975,*109*, 83–92.

Caspari, E. Pleiotropic gene action. *Evolution*, 1952, *6*, 1–18.

Caspari, E. Selective forces in the evolution of man. *American Naturalist*, 1963, *97*, 5–14.

Chetverikov, S. S. On certain aspects of the evolutionary process from the standpoint of modern genetics. *Journal of Experimental Biology*, 1926, *A2*, 3–54. (In Russian—English translation: *Proceedings of the American Philosophical Society*, 1961, *105*, 167–195.)

Dobzhansky, T. *Genetics and the origin of species*. (1st Ed.). New York: Columbia University Press, 1937.

Eden, F. C., Hendrick, J. P., & Gottlieb, S. S. Homology of single copy and repeat sequences in chicken, duck, Japanese quail and ostrich DNA. *Biochemistry*, 1978, *17*, 5113–5121.

Fitch, W. M. & Langley, C. M. Protein evolution and the molecular clock. *Federation Proceedings*, 1976, *35*, 2092–2097.

Friedenthal, M. Ueber die Gültigkeit der Massenwirkung für den Energieumsatz der lebendigen Substanz. *Zentralblatt für Physiologie*, 1910, *24*, 321–327.

Fuller, J. L. From genes to behavioral traits. In S. J. Geerts (Ed.), *Genetics today*: Proceedings XI, International Congress of Genetics, Vol. 3. Oxford: Pergamon Press, 1963. Pp. 789–794.

Goldschmidt, R. *The material basis of evolution*. New Haven: Yale University Press, 1940.

Gould, S. J., & Eldredge, N. Punctuated equilibria: The tempo and mode of evolution reconsidered. *Paleobiology*, 1977, *3*, 115–151.

Grunstein, M., Schedl, P., & Kedes, L. Sequence analysis and evolution of sea urchin (*Lytechinus pictus* and *Strongylocentrotus purpuratus*) histone H4 messenger RNAs. *Journal of Molecular Biology*, 1976, *104*, 351–369.

Harris, H. Enzyme polymorphism in man. *Proceedings of the Royal Society of London*, 1966, Ser. B *164*, 298–310.

Johanson, D. C. & White, T. D. A systematic assessment of early African Hominids. *Science* 1979, *203*: 321–330.

Kimura, M. The rate of molecular evolution considered from the standpoint of population genetics. *Proceedings of the National Academy of Science, U.S.A.*, 1969, *63*, 1181–1188.

Kimura, M., & Ohta, T. *Theoretical aspects of population genetics*. Princeton, N.J.: Princeton University Press, 1971.

Kimura, M., & Ohta, T. On some principles governing molecular evolution. *Proceedings of the National Academy of Science, U.S.A.*, 1974, *71*, 2848–2852.

King, J. L., & Jukes, T. H. Non-Darwinian evolution. *Science*, 1969, *164*, 788–798.

King, M. C., & Wilson, A. C. Evolution at two levels in humans and chimpanzees. *Science*, 1975, *188*, 107–116.

Kohne, D. E. Evolution of higher-organism DNA. *Quarterly Review of Biophysiology*, 1970, *33*, 327–375.

Kohne, D. E., Chiscon, J. A. & Hoyer, B. H. Evolution of primate DNA: A summary. In S. L. Washburn & P. Dobriner (Eds.), *Perspectives on human evolution 2*. New York: Holt, Rinehart and Winston, 1972. Pp. 166–168.

Lewontin, R. C. *The genetic basis of evolutionary change*. New York: Columbia University Press, 1974.

Lewontin, R. C., Ginzburg, L. R., & Tuljapurkar, S. D. Heterosis as an explanation for large amounts of genic polymorphism. *Genetics*, 1978, *88*, 149–169.

Lewontin, R. C., & Hubby, J. L. A molecular approach to the study of genic heterozygosity in natural populations. II. Amount of variation and degree of heterozygosity in natural populations of *Drosophila pseudoobscura*. *Genetics*, 1966, *54*, 595–609.

L'Héritier, P., & Teissier, G. Une expérience de sélection naturelle. Courbe d' élimination du gène "Bar" dans une population de Drosophiles en équilibre. *Comptes Rendus Des Séances de la Société de Biologie et de ses Filiales*, 1934, *117*, 1049–1051.

Margoliash, E. & Fitch, W. M. Evolutionary variability of cytochrome c primary structures. *Annals of the New York Academy of Science*, 1968, *151*, 359–881.

Mather, K. Polygenic inheritance and natural selection. *Biological Review*, 1943, *18*, 32–64.

Mayr, E. *Systematics and the origin of species*. New York: Columbia University Press, 1942.

Mayr, E. *Animal species and evolution*. Boston: Belknap, 1963.

McClintock, B. The control of gene action in maize. In H. H. Smith (Ed.), *Genetic control of differentiation*. Brookhaven Symposium of Biology, No. 18, 1965. Pp. 162–184.

Moore, G. P., Scheller, R. H., Davidson, E. H. & Britten, R. J. Evolutionary change in the repetition frequency of sea urchin DNA sequences, 1978, *15*, 649–660.

Nuttall, G. H. F. *Blood immunity and blood relationship*. Cambridge: Cambridge University Press, 1904.

Ohta, T., & Kimura, M. On the constancy of the evolutionary rate of cistrons. *Journal of Molecular Evolution*, 1971, *1*, 18–25.

Sacher, G. A. Relation of life span to brain weight and body weight in mammals. In G. E. W. Wolstenholme & M. O'Connor (Eds.), *CIBA colloquium on aging. The lifespan of animals*, Vol. 5. Boston: Brown, Little, 1959. Pp. 115–133.

Sarich, V. M. Primate systematics with special reference to Old World Monkeys. In J. R. Napier & P. H. Napier (Eds.), *Old world monkeys: Evolution, systematics and behavior*. New York: Academic Press, 1970. Pp. 175–226.

Simpson, G. G. *Time and mode in evolution*. New York: Columbia University Press, 1944.

Thoday, J. M. Location of polygenes. *Nature* (London), 1961, *191*, 368–370.

Van Valen, L. A new evolutionary law. *Evolutionary Theory*, 1973, *1*, 1–30.

Weinberg, A. M. The limits of science and transcience. *Interdisciplinary Science Review*, 1977, *2*, 337–342.

Wilson, A. C., & Sarich, V. M. A molecular time scale for human evolution. *Proceedings of the National Academy of Science, U.S.A.*, 1969, *63*, 1088–1093.

Wilson, A. C., Sarich, V. M. & Maxson, L. The importance of gene rearrangement in evolution: Evidence from studies of chromosomal, protein and anatomical evolution. *Proceedings of the National Academy of Science, U.S.A.*, 1974, *71*, 3028–3030.

The Evolution of Diversity in Brain Size

HARRY J. JERISON

The size of the brain—its weight or volume—is an extraordinarily useful measure in neurobiology. Other chapters in this volume show many of the ways in which it is useful. In this chapter I will discuss aspects of the "why" of it. There is order even in diversity, a well known fact in analysis above the species level. I will review that interspecific orderliness as background for the main theme of this chapter, which emphasizes diversity in brain size at the intraspecific level, at the level of individual differences.

Toward the end of this chapter, data to justify the "evolution" in my title will be presented. Those are exciting data, covered only in summary form here; detailed statements must be reserved for other publications in which each result receives a properly complete treatment. I will analyze the evolution of diversity by considering the pattern of individual differences in brain size in each of the presently recognized hominid species or genera. To see those results in context, I will also review new data on diversity in brain size within an ancient species of mammal that lived about 35 million years ago. But first I must consider interspecific diversity.

There are three points to be made above the species level. First, brain size is a dependent variable determined by two major factors: allometry and encephalization. In the analysis of encephalization, both factors must be considered in depth. Second, brain size is an independent

29

DEVELOPMENT AND EVOLUTION
OF BRAIN SIZE

variable. It acts as a statistic that enables us to estimate more obviously fundamental parameters of the brain. Finally, brain size can operate as an intervening variable for general theory. Multivariate methods have been introduced for analyses of the first and second type. I present a multivariate analysis of intraspecific data at the end of this chapter, and discuss its role for interspecific analysis at that time.

Above the Species Level

Geometry and evolutionary history impose two basic constraints on the structure and function of the vertebrate brain. It is very likely that all living mammals are descended from a common ancestor among the mammallike reptiles of about 200 million years ago, and in the evolutionary diversification of the brain, in speciation, in adaptive radiation, a common pattern remained. Forebrain, midbrain, and hindbrain are distinguishable in all vertebrates, and the basic circuitry of mammalian brains is detectable in all mammalian species. The description of the relationships has been the task of comparative neurology.

Given the common structural pattern, there is also the constraint of geometry. Mammalian brains, and especially the brains of placental mammals, have essentially the same assortment of nuclear masses of neurons, differing primarily in the relative contributions of each nuclear mass to the brain as a whole. The various kinds of neurons in the brain are present in quantity in all brains, one supposes, and an alternative way of analyzing a brain is to emphasize the problem of packing neurons into the available space.

Such an analysis leads eventually to a notion of a statistical, rather than morphological, neuron which represents an average neuron with respect to size, packing density, and the average amount of glial cells that it encumbers. This approach clarifies the statistical analysis of brain size, in which an allometric component is associated with body size and the remainder, or residual, is associated with encephalization.

Allometry and Encephalization

The empirical definition of encephalization is derived from the double logarithmic graph of the brain and body weights of species. The regression of log brain weight on log body weight is the allometric equation. It accounts for about 80% of the variance in interspecific brain/body data. Encephalization is the residual from this regression. We do not have to be satisfied with this purely empirical definition, however; the orderly data of allometry and encephalization cry out for a reasonable theoretical analysis. I will outline such a theory. (See Jerison, 1977, for a more complete statement.)

The theory is based on a fundamental feature of all vertebrates: sensory and motor surfaces of the body are represented as maps in the brain, and the maps are repeated again and again in different parts of the brain. To the extent that bodily structures are similar, there are inevitable similarities in the brain maps of different species. When there are also important functional differences among species, these may be reflected in the brain as differences in the number of maps and the amount of detail in a map. Rhesus monkeys, for example, probably have at least 12 separable and differently specialized maps of their retinas at the level of the visual cortex alone (Zeki, 1978). Mammals less reliant on vision probably have fewer and less detailed maps, and, consequently, less extensive visual cortex.

When functional differences are less important, as in related species that are similar behaviorally but differ in body size, the theory posits a different kind of enlargement of the brain. The number of maps and their detailed organization are considered to be more or less the same, but they are assumed to be enlarged in the larger species, following the enlargement of the body surfaces that are represented. Differentiation of this type appears to occur in at least some rodents (Campos & Welker, 1976; Welker, 1976).

The distinction between the two kinds of enlargement of the brain and its maps is a distinction between amplification and mere representation. A difference in amplification in two species implies a difference in their capacities to process information derived from a bodily surface such as retina, basilar membrane, muscle, or skin. When brains differ in size but not in amplification, the species should be similar in their behavioral capacities despite differences in body size.

In its quantitative statement, the theory leads to the identification of encephalization with the amplification factor and allometry with the consistency, or conservation, of representation in species that differ in body size but are similar in information-processing capacity. The amplification factor turns out to be essentially the same as the encephalization quotient, and the requirement for consistency in the mapping explains the appearance of the two-thirds exponent (slope on a log-log plot) for the allometric equation. Furthermore, when there are significant amounts of brain tissue not related in any way to the mapping functions, this nonmapped tissue accounts for the empirical exponents of less than two-thirds that are found in curve fitting with data from closely related species.

That species differ in their encephalization, whether defined theoretically or empirically, may raise questions for intraspecific analysis of diversity. Should highly encephalized species be more (or less) variable in brain size than less encephalized species? That is the sort of issue that will be considered in the second half of this chapter under the heading, "Diversity within Species."

Brain Size as an Independent Variable

The most accepted justification for the use of brain size as a neurobiological measure is its role as a statistic in estimating parameters. This role is clearest when equations can be formulated to relate measures such as the packing density of cortical neurons to brain size. I found correlations ranging from .9 to 1.0 in eight such equations, in which cortical volume, cortical surface, neuron/glia ratio, length of dendritic arborization, and several neurochemical measures were treated as dependent variables (Jerison, 1977).

These equations emphasize the orderliness in the system. It is possible to highlight differences among species, however, by selecting species that are specialists in one adaptation or another. The equation for neuron density as a function of brain size, for example, looks very different if it is based on a relatively homogeneous and nonspecialized somatosensory area as opposed to a visual area, especially if the highly visual primates are included in the analysis. The equation, developed from work by Tower and his associates (see Tower & Young, 1973) on 11 species, from mouse to whale, is

$$N/V = K_1 E^{-1/3} \tag{1}$$

The correlation between log N/V (neurons per ccm of cortical volume) and log E (weight of the brain in grams) was $-.99$, an essentially perfect correlation, negative to reflect the negative value of the exponent. This orderliness is only vaguely present in the visual system; the striate cortex of large-brained monkeys and humans is significantly more densely packed relatively to that of smaller brained mammals than would be anticipated from this negative correlation (Cragg, 1967). There is, therefore, uncertainty associated with functions such as Eq. 1. But their orderliness and the orderliness of many other functions of brain size encourages one to work with them.

The most impressively orderly function of brain size that I have seen relates the surface area of the cortex to the weight of the brain. Elias and Schwartz (1969, 1971) provided data on 15 species of mammals, and Brodmann (1913) reported data on 32 other mammalian species. The correlation between log surface and log brain volume for the 47 species is .997. To two significant figures the correlation is 1.00. Because of the high correlation we should treat the regression equation as a functional equation. The relationship determined empirically between cortical surface S and brain size E is formally comparable to the kind of empirical law that led to major advances in other sciences, Kepler's laws, for example. The equation is

$$S = 4E^{.91} \tag{2}$$

The dimensional implications of the strange exponent will be developed in the next section.

The quantity of cortical neurons N in the brain appears to be related to brain size in proportion to a surface, as evidenced by the two-thirds exponent in the following equation from Shariff's (1953) data:

$$N = 10^8 E^{2/3} \tag{3}$$

Equation 3 is based on a correlation of .96 for log data on five primate species.

A dimensionally curious equation results from the analysis of cortical volume V as a function of brain size (Harman, 1947). Based on the data of 21 species, the log V versus log E correlation is .93. The equation is approximately:

$$V = .4E \tag{4}$$

This looks right for dimensional purposes because the equation is dimensionally balanced. But all is not quite so dainty, as we shall see in the next section.

Recognizing that longer dendritic arborizations imply more connections and that longer dendritic arborizations require more glial cells placed about the dendrites, we seek equations relating the length of the dendrite tree L (Bok, 1959) and the glia/neuron ration G/N (Tower and Young, 1973) to brain size E:

$$L = .1E^{1/3} \tag{5}$$

$$G/N = E^{1/3} \tag{6}$$

Equation 5 is based on four species, six neurons per species, as reported by Bok, and the correlation for the log data is .99 (not excessively high for so few measures). The correlation supporting Eq. 6, based on six species, is $r = .95$.

In summarizing these relationships I have presented them in their dimensionally simplest form. A more complete summary statement, which included least-squares fits in every instance, was presented in Jerison (1977). In each instance the equations are in the centimeter-grams-second (cgs) system. This is necessary because some of the constants in the equations are not dimensionless.

The parameters of the brain, as estimated by brain size, are precisely those that should be associated with its overall capacity to process information: the number of elements (Eq. 3) and the complexity of their interconnections (Eqs. 5 and 6). Recent advances in neuroanatomy and neurophysiology emphasize the vertical or columnar organization of the cerebral cortex. The unit may be a module of a few hundred neurons contained in a column of cortex about .1 cm deep that look like adjacent circles (the tops of cylinders) when the cortex is viewed from above Surface (Eccles, 1979; Szentágothai, 1978). Surface may, therefore, be fundamental, and it, too, is determined by brain size above the species level (Eq. 2).

None of these functions of brain size is significantly affected by encephalization. The statistics of the brain are determined by its size, but not by how it came by its size. Whether enlargement of the brain is by allometry or by encephalization it has the consequences indicated by Equations 1–6.

Theory: Braininess and Convolutedness

With the help of a bit of geometry, the functions of the brain size presented in the previous section explain why mammalian brains are as convoluted, or fissured, as they are. The explanation ties gross and microscopic and even submicroscopic anatomy together in a simple statement about the way brains are built.

The geometry is on the necessary relationship between surface and volume in similar solids. This must be of the form

$$Y = aX^{2/3} \tag{7}$$

The surface Y of any solid of a particular shape is related to the volume X of that solid, as shown by Eq. 7. This is a dimensionally balanced equation in that the square units of Y on the left are equated to square units on the right because the two-thirds power reduces the dimensionality of the volume from cubic to square units: $(U^3)^{2/3} = U^2$. The value a in Eq. 7 is determined by shape. In the sphere, which is the solid that minimizes surface per unit volume, $a = 4.84$. In cubes, $a = 6$. One of the solids that will interest us is a sectored sphere, which has a surface area equal to the sum of the external surface plus the flat areas of the sectors. When sectors are placed through the centroid, a sphere divided into two sectors (two hemispheres) has a value of $a = 7.26$. A four-sectored sphere has a value of $a = 9.68$.

To study the geometry of the brain and interpret some of the equations of the previous section dimensionally, we must have a consistent set of units. Some of the equations are not dimensionally balanced, and in those instances a geometric interpretation may be maintained if the constants are not dimensionless. All of the equations are in the centimeter-gram-second system for this reason. In living tissues such as brain, grams, milliliters, and cubic centimeters (weight, displacement, and volume) are dimensionally equivalent and will be treated as cubic units.

The surface/volume relationship for the brain given by Eq. 2 has an exponent of $.91 \pm .02$. This exponent, which is greater than two-thirds, coupled with the essentially perfect correlation between the logarithms of the measures, shows that the brain's shape changes in a extraordinarily orderly way when its size changes. The change is equivalent to an orangelike object without sectors becoming fissured into two sectors, then four sectors, and finally (for human, whale, and elephant brains) between eight and sixteen sectors. Imagine Equations 2 and 7, both graphed on log-log paper, with Eq. 7 represented in parametric form as a series of parallel lines at slope $2/3$ with values of a at 4.84, 7.26, 9.68, ... Eq. 2 would be a line with slope .91, crossing the set of parallel lines. Eq. 2 is, thus, an empirical representation of a discontinuous shift from value to value of a, a graphic representation of the changing shape of the brain. The increase in the amount of surface associated with the volume of the brain is produced by folding or fissuring the surface to an extent that is rigidly determined, or constrained, by the volume of the brain.

An empirical implication is that convolutedness, expressed as total surface area and braininess, or absolute brain size (across species), are equivalent measures. Neither is more important than the other empirically, because each can be estimated from the other by treating Eq. 2 as a regression equation. The estimate is almost free of error.

Why did extra fissurization and convolutions evolve? We know that the cerebral cortex is organized into columns, or modules, of neurons, and that fissures and convolutions allow more of these to be packed under the more extended surface. But Eq. 3 showed that the number of neurons in the cortex was related to the two-thirds power of brain size, and the neurons of a larger brain should fit under a surface generated by brain size without a change of shape.

The paradox is made more strange by the linear (though dimensionally clean) relationship between cortical volume V and brain size E in Eq. 4. The oddity of Eq. 4 is evident when we recognize that *cortex* means rind, or outer shell. The cortex is actually only a millimeter or so thick. If the brain had conserved its shape, rather than becoming convoluted, and if the cortex were compressed to zero thickness, then its area would be a function of the two-thirds power of E. As the thickness of the cortex increased slightly the very small volume would be a function of E raised to a power slightly greater than two-thirds. Only if the thickness of the cortex were so great that all of the brain were cortex would we expect a power of 1 (least-squares fitting for Eq. 4 actually resulted in $V = 0.31$ $E^{1.09}$, a still odder dimensional situation). The explanation must be that Eq. 4 is comparable to Eq. 2 in that it is a result of the changing shape of the cortical mass and the disproportionate increase in surface. It can, in fact, be shown that the cortex becomes slightly thicker in larger brains (proportional, approximately, to the one-sixth power of E). By taking the measures mentioned parenthetically in this paragraph, we see that the volume of the cortex should be determined by the product of its surface and thickness and thus be proportional to $E^{(.91 + .17)}$ or $E^{1.08}$.

The idea of dimensional cleanliness in interpreting equations 1–6 may be inappropriate. Curve-fitting seems to make better sense here since apparent changes in dimensionality are really changes in shape with changes in size, and can be represented by moving a function from one dimensionally clean equation to another, where the parameter is shape (e.g., sectors of a sphere). The unusual thing is the orderliness of the shift from one level to another.

We see now that the volume of cortex increased disproportionately in spite of the apparently dimensionally clean Eq. 4. Since from Eq. 3 it is evident that this was not necessary to pack the right number of neurons into the cortex, it must be the case that fewer neurons are packed into a unit amount of cortex in larger brained species. (We know that to be so from Eq. 1.) And we can now see the resolution of the paradox between Equations 2 and 3. The number of neurons is arrived at by counting Nissl-stained neurons; in effect by counting nuclei of cells. If nuclei were all that had to be packed into the cerebral cortex, Eq. 3 tells us that there would be no need for (and presumably no development of) convolutions. But a neuron is more than its nucleus, or even its cell body. Most of its mass is in its dendritic arborization. When we see pictures of neurons that show the arborization, the dendrites appear as almost Euclidian lines, and we may be tempted to think of them as massless lines. But they are solid objects that take up space. Convolutions evolved to provide space for the increased arborization in larger brains; we can read the increase from Equations 5 and 6. And the amount of convolutedness is exactly right for packing the arborization. No space is wasted.

As a final exercise, let us calculate the amount of space occupied by the arborization of one neuron. Note, first, that dividing Eq. 3 by Eq. 4 provides the value $K_1 = 2.5 \times 10^8$ for Eq. 1. Though a bit high for Tower's data, this is a reasonable one for Shariff's (1953). The reciprocal of Eq. 1 can now be written to give the volume of cortex for a neuron:

$$V/N = 4 \times 10^{-9} E^{1/3} \tag{8}$$

The constant in Eq. 8 has the dimension U^2, when U is "length." If we now imagine the space occupied by a single neuron as made up of a long shaft of length L given by Eq. 5 and of (equal) width and height, w, this volume would be

$$
\begin{aligned}
w^2 L &= V/N & (9) \\
w^2 &= (V/N)/L \\
&= (4 \times 10^{-9} E^{1/3})/10^{-1} E^{1/3} \\
w^2 &= 4 \times 10^{-8} \text{ cm}^2 & (10)
\end{aligned}
$$

(Recall that the constant has the dimension U^2.) This is the cross-sectional area that we should expect to find for a dendrite in a photomicrograph. We are more accustomed to linear statements of this dimension. Thus, we note that

$$
\begin{aligned}
w &= 2 \times 10^{-4} \text{ cm} \\
w &= 2 \text{ microns} & (11)
\end{aligned}
$$

Although this has been little more than an exercise in geometry, an analysis of how the space of the brain is filled by material, this last result must be gratifying. With the exception of the length of the dendritic arborization (Eq. 5), all of the calculations involved only gross measures of the brain. Counting neurons for Eq. 1 or Eq. 3 does not qualify as measurement for this purpose. And the fact that the order of magnitude of the dendritic arborization averages no more than a few millimeters and is partially determined by the size of the brain is hardly a surprise. Yet the final analysis enabled us to establish the order of magnitude of the diameter of a dendrite, a reasonable number in the light of electron microscopy. It suggests that this game can pay off in surprising ways.

Diversity within Species

This discussion of individual differences begins with a new look at brain/body relations in the human species. It is important to do this because of the mistaken consensus that certain differences in brain size, in particular those related to sex differences, can be accounted for by differences in body size. I will not review the matter in full, but will, instead, present a graphic reanalysis of what is perhaps the best available set of data in the present variability of human brain size (Pakkenberg & Voigt, 1964). Most of the discussion is on the evolution of within-species diversity in brain size as indicated by the fossil record and by several living species of mammals. I conclude the discussion and the chapter with the results of a multivariate analysis of some of the fossil materials that are available. At that point I will also review critically the application of multivariate methods to interspecific as well as intra-specific data.

The orderly pattern of variation is one of the aspects of brain size that makes it an important measure in quantitative neurobiology as well as in theoretical biology.

Brain: Body Relations

Body size has been overemphasized as a factor in brain size within species. In the early days of allometric analysis of brain/body relations, Lapique (1898, 1907) reported an exponent of about one-fourth for comparisons among different breeds of dogs. The interesting point to him was that this value was significantly lower than that found earlier by Dubois (1897) in fitting lines to pairs of points representing equally "intelligent" species that differed grossly in body size (e.g., cat and puma). Although it is clearly true that closely related species, such as the several species of macaques, do show some allometric brain/body relation, with an exponent of the order of .2, within-species data from homogeneous sample (i.e., controlling sex, breed, and age), often do not show impressive relationships. In the human species it is likely that there is no relationship at all between brain size and body size in healthy adults of the same sex and ethnic group.

Pakkenberg and Voigt (1964) summarized data on relatively normal brains and bodies from cadavers dissected at the University Institute of Forensic Medicine, University of Copenhagen. Their summary statistics were on brain weight, body weight, height, sex, and age. They reported brain weights consistently higher than those found in other populations, such as that from the Institute of Pathological Anatomy, Zagreb, Yugoslavia (Gjukic, 1955), and suggested that the Danish population was more nearly normal, since deaths were generally not preceded by prolonged illness and consequent emaciation. The differences were great enough to suggest the possibility of different procedures at autopsy and weighing of the brain, and it should be kept in mind that there is a possibility of real differences in the living brains of these ethnically different populations. The two sets of brain weights are summarized in Table III.1.

There are two other points of special interest. First, the differences between the sexes are obviously major. According to these data there is a 158 gm advantage of the Danish male over the female and a 130 gm advantage in the Yugoslavian sample. Gjukic (1955) reports the standard deviations for the latter population as 119 gm for males and 115 gm for females. From this we can calculate a combined standard deviation for the entire Yugoslavian sample of 1901 as 133.5 gm. It is evident that the coefficient of variation in this human population is of the order of 10% (119/1358 = 8.8% for the male sample; 115/1228 = 9.4% for the Yugoslavian population). (The value of the coefficient of variation will be a major concern in the analysis of the evolutionary problem to be pre-

TABLE III.1
Mean Brain Weight in Human Populations[a]

Investigator	Males	Females	Total
Pakkenberg and Voigt (1964)	1440 gm (724)	1282 gm (302)	1393 gm (1026)
Gjukic (1955)	1358 gm (852)	1228 gm (1049)	1286 gm (1901)

[a]Number of cases for each mean is in parentheses.

sented later.) It may be appropriate to point out here that the problem of combining two "normal" (Gaussian) samples to produce a third "normal" sample is a methodological oddity, since the third sample is known to be bimodal. In fact, bimodality (as opposed to nonnormality) cannot be detected with known statistical tests unless the means of the samples producing the two modes are at least two standard deviations apart (Cox, 1966).

The second point of interest about the human brain sizes in Table III.1 is methodological. The apparent difference between the Danish and the Yugoslavian populations is 107 gm, almost a full standard deviation (assuming these equal for the two populations). But none of the samples contributing to the populations are as different as that. The male samples are 82gm apart, and the females are 54 gm apart, differences of the order of one-half a standard deviation. The inflated difference between the total populations is an artifact of the true sex difference and the different contributions of male and female brains to the population means. The Danish population has more than twice as many men as women, and so has a population mean artifactually close to the male mean; the Yugoslavian population has about four-fifths as many men as women, and thus has a mean somewhat too close to that of the female sample. A correct view would thus place the Danish population at about one-half a standard deviation above the Yugoslavian, and that is the difference that has to be explained, either on the basis of the condition of the brain at death (edema, emaciation, etc.); on the basis of differences in dissection, weighing, or other technical, procedural matters; or as indicating a true difference between the groups from which these samples were obtained. It is not presently possible to choose among the alternatives.

The population differences that resulted from unequal sampling of the sexes in the two groups alerts us to other artifacts of a related sort. The previous artifact is a statistical confounding in which sex is a hidden variable. The most frequently cited aspect of Pakkenberg and Voigt's (1964) work is on another effect, the brain/body relationship within the human species: "Brain weight depends significantly on height, but not on body weight [p. 303]." This conclusion is wrong on two counts. An inappropriate regression analysis seems to have been used; at least, no clearly interpretable regression analysis is presented. However, this criticism is minor; even on the basis of the reported data a more correct conclusion would be: *Brain weight depends neither on height nor weight, but a brain/body relationship may appear if age is permitted to enter into an analysis as an uncontrolled or "hidden," variable.*

That this is the case is evident from Figure III.1, which is based on Pakkenberg and Voigt's male sample. If one examines only the left-hand histogram in Figure III.1, Pakkenberg and Voigt's conclusion about brain weight and height appears to be amply justified. It is only when the companion data in the right-hand histogram are seen, with the knowledge that these are from the same sample, that we suspect a possible artifact. Can it be that the effect of height is really a hidden effect of age? Their data strongly suggest that this is precisely the case.

The crux of the matter is in the nature of their sample. The data were collected between 1959 and 1962, which means that the oldest men, the 32 who were more than 79 years old, were born in the year 1882 or earlier. The youngest men were 19 years old, and may have been born as recently as 1943. One of the major trends during that 60 year interval has been the steady increase in height, and in a large sample of individuals of different ages taken in the year 1960 we can predict with confidence that an age-height correlation of exactly the same appearance as the age-brain-weight histogram of Figure III.1 would be found. This reasoning from anthropometric data also helps explain the poorer correlation between brain weight and body weight in the Danish population of men. Although there is a secular trend toward increased height during the past century, there is another correlate of aging: putting on weight. So we can assume that the increase in body weight with age (if it occurred in this population) would have counteracted somewhat the effect of increased height in younger men.

The role of aging indicated in Figure III.1 has been known for many years. The right-hand histogram very likely represents a real reduction in brain size as we age, but one may question whether the effect among

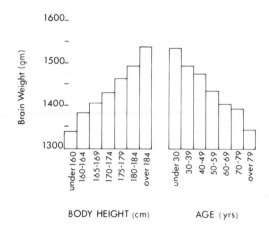

FIGURE III.1. Frequency distributions of brain weight in 724 Danish men classified with respect to height (left) and age (right) [Data from Pakkenberg and Voigt, 1964.]

younger men (under 40 or 50 in Figure III.1) is due to aging. Perhaps here the causal sequence is reversed and the apparent effect of age is due to a contribution of a true effect of height as a hidden variable. It seems hard to honor the idea that we lose as much brain weight between our 20s and our 30s as is indicated in the histogram. The question cannot be answered on the basis of the published data.

Pakkenberg has kindly provided me with raw data on his group, and I examined the relationship in younger men, ranging from 28 to 41 years of age. The sample was chosen to match 80 men with a comparable sample of women with about that range of ages. I assumed that the effect of age would be minimal in this sample, and that any effect of height would be evident. None of the correlations within this sample of 80 was significantly different from zero. No effect of height, no effect of weight, and no effect of age on brain weight was evident.

Given the underlying variation of the measures, a sample size of 80 is large enough to produce a significant effect by usual criteria ($p < .05$) if the effect of height indicated by Figure III.1 is still present when the effect of age is controlled. (The statistical control by partial regression techniques fails in this instance because of nonlinearities.) The effect of age is controlled by selecting a sample that is homogeneous in age. Although this restricts the range of heights, the restriction is not very great, and almost the full range of heights of the original population was represented. The correlations within the sample of 80 were as follows: for age-height, $r = -.08$; for age-brain-weight, $r = .02$ (i.e., the control was effective); for height-brain-weight, $r = .05$.

Sex differences in brain weight in samples of 80 younger men and women were significant, and, as in the population, the difference was about one standard deviation. It is not explained by a body size effect, since the effect is absent in these samples. There is more to be said on this matter, but it can be summed up by admitting that we have no explanation for the difference between the sexes in brain weight.

The History of Diversity

We are now ready to review the fossil record of diversity in brain size. Our perspective is that developed in the previous pages. The fossil record of diversity above the species level was the main topic of Jerison (1973). It can be summed up briefly as indicating that body size has played more or less the same role in determining brain size throughout the history of the vertebrates. Thus, an allometric analysis of brain/body relations reveals comparable trends throughout vertebrate history. The picture for living fish and reptiles is also the same as that found for fossil fish and reptiles, although we now have evidence of some groups, living and fossil, that strain the orderly analysis first presented (see Ebbesson & Northcutt, 1976, for evidence of the lower grade of encephalization in agnathans; Hopson, 1977, for evidence of a higher-than-reptilian grade in the ostrich-like dinosaurs; and Platel, 1974, for evidence of living lizards that appear to be more encephalized than any other living reptiles, and close to the mammalian grade).

The history of diversity in encephalization above the species level indicates that when a particular grade of encephalization was achieved within an adaptive zone, the taxon (family or higher) achieving that grade tended to conserve it in further evolution. There are few instances of continued progressive evolution within an adaptive zone, even in the class of vertebrates that "specialized" in encephalization, the mammals. Generally, the early mammals were less encephalized than their descendants, which presumably reflects the more diverse adaptive modes in later taxa. The interspecific picture is generally one of conservative evolution for the brain. Most adaptations are accomplished without a heavy demand for mass of neural control tissues, and evolution does not "progress" without appropriate value for the investment in neural expansion.

Most of the evidence of intraspecific evolution of diversity is from the history of the primates—specifically of the hominids. There is now a fairly large literature on hominid endocranial casts (Tobias, 1975), which is summarized in Figure III.2. This graph is the centerpiece of my contribution, and I want to analyze it with you in some detail.

Figure III.2 is a graph that "grew." It began as an illustration of the fossil evidence on the history of the human brain. For that analysis (Jerison, 1975) I used Tobias's review (1975) as a point of departure. Tobias had summarized the evidence on 10 australopithecine endocasts, 15 endocasts of *Homo erectus*, and 5 endocasts attributed to *Homo habilis*. To those data I added Gjukic's (1955), in order to suggest a progression from an australopithecine (*A* in Figure III.2) to habiline (*H*) to erectus, or pithecanthropine (*P*), and to a sapient (*S*) grade. Originally I provided the data in the form of cumulative frequency distributions of brain size. Graphed on "probability paper," such distributions are fitted by straight lines, the slopes of which are proportional to the standard deviations. In reviewing these lines for Tobias's summary of hominid data, it was clear that the standard deviations increased as the means of the distributions increased. I therefore regraphed the data, taking the cumulative frequencies as functions of the logarithms of brain size. If the standard

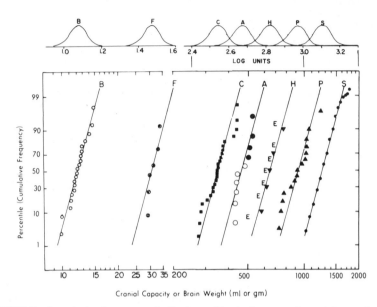

Cranial Capacity or Brain Weight (ml or gm)

FIGURE III.2. Cumulative frequency distributions of brain size or endocranial capacity seen in eight mammalian species. When a measure from a normally distributed variate is graphed in this way, on probability paper, the slope of the fitted line is proportional to the standard deviation. Standard deviations may be read directly by subtracting the 16th from the 50th percentile. The abcissa in this graph is scaled logarithmically, hence standard deviations are in log-units. The first derivatives of the "lines" are shown above the graph—as normal curves. When parallel lines can be drawn for log—normal data (as in this case), it signifies equal coefficients of variation for the samples. Groups are *B—Barthygenys reevesi* (Wilson, 1971); *F—Felis domestica* (Weber, 1896); *C—Pan troglodytes* (25 male and female chimpanzees weighing 35 kg or more, from Bauchot & Stephan, 1969); *A—Australopithecus* (filled circles are robust, open are gracile specimens; Tobias, 1975); *H—Homo habilis* (Tobias, 1975); *P—Homo erectus* (pithecanthropines, Tobias, 1975); *S—Homo sapiens* (Gjukic, 1955); *E—Equus caballus* (horse; Count, 1947). Note that log-units corresponding to linear measures of brain size are shown with the bell-shaped curves at top. From Jerison, 1979, reprinted by permission.

deviation is proportional to the mean, the data should be fitted by a set of parallel lines.

The four lines marked *A*, *H*, *P*, and *S* in Figure III.2 are the ones drawn in the log-frequency graph that I originally prepared; the lines can indeed be parallel and fit these data. The lines are actually drawn by visual inspection, and my procedure was to use the remarkably "linear" arrangement that resulted from casting Gjukic's data on *Homo sapiens* into the form of a cumulative frequency distribution graphed on probability paper. I simply drew a set of lines through the three other sets of points that would be parallel to the line through Gjukic's data. Before going on to the remaining data in Figure III.2, I wish to comment in more detail on the method of graphing, its validity and utility, and on the reliability of the data.

The method of graphing is borrowed from classical psychophysics. Assuming that measures are randomly derived from an underlying population, the graph provides a way of testing the reasonableness of the assumption that the population is normal (Gaussian). To illustrate with the habiline data: Five values are available from Tobias's review. If these are truly random samples from a normal population, the lowest value may be taken to represent the lowest 20% of the population, the next higher as representing the twenty-forty percentile range of the population, and so on. The graphic procedure assigns each point to the midpoint of the range; thus the lowest habiline value is assigned to the tenth percentile (midpoint between 0-20), the next to the thirtieth percentile, then fiftieth, seventieth, and ninetieth. Although there are a few assumptions about the distribution hidden in this procedure, the end result does no violence to the facts.

In the case of Gjukic's data on *Homo sapiens*, the graphing followed a somewhat different procedure, since the published data were in the form of a frequency distribution. Gjukic tallied the brain sizes of his population within class intervals of 50 gm for the range from 1000 gm to 1800 gm, resulting in 16 class intervals. The mean within each class interval was taken as a percentile value in the same way that individual data were used in the other curves of Figure III.2.

The preparation of the present form of Figure III.2 was a kind of experimental analysis of intraspecific diversity, in which, as additional data were collected, they were added to an earlier graph. Each increment of data was a kind of experiment. The first of these experiments was on hominid evolution, as noted before. My basic motive was to summarize the available data, but in the summarization, there appeared the serendipitous result that the intraspecific diversity of brain size in the homind data was consistent with the idea that diversity was proportional to the mean brain size. In the original graph (Jerison, 1975) only lines A, H, P, and S were drawn. The constant proportionality of diversity to mean is reflected in the reasonableness of drawing the diagonal lines for these groups parallel to one another. Among the more interesting aspects of this conclusion is that the much vaunted variability of living human brain sizes turns out to be an artifact, an instance of the selection of very unusual brains from the extremes of a normal, or at least not unusual, distribution. The famous cases of Anatole France (with a

1050gm brain) and Turgenev (with a 1900gm brain) appear as odd cases. In France's case, the brain was a reasonably normal one for an aged person—at the lower end of one's normal expectations. Turgenev's brain, on the other hand, must have been of the type seen at the upper tail of Gjukic's distribution; it is probably a sample from a different population. The best guess is that Turgenev suffered from and recovered from a subclinical hydrocephalus, presumably during infancy.

Following the unusual result on living and fossil hominids, it occurred to me to consider whether the unusual evolution of the human brain was peculiarly related to the evolution of language (Jerison, 1976). It is important to appreciate here that it is only when a particular behavioral adaptation is known to require large amounts of brain tissue that one may look at gross effects of the type to be found in this analysis of diversity for evidence directly connected to the behavior. I reasoned that if the enlargement of the hominid brain to the grade of *Homo sapiens* was related to the evolution of verbal language, it was conceivable that there would be different diversity in the hominid lineage than in mammals of comparable brain size that did not have language. More specifically, I considered the chimpanzee as a control for encephalization associated with verbal language. It is a species in which encephalization is related to other behavioral adaptations. I therefore added the chimpanzee data (C) to the graph. As you can see, these data are also adequately fitted by a normal curve showing the same diversity (same slope) as that for living and fossil humans.

In the complete form of Figure III.2 you see the results of further "experiments" to determine whether encephalization can be identified as the source of the pattern of diversity; that is, whether less encephalized species would be as diverse in brain size as the highly encephalized hominoids.

This test could be undertaken because of the lucky discovery of the 20 endocasts of *Bathygenys reevesi* (Wilson, 1971). These represent a grade of brain evolution, encephalization, achieved about 35 million years ago in a relatively unencephalized family of ungulates. There are no data on body size in *Bathygenys*, which makes it impossible to estimate its encephalization. But no species from its geological stratum and from its superfamily (entirely extinct today) has yet been discovered that was even close to the present average mammalian grade of encephalization. I analyzed the data from this sample and added these to the graph. As you can see, this sample, too, could be fitted by a line parallel to that of living humans.

Finally, data from six living cats (F) and seven living horses (E) were added as controls for known species with brain sizes at an essentially average mammalian grade, and yet differ in mean brain sizes as indicated. Horses were chosen as an average species that has a large brain as a result of the allometric relationship between brain and body size—that is, horses are relatively large-bodied and consequently have appropriately large brains.

The data on cats are interesting for methodological reasons, since this particular sample, though fitted reasonably by a line of the same slope as that for living humans, would actually be fitted by a steeper line if an "objective" method such as least-squares were used. The extreme values, the lightest and heaviest brain in the sample, are less extreme than they should be were the normality suggested by the middle four values retained. The line parallel to that for living humans fits the middle four values better than would an "objectively" determined least-squares fit. The objective fit would be distorted by the outliers if the visual fit is correct. In the horses, the least-squares and visual fits agree. Here it was impossible to draw a line for the horses and distinguish them from *Homo habilis* line. I therefore simply indicate the place of the horses by drawing their Es on the graph.

We will shortly consider the possible partitioning of diversity into contributions by various factors of brain size. Overall diversity, however, appears to be robust in the face of several evolutionary contributions to brain size. Species may be highly encephalized or relatively unencephalized and be equally diverse in brain size. Thus, the ancient ungulate species, *Bathygenys reevesi*, which could not have been especially encephalized, is comparable to the most encephalized of living mammals, *Homo sapiens*, in the diversity of brain size. Given that, it is less surprising to discover that it does not seem to matter why species are encephalized. The hominids, evolving toward a grade in which language and associated massive encephalization is characteristic, are comparable to their close relatives among the primates in the diversity of brain size within the species. This constancy of diversity, its conservation in the evolution of the mammalian brain, is the most important discovery that I have to report. It is a useful discovery for further evolutionary analysis (Lande, 1979).

The "objective" way of stating the idea that diversity remained constant is that the coefficient of variation remains the same. Here we normally compute a standard deviation from the actual values, a mean from the actual values, and divide the standard deviation by the mean. For such a computation, each datum is as heavily loaded as every other one, and there is no place for either art or subjectivity. The coefficients of variation as percentages V_i for the eight groups in Figure III.2, are subscripted as in the graph; $V_B = 10.2$, $V_F = 6.4$; $V_E = 10.9$, $V_C = 13.8$, $V_A = 9.2$, $V_H = 9.2$, $V_P = 15.0$, $V_S = 10.4$.

The graphic analysis of Figure III.2 indicates equal values for coefficients of variation. In a sense, the graph is a test of this equality, and I have asked you to join in a subjective judgment of the adequacy of the fit. I have suggested that the hypothesis of equality is reasonable— that is, the fit of all the sets of data by a set of parallel lines does not do violence to the data. Comparing this with the "objective analysis" just presented, we might be concerned by the too-small value for cats and the too-large values for chimps and pithecanthropines. The real problem is best seen by looking more closely at Figure III.2. The cat problem is resolved, I have suggested, by the outliers not lying far enough out. The opposite is evidently true for chimpanzees, with three of the upper points being "too heavy" and four of the lower points "too light." A slope of 13.8 on Figure III.2 would miss the mark for the sixteen central points in the chimpanzee distribution. It is clear that an "objective" analysis may be as misleading as a subjective one.

The pithecanthropine case may be a true misfit; that is, it may be that the pithecanthropines are actually sampled from two populations. If such sampling occurs, it appears in this kind of graphic analysis as an inflection point, a more or less horizontal array of points between the means of the two populations. In Figure III.2, such an inflection point may occur in the pithecanthropine data at about the thirtieth percentile— at an endocranial volume of about 850ml. Note that this interpretation is available if one graphs the data. It is masked in an "objective" calculation of a coefficient of variation or a standard deviation. I should note here that one can perform significance tests on data like these, and the pithecanthropine distribution is not statistically nonnormal by conventional criteria ($p < .05$) according to such tests. In fact, the only nonnormal distribution is that of *Homo sapiens*. The very large sample that is available enables one to reject the hypothesis of normality in living humans with great confidence: $\chi^2 = 363.8556$; $df = 13$; $p = .0000000016$.

In view of the difficulty normally involved in rejecting a false hypothesis of normality, the rejection of this hypothesis for Gjukic's human population may seem surprising, especially in view of the graphic data in Figure III.2 (S). It is not only the upper tail that forces the rejection. Examining the theoretical and actual distributions makes it clear that there are deviations from the predicted values throughout the distribution. The statistical test of goodness-of-fit was apparently adequate for picking up the effect of the bimodality of the population, consisting of combined male and female data. When the test was performed on only one sex, the sample size was still large enough to reject the hypothesis of normality, but in these instances the rejection is a result of the large number of outliers at the upper end of the distribution in both sexes. I assume that these outliers represent a different population, including subclinical hydrocephalus, post mortem edema, and so on.

Although the other data sets meet the criterion of normality according to statistical tests, it is worth noting how inadequate the raw data are. Hints about these data are available from the graphic analysis of Figure III.2. The situation of the pithecanthropines has already been noted. The hypothesis of two populations of this species—perhaps two species or subspecies—cannot be discounted, though there is nothing in Tobias's (1975) samples graphed here to suggest a basis for distinguishing a small-brained population from a large-brained one on biological or geological grounds.

The most unusual group in Figure III.2 is the australopithecines. It is assumed, conventionally, that at least two good species are involved here, gracile *Australopithecus africanus* contributing the lower six points and *Australopithecus robustus* (or *boisei*) contributing the upper four. These groups were combined in this analysis when it became clear that the coefficient of variation for brain (in the size range covered in Figure III.2) was likely to deviate from the 10% value of the graph had we separated the gracile from the robust australopithecines. With such small samples (four cases and six cases, respectively) there would have been little difficulty in satisfying ourselves with a fit by a straight line, but we would have been unhappy with a line parallel to the other lines in Figure III.2. Computing the coefficient of variation we would have found values of 4.4% for the gracile and 2.5% for the robust species. Since the combined data gave the "good" value of 9.2% we have, in effect, used the circular argument of "good" diversity to justify this particular grouping of data for Figure III.2. It should, perhaps, be noted that the situation in paleoanthropology and primate taxonomy is sufficiently fluid that this grouping may turn out to be acceptable (Wolpoff, 1976), that is, that our australopithecines constitute only one "good" species.

On the other hand, the australopithecine situation may be an artifact of the way brain size was measured in these specimens. Because of the great interest in the evolution of the human brain, the analysis of the fossil record has been unusually complete. Some of the specimens that have contributed data for this purpose have been quite fragmentary, and the endocranial volumes cited by Tobias (and copied for Figure III.2) often involved considerable reconstruction and conjecture. The method of reconstruction was to fill in gaps in an endocast with material modeled on known brains and endocasts. The result has been to make the "different" specimens partial models of one another in some instances. This results in a systematic reduction in measured diversity, and the calculated coefficients of variation among the australopithecines may be correctly low, because the diversity of this particular sample is low—the endocasts are not independently reconstructed. The habiline data (H) are comparably flawed, since the lower four points are all based on considerable, and imaginative, reconstruction. One recent text (Kochetkova, 1978) sees the habilines as modeled by australopithecines, and reconstructs the point shown as being at the seventieth percentile in Figure III.2 as so much smaller that it would fall at the tenth percentile with the smallest volume in the sample (560 ml). I believe the reconstruction by Tobias to be better, but the uncertainty about this and several other australopithecine and habiline endocasts is very great. In the habiline group, only the largest endocast, shown at the nineteenth percentile, is a value that most paleoanthropologists would accept with confidence. This is the well known KNM ER 1470, the specimen from East Rudolph (Koobi Fora) that displaces about 775 ml of water.

I hope you sense some of the uncertainties in the data and the analysis, but these uncertainties should not hide the orderliness evident in Figure III.2. The orderliness is apparent in the ease with which the lines in Figure III.2 can be drawn parallel to one another. And the orderliness consists in the conservation of diversity. Present diversity of brain size in mammalian species reflects past diversity. The amount of diversity (like the interspecific functions of brain size) is determined by the average brain size of a species, regardless of whether that size resulted from encephalization or allometry.

Multivariate Analysis

Among the methodological advances in the study of brain size, the application of multivariate methods is certain to have important effects. There have been several critical discussions of this issue (see Gould, 1975; Jerison, 1975 for reviews). Most of the applications of multivariate methods have been to interspecific diversity in brain size. Before presenting an analysis at the intraspecific level, a few critical comments on its application above the species level are in order.

The first comprehensive analysis (Sacher, 1970) was a factor analysis of the logarithms of the volume of various structures in the brain, the whole brain weight, body weight, and various ratios among those measures, as well as a "phyletic variate." The last was a subjectively assigned rank for each species with respect to degree of progressiveness of the brain. The most parsimonious interpretation of the results recognizes a general size factor that accounts for almost all (about 95%) of the variance in the data, and at least one additional factor related to the development of the olfactory system. As might be expected, the size factor contributes both to the encephalized and unencephalized fraction of the brain weight, the latter appearing as a contribution to total brain weight. In view of the correlation of the parts of the brain with the whole brain weight, and of the correlation of brain weight with body weight, it is not surprising that the inferences consistent with the factor analysis are complex. But the outstanding result was clearly that the first principal component in the analysis accounted for nearly all of the variance. This is particularly interesting in view of the population that provided data: 39 primate species and 24 insectivore species. The olfactory system factor was probably enhanced by the difference between these orders in the extent to which the olfactory (paleocortical), as opposed to visual and somatosensory (neocortical), systems are represented differentially.

Sacher's article is a landmark in multivariate analysis. However, an important artifact in his data has been consistently overlooked by most other researchers. The volume of the "neocortex" in his sample was actually the volume of the entire telencephalon from which was subtracted the volume of the several telencephalic systems that had been measured (schizocortex, hippocampus, etc.). The "neocortex" had originally been described as including the adjacent white matter (Stephan, Bauchot, & Andy, 1970). This volume of neocortex is not closely related to the "cortical volume" of Eq. 4.

We do an injustice to the organization of the brain by emphasizing the *multi* in multivariate analysis. This emphasis might lead one to expect many important factors, more or less independent of one another, to be contributing to brain size. It is important (even if surprising) that as a first approximation the reverse is the case. If total brain size is known, many of the other sizes can be estimated with remarkable accuracy. The situation is almost as rigidly determined as the cortical surface is by the brain volume (Eq. 2).

Intraspecific Analysis: *Bathygenys reevesi*

The primary objective of the following analysis was to relate measures of the foramen magnum to other measures that are taken on the endocasts. The issue is the incompletely resolved one of the place of the foramen magnum as an estimator of body size (Jerison, 1973, 1975). I present the graphic version of the analysis, performed on the 20 endocasts of *Bathygenys reevesi,* as a methodological exercise.

In this factor analysis I extracted two or three factors from a matrix of 10 measures × 20 individual endocasts. The measures are illustrated in Figure III.3,which also shows the positions of the measures in a two-factor space (varimax rotation). *Bathygenys* was probably a relatively small mammal, about the size of a living cat and smaller than any living ungulate. In appearance it may have resembled a miniaturized sheep. The mean volume of the 20 endocasts was 12.2 ml; the value of *L* in Figure III.3 averages 4.3 cm.

The first point about Figure III.3 is the independence of the size of the foramen magnum from the size of other structures or measures on the endocast. Factor II is a foramen magnum factor and Factor I is the general brain size factor. In view of the apparent independence of the measures, it is not surprising to find the first factor accounting for about 70% of the explained variance and the second factor for about 30%.

An unusual feature revealed by the analysis is the distinction between height and width of the foramen magnum. Furthermore, most of the cross-sectional area variance for the foramen magnum is accounted for by width variations. Height remains incompletely accounted for by these two factors.

Although the situation is too underdetermined to extract three factors, I was curious about the fate of the height of the foramen magnum if a third factor were extracted and performed the analysis summarized in Figure IV.4. Factor I remains the general size factor and is shown in

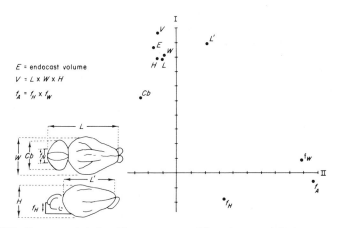

FIGURE III.3. Factor analysis for 10 measures on 20 endocasts of *Bathygenys reevesi,* a small oreodon from the Lower Oligocene of Big Bend, Texas. Varimax rotation has two factors extracted (cf. Fig. 4). Measures indicated on inset sketches of endocast: dorsal view above and lateral view below.

Figure IV.4 as the height of the vertical column for each measure. The relationship between the two linear measures of the foramen magnum and its area are clarified here; the linear measures were apparently independent but both contribute to the area factor although width contributes more.

Within a species—at least within *Bathygenys*—foramen magnum may be less associated with gross brain size than in interspecific analyses. Across species, the measure appears to estimate both body size and total brain size rather well. As an estimator its utility for the analysis of encephalization is limited, however, because in estimating total brain size it leaves almost no residuals that can be related to encephalization. There are presumably no intraspecific differences in encephalization— at least, no measurable ones. The low common variance of brain size and the size of the foramen magnum is therefore not surprising. We lack data on body size in *Bathygenys*, but the low intraspecific correlation between brain and body size (except where different breeding populations are compared) suggests that here the foramen magnum may be correlated with body size. It is a relationship worth looking at in paleoneurology.

Summary and Conclusions

Intraspecific diversity in brain size is significantly different from interspecific diversity. The common roots in diversity are certain to be a

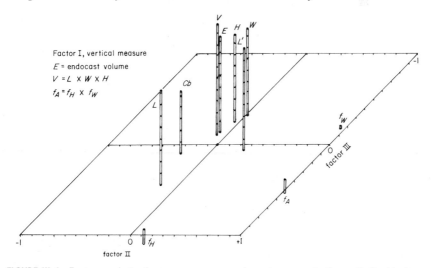

FIGURE III.4. Factor analysis of same measures and specimens as in Figure III. 3 with three factors extracted. Note that Factor I of Figure III. 3 is represented here as the height of the column, indicating the factor loading of each measure.

major topic of future analyses in paleoneurology. The interspecific problem has hardly been touched by geneticists, although its relationship to individual differences within a species is certain to be an important concern for those who suggest an evolutionary analysis based on models from population genetics (Lande, 1979).

At all levels of analysis, the most encouraging element is the orderly structure of the brain and the frequency with which metrical features of the brain have been conserved in evolution. The brain is a physical structure that exists in three dimensions. Its contents, at least those that are cellular or more massive, are also three dimensional structures. This poses constraints that make certain relationships unavoidable. When it must seem that a dimensional requirement is not met, there is usually a clue in the failure that can lead to the discovery of some unsuspected structural feature. One such "failure" led to our discussion here of the significance of convolutedness.

Convolutedness is a simple adaptation to brain size, made to accommodate the additional neurons needed by larger brains. If these additional neurons are to connect to other neurons, including those homologous with neurons of smaller brains, they must have more extensive dendritic arborizations than do neurons in smaller brains, at least on the average. The arborization requires space, and the convoluting of brains permits brains to add more space for neurons. The addition is exactly appropriate for the extra arborization. The metric analysis incidentally enables one to calculate the average diameter of a dendrite—two microns in the calculation presented here—an illustration of the orderliness of brain structure in neurobiology. It is great enough to permit easy transfer from the most gross level to the ultramicroscopic level of analysis.

In our analysis of convolutedness the aim was to account for quantitative rather than qualitative differences. The *pattern* of convolutions in a species is relatively fixed and is determined by a complex interaction between genetic programs for the growth of the brain and its coverings, and the environment within which the growth takes place. The issue has been reviewed in recent years by Richman, Stewart, Hutchinson, and Caviness (1975) and by Welker (1976).

Much of the orderliness of the functions of brain size is inherent in the brain's characteristics as tissue. For most metrical analyses it makes little or no difference whether brains differ in size because of allometry, encephalization, or differential specializations. In most instances, all that seems to count is that a brain is a particular size. The orderliness that I have stressed may have exceptions, however. Several were noted in connection with Eq. 1. They may also occur in the conservation of intraspecific diversity in that the coefficient of variation in species with brains weighing 5 or 10 gm or less may be significantly less than 10%. In laboratory rats it appears to be of the order of 5%. This may also be true of several insectivore species (Bauchot & Stephan, 1966).

This has been a chapter on orderliness and constraints. As noted several times, the emphasis on order may mask disorder inherent in some systems. But the evidence of order in the brain viewed from a geometer's perspective must certainly lead to a true picture of the brain. As a neurobiological variable, brain size is especially useful in enabling us to see that order.

References

Bauchot, R. & Stephan, H. Données nouvelles sur l'encéphalisation des insectivores et des prosimiens. *Mammalia, 1966, 30,* 160–196.

Bauchot, R. & Stephan, H. Encéphalisation et niveau evolutif chez les Simiens. *Mammalia,* 1969, 33, 225–275.

Bok, S. T. *Histonomy of the Cerebral Cortex.* New Jersey: Van Nostrand-Reinhold, 1959.

Brodmann, K. Neue Forschungsergebnisse der Grosshirnrindenanatomie mit besonderer Berucksichtigung anthropologischer Fragen. *Verh. 85 Vers. Deutsch, Naturf, and Aertze in Wien,* 1913.

Campos, G. B. & Welker, W. I. Comparisons between brains of a large and small hystricomorph rodent: Capybara, *Hydrochoerus* and Guinea Pig, *Cavia;* neocortical projection regions and measurements of brain subdivisions. *Brain, Behavior and Evolution,* 1976, 13, 243–306.

Count, E. W. Brain and body weight in man: Their antecedents in growth and evolution. *Annals of the New York Academy of Science,* 1947, 46, 993–1122.

Cox, D. R. Notes on the analysis of mixed frequency distributions. *British Journal of Mathematical and Statistical Psychology,* 1966, 19, 39–47.

Cragg, B. G. The density of synapses and neurones in the motor and visual areas of the cerebral cortex. *Journal of Anatomy,* 1967, 101, 639–654.

Dubois, E. Sur le rapport du poids de l'encéphale avec la grandeur du corps chez les mammifères. *Bulletins de la Société d'Anthropologie de Paris,* 1897, 8, 337–376.

Ebbesson, S. O. E., & Northcutt, R. G. Neurology of anamniotic vertebrates. In R. B. Masterton, M. E. Bitterman, C. B. G. Campbell, & N. Hotton (Eds.), *Evolution of Brain and Behavior in Vertebrates.* Hillsdale, N.J.: Erlbaum-Wiley, 1976. Pp. 115–146.

Eccles, J. C. *The human mystery.* New York: Springer-Verlag, 1979.

Elias, H., & Schwartz, D. Surface areas of the cerebral cortex of mammals determined by stereological methods. *Science,* 1969, 166, 111–113.

Elias, H. & Schwartz, D. Cerebro-cortical surface areas, volumes, lengths of gyri and their interdependence in mammals, including man. *Zeitschrift für Saugetierkunde,* 1971, 36, 147–163.

Gjukic, M. Ein Beitrag zum Problem der Korrelation zwischen Hirngewicht and Körpergewicht. *Zeitschrift für Morphologie and Anthropologie*, 1955, *47*, 43–57.

Gould, S. J. Allometry in Primates, With Emphasis of Scaling and the Evolution of the Brain. *Contributions to primatology*, 1975, *5*, 244–292.

Harman, P. J. Quantitative analysis of the brain-isocortex relationship in Mammalia. *Anatomical Record*, 1947, *97*, 342.

Hopson, J. A. Relative brain size and behavior in archosaurian reptiles. *Annual Review of Ecology and Systematics*, 1977, *8*, 429–448.

Jerison, H. J. *Evolution of the brain and intelligence*. New York: Academic Press, 1973.

Jerison, H. J. Fossil evidence of the evolution of the human brain. *Annual Review of Anthropology*, 1975, *4*, 27–58.

Jerison, H. J. Discussion paper: The paleoneurology of language. *Annals of the New York Academy of Science*, 1976, *280*, 370–382.

Jerison, H. J. The theory of encephalization. *Annals of the New York Academy of Science*, 1977, *299*, 146–160.

Jerison, H. J. On the evolution of neurolinguistic diversity: Fossil brains speak. In. C. J. Fillmore, & W. S-Y. Wang, (Eds.), *Individual differences in language ability and language behavior*. New York: Academic Press, 1979, Pp. 277–287.

Kochetkova, V. I. *Paleoneurology*. New York: Halsted Press, 1978.

Lapique, L. Sur la relation du poids de l'encéphale au poids du corps. *Comptes Rendus des séances de la Société de Biologie et de ses Filiales*, 1898, *50*, 62–63.

Lapique, L. Tableau générale des poids somatique et encéphalique dans les especes animales. *Bulletins de la Société d'Anthropologie de Paris*, 1907, *8*, 248–262.

Lande, R. Quantitative genetic analysis of multivariate evolution, applied to brain:body size allometry. *Evolution*, 1979, *33*,(1), 402–416.

Pakkenberg, H. & Voigt, J. Brain weights of Danes. *Acta Anatomica*, 1964, *56*, 297–307.

Platel, R. Poids encéphalique et indice d'encéphalisation chez les reptiles sauriens. *Zoologica Anzeiger, Jena*, 1974, *192*, 332–382.

Richman, D. P., Stewart, R. M., Hutchinson, J. W. & Caviness, V. S., Jr. Mechanical model of brain convolutional development. *Science*, 1975, *189*, 18–21.

Sacher, G. A. Allometric and factorial analysis of brain structure in insectivores and primates. In C. R. Noback & W. Montagna (Eds.), *The Primate Brain*. New York: Appleton, 1970. Pp. 245–287.

Shariff, G. A. Cell counts in the primate cerebral cortex. *Journal of Comparative Neurology*, 1953, *98*, 381–400.

Stephan, H., Bauchot, R. & Andy, O. J. Data on size of the brain and of various parts in insectivores and primates. In C. R. Noback, & W. Montagna (Eds.), *The Primate Brain*. New York: Appleton, 1970. Pp. 289–297.

Szentágothai, J. The neuron network of the cerebral cortex: A functional interpretation. *Proceedings of the Royal Society (London)* Series B, 1978, *201*, 219–248.

Tobias, P. V. Brain evolution in the Hominoidea. In R. H. Tuttle. (Eds.), *Primate Functional Morphology and Evolution*. The Hague: Mouton, 1975. Pp. 353–392.

Tower, D. B. & Young, O. M. The activities of butyrylcholinesterase and carbonic anhydrase, the rate of anaerobic glycolysis, and the question of a constant density of flial cells in cerebral cortices of mammalian species from mouse to whale. *Journal of Neurochemistry*, 1973, *20*, 269–278.

Weber, M. Vorstudien über das Hirngewicht der Säugethiere. *Festchrift für Carl Gebenbauer*, 1896, *3*, 105–123.

Welker, W. I. Brain evolution in mammals. In R. B. Masterton, M. E. Bitterman, C. B. G.

Campbell, & N. Hotton (Eds.), *Evolution of brain and behavior in vertebrates.* Hillsdale, New Jersey: Erlbaum–Wiley, 1976. Pp. 251–344.

Wilson, J. A. Early Tertiary vertebrate faunas, Vieja Group. Trans-Pecos Texas: Agriochoeridae and Merycoidodontidae. *Texas Memorial Museum Bulletin 18,* 1971. PP. 1–83.

Wolpoff, M. H. Some aspects of the evolution of early hominid sexual dimorphism. *Current Anthropology,* 1976, *17,* 579–606.

Zeki, S. M. Functional specialization in the visual cortex of the rhesus monkey. *Nature,* 1978, *274,* 423–428.

Chapter IV

Brain Size, Allometry, and Reorganization: Toward a Synthesis

Ralph L. Holloway

Few would doubt that the brain is one of the major organs most responsible for human behavioral adaptation, and that by better understanding the evolutionary development of this organ, we increase our chances of finding a scientific explanation of what we are and how we came to be. The study of brain evolution, particularly in higher[1] primates, presents enormous difficulties, however. Such study can only be approached in a synthetic manner, relying strongly on both comparative neuroanatomy and paleoneurology, which must in turn be integrated with ever-expanding knowledge in genetics, evolutionary theory, ecology and adaptation, the fossil and archaeological records of hominid evolution, and all aspects of neurobiology that provide insights into structural–functional relationships. Aside from the difficulties residing in the synthetic approach, evidential problems exist regarding the question of which neurological structural units are most appropriate for studying brain evolution (see Welker, 1976 for a review of many of these epistemological problems; also Edinger, 1949; Gould, 1975; Holloway, 1968, 1969, 1975, 1976a, 1976b; Jerison, 1973, 1975, 1976; Radinsky, 1974, 1975, 1977; Passingham & Ettlinger, 1973; Sacher, 1970, 1973; and Sacher & Staffeldt, 1974).

[1]Many of these data were collected and analyzed concurrently while working on stereometric analyses of hominoid endocasts, research funded by the National Science Foundation SOC-74-20149 and BNS 78-05651, for which support I am most grateful.

59

DEVELOPMENT AND EVOLUTION
OF BRAIN SIZE

Two issues are of particular importance in understanding any taxon's neural evolutionary development: How have neural mass and neural "wiring" changed through time? Neural mass refers to gross weight or volume of functioning neural tissue, and neural "wiring" refers to how the substructural components of the whole brain are interconnected; that is, how the brain is organized. It is unfortunate that much of the literature on brain evolution reflects · a single-minded approach on the part of various investigators to the exclusion of others. Regarding the concepts of reorganization and allometry (as, for example between Holloway, 1968, 1969, 1975, and Jerison, 1973, 1975), clearly both neural mass and wiring must be considered together in any attempt to unravel the mysteries of neural evolution.

I have emphasized the concept of *reorganization*, by which I mean that the study of quantitative shifts among the components (nuclei + fiber tracts, minimally) of the brains will eventually be useful in understanding the selection forces that operated to produce for each species a unique (species-specific) structural–behavioral adaptational amalgam.

It is true that I did not attempt until 1972 a synthesis between reorganizational changes and the more general relationships between brain and body sizes. I had honestly believed the latter to be trivial and reasonably well understood since the time of Snell (1892) and Dubois (1897), and placed much of my "faith" in the critical analyses of Sholl (1956). And here perhaps, Jerison (1973) and I are in conflict because our purposes appear so diverse, although certainly equally legitimate.

Jerison is interested in a more general theory of brain size for all animals that will also be useful in explaining taxa shifts in behavioral and structural adaptations above the species level, and in which the species-specific "wiring plans," or reorganization, are simply "trivial," or unnecessary to his theory. In 1973 Jerison specifically enjoined a "reorganizationist" approach that he labeled "the additive hypothesis" (pp. 361–362, 395).

In addition, Jerison is reasonably (and with reason) adamant that brain size per se may have considerable utility as a way of predicting more interesting and relevant parameters or variables for understanding brain and behavior evolution. As I hope to show, the present neuroanatomical comparative data on primates does not always permit such predictive power.

On the other hand, my purpose as a physical anthropologist is to understand the evolutionary development of our own peculiar species, and in that quest *both size and organization* are important. Size, however, is insufficient taken alone. Thus, in some ways at least, a general *con-*

straint[2] of brain–body weight relationships, described by Jerison's formula (1973, p. 61): Brain size = .12 Body weight·[66] is trivial to my interests.[3] Incidentally, I would make the same statement whether I specialized in humans, australopithecines, aardvarks, or bats!

Since the "additive hypothesis" is much the same as what I meant by "reorganization" from 1964 on, and since I too agree that size is important in understanding human evolution, one might ask just how Jerison and I disagree. I believe the answer lies partly in our diverse purposes, and in our approaches to theory, and our expectations or faith in prediction, extrapolation, and hypotheses testing. Actually, I think Jerison and I are far closer in our purposes than many realize or we ourselves have believed, and I specifically hope that this contribution will be a beginning to our joint appreciation of common goals.

Scope and Purpose

In this paper I would like to suggest a general model for brain evolution that offers some synthetic possibilities for approaching the questions of general and specific brain evolution, size, organization, and hierarchy. I must emphatically stress that these thoughts are not purely a rebuttal to the criticism provided by Jerison (1973, 1975), Sacher (1970), Passingham (1973), or Gould (1975). I am more concerned with showing the limitations of certain models of neural evolution (my own as well); and the limitations of the present data base, particularly for the Primates; and some directions for future research that appear promising at this time. To do this I will first concern myself with an appropriate although

[2] Perhaps the term "constraint" is confusing. Its use here implies some analogy, or indeed homology, with Dobzhansky's well known phrase, "norm of reaction." "Trend" might be a better term, except for its evolutionary context of necessary progress. All I mean really is that there is some lawful relationship between brain weight and body size in all animal groups, and these "lawful" relationships can be expressed mathematically, but are relational to the data base assumed. Thus animal groupings at the species level, that is, the same genus, show a variable "constraint" of about .3, as measured by the slope of least-squares line drawn through their $\log_{10}$ values for brain and body weights. At the genus level, or above, the "constraint" appears about .6; within the species, the "constraint" is seldom apparent, but when existent, is low, perhaps .1–.2. Unfortunately, the published primate data for healthy known-sex adults is insufficient, although my (unpublished) results show definite, significant, relationships *in males,* for *Homo sapiens, Pan troglodytes, Gorilla, Pongo, Macaca.*

[3] I think the use of this term is unfortunate, since it has inescapable pejorative connotations. The constraints are not "trivial," but their importance varies with the concern and goals of the research person.

insufficient and awkward model, and will then examine the data base, mainly for primates, as an almost purely quantitiative increase in size alone, with neither reorganization nor hierarchical changes.

Toward a Model

Figure IV.1 depicts a model, which, as all models, is oversimplistic, incomplete, and merely suggestive of the kinds of relationships I believe should be considered when brain size is discussed as if it were the brain.[4] I see three basic aspects of the brain, whether we are discussing it at generic or specific levels. Brains have *size, organizational components* (which also vary in size, phylogenetically), and *hierarchy*. Hierarchy refers to the unique timing of embryological and all further ontogenetic development of brain processes; that is, myelinization, neural nuclei, and fiber tract maturational interactions, and transactions with the rest of the organism and environment. It is essentially hierarchy that results in species-specific patterns of maturation of different parts of the brain at different times in relationship to some ethological paradigm of infant–mature interaction (particularly in social animals).

Hierarchy here refers mainly, but not exclusively, to maturational changes. Examples include such studies as: Flechsig's (1876) early studies in cortical myelogenesis; Salamy's (1978) recent findings on modality-specific projection through the corpus callosum as shown by latency differences between ipsilateral and contralateral somatosensory evoked potentials; the findings by Oke, Keller, Meford, and Adams (1978) of norepinephrine lateralization in the human thalamus; Denenberg, Garbanati, Sherman, Yutzey, and Kaplan's (1978) report of brain lateralization in rats given infantile stimulation; numerous reports of cerebral asymmetries in man and chimp (see Molfese, 1977), or Harnard, Steklis, & Lancaster, 1976, for reviews); Goldman, Crawford, Stokes, Galkin, and Rosvold's (1974) observations on sex differences in young and older juvenile rhesus monkeys regarding earlier maturation of fronto-orbital cortex, and earlier impairment of discrimination-reversal, or delayed response tasks in males; the purported differences in human male and

---

[4]Nobody knows how many genes help to control the ontogenetic unfolding of size, organization, and hierarchy of the brain. One estimate, based on DNA recombinant research, is that about 10–12% of the genetic material in brain cells is operative. My reasons for dissatisfaction with much of the work done on various genetic strains of mice, rats, cats, dogs, etc., were spelled out before (Holloway, 1969, 1970). We all realize the labors involved in dissecting microscopically and *quantitatively*, brain regions, but until those investments are made, we should be more humble, and not speak of brain weight as if it were "the brain."

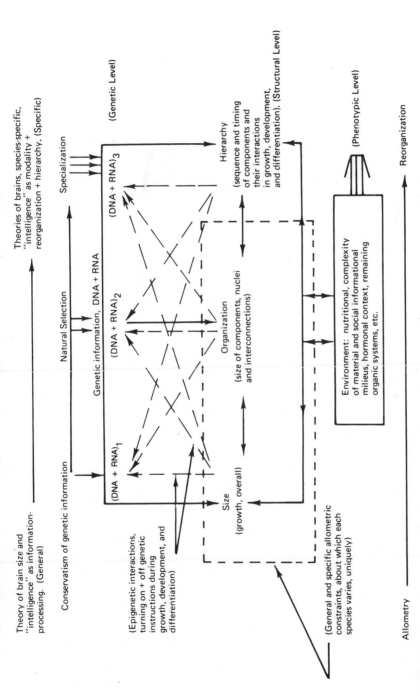

FIGURE IV.1. The brain is a composite of size, organization, and hierarchy, which is acted upon at the phenotypic level by natural selection *throughout* the life of the organism. Mathematical formulations and prediction tests are so far only applied to the box (dotted line) containing size and organization. This model conceives of natural selection variously acting on three subsets of genetic information (DNA + RNA$_{1,2,3}$), which also interact between each other, and the developing and differentiating organism in epigenetic fashion. Allometrists and brain mass theorists are almost totally working within the framework of the left-hand size of the diagram.

female performances for linguistic and spatial skill tasks (Harris, 1976); Dewson's (1976) work on auditory asymmetry in monkeys. These are only a sample, but each points to a set of complex genetic–environmental interactions that have variable maturational onsets and delays, and which are probably species-specific, particularly when placed in a truly ethological context. These are not trivia: they are the "very stuff" that natural selection acts upon. Nor do I believe that these considerations are in any way competitive with the "cortical column" module of cerebral organization elaborated by Mountcastle (1978) and Szentagothai (1975), who view most of neural evolution as additions of such units.

⌐   This model suggests that there are at least three subsets of genetic information involved with the expression of DNA and RNA information associated with size, organization, and hierarchy, and that these interact through ontogenetic time (as the solid and dashed lines indicate), as the process is *epigenetic*, (i.e., information about the state of the developing structures' feedback to the genetic level). Imposed on this model are my
∟   conceptualizations of existing theory and what these theoretical biases tend to emphasize. For example, the dotted line surrounding *size* and *organization* is my perception of the basic concerns of Jerison's (1973) argument. My own writings have focused on *organization*, have inadequately accounted for *size*, and have only treated the isssue of *hierarchy* in a conceptual way (Holloway, 1968, 1969, 1970, 1975, 1976a, 1976b).

Tentatively, I would like to suggest that the differences between Jerison's concerns and mine more or less move from left to right on the model. My occupation as a physical anthropologist concerned specifically with human evolution leaves me very concerned, perhaps preoccupied, with the right half of the model. Thus, I perceive the general constraint, basically allometric of surface to volume, as represented by the .666 two-thirds exponent, as one that is conservative in the evolutionary sense, and therefore "trivial" to understanding how brains in specific animals undergo evolutionary change.[5] Obversely, as Jerison has stated it, the right hand of the model is "trivial" to his interests.

Unfortunately, the present model is already too complex for mathematical testing, except in certain parts. Our knowledge regarding *size* is relatively good, as Jerison's (1973) book and references makes clear.[6]

[5]This comment follows my position in footnote 2, and is based on my perception of how many people seem to regard the slope as a genetic law. While I have never seen reference to a ".66 gene," I believe most people think in those terms.

[6]I am referring here to the data of Stephan, Bauchot, and Andy (1970) for example. Within-species variability, for healthy, mature, known-sex specimens, presently available from the literature is insufficient, and in some cases, wrongly reported. Considering all the primatological works done over the past two decades at many centers, plus the forensic potentials from autopsies, this hiatus is indeed a pity.

Our knowledge regarding *organization* (in the quantitative sense) is only beginning to develop, thanks to the empirical works of Stephan and his associates on the Insectivora, Primates, and Chiroptera. This level of structural investigation has yet to be carried out for the rodent strains discussed in this volume. Our knowledge of *hierarchy* is strong within only a very few species, and is not truly comparative as of yet.

Not reflected in this model is the role that brain size alone can play in *predicting* other neural statistics, or variables, of greater relevancy to behavior, and thus to evolutionary development. Here, I am skeptical, as I will make clear.

To sum-up the model, I believe that the brain and behavior within each species, and eventually among them, evolves within the constraints of allometry, which provides metabolical, size-determined, biologically based limits on growth, *but that within those constraints, organization and hierarchy can and do vary. Furthermore, some of that latter variation can be measured by examining the residuals of deviations from the allometric constraints.* The synthesis lies in the fact that reorganization occurs through the positive and negative increments of mitotic divisions and cell migrations, which are surely controlled to varying degrees by allometric considerations. The reorganization lies in natural selection favoring certain patterns or matrices of growth rates within and between neural nuclei, and their behavioral effectiveness, which is dependent upon the integrative success of parental members relative to behavioral patterns that prolong reproductive life, or efficiency. The allometry lies in the fact that mitotic divisions and thus growth rates are exponential or power-curved in mathematical expression, and regulated by factors of general size of the total nervous system in relationship to metabolism, among other things. And it is here that the units of neural variability become phenotypically manifested, so that eventually natural selection has something to work upon. In this model, it is these shifts in maturational speeds that contribute most proximally to both hierarchy and organization, and provide the intrapopulational variability upon which natural selection operates, both with regard to social behavior and to individual responses to environmental (nonsocial) variances. Brain size per se is in part the outward manifestion of these other units, and not the phenotypic unit or level most appropriately translated into genetic selection paradigms. But as long as we are only willing to look at straight-line log–log plots between gross size (whether brain or body weights) and substructures, and *not* to examine patterns of residuals in related species, the reorganizational shifts cannot be detected and will continue to be glossed over in analyses that account solely for variance or in log–log regressions per se.

How Good Are the Primate Data?

"Extra" Neurons

In my review (Holloway, 1974) of Jerison's (1973) book, I suggested that the concept of "extra neurons" measured by the formula,

$$Nc = (8 \times 10^7) \, [\text{Brain weight}^{.66} - (.03 \text{ Body weight}^{.66})^{.66}]$$

resulted in essentially fictional numbers. For the time being, I will avoid any argument regarding just what "extra" means. My question is, simply: How do the resulting figures match empirical reality as we *presently* know it?

Figure IV.2 is a representation of Nc values for populations of adult healthy primates that shows the ranges, means, and S.D.s of the Nc values. These are arranged vertically, whereas the actual, empirically determined number of total nerve cells in the brain are represented horizontally. *Homo sapiens* has more extra neurons than all other neurons in its brain, according to Pakkenberg's (1966) and Shariff's (1953) data. The gorilla, which has a lower EQ than either chimpanzee or orangutan, has more extra neurons than either the chimpanzee or the orangutan. Jerison's derivation of the constants, 8×10^7 and .03, are based on his acceptance and application of Shariff's (1953) data on neuron density, as well as those of Bok (1959), and Tower (1953), to a primitive ancestral form of mammal. Bok's work was on rodents and cats, and his earlier works can be found critically assayed in Sholl's (1956) book. Tower's (1953) measurements go from mouse to whale, neuron density varying by a factor of 10, brain weight by a factor of more than 10,000![7]

I am aware that Jerison's meaning of extra neurons (Nc), does not necessarily substitute as a measure for intelligence, but is a residual term in an equation using the .66 power of body weight and a theoretically derived estimate of density extrapolated for a primitive mammal, with a resultant estimate of its extra neurons. Thus, heavier-bodied animals will obviously have more Nc's than lighter ones. The question one should ask is why, if the theory is good, and the empirical claims of brain–body scaling so accurate, the predictions of Nc appear so inconsistent with our present empirical base? Is the theory wrong, too

---

[7]As one participant in this conference put it, anytime one starts with mice and ends up with whales, one gets a regression line of satisfying straightness, particularly when the data is plotted in log terms. These methods militate against discovering patterns of residuals that could be taxon-specific, and thus "informative." These relationships might be useful for prediction or retrodiction, or interpolation, of some species, but "individual" specimens?

gross, or is the empirical data base inaccurate? Frankly, I do not know, but suspect both. This should be clearer from reading my critique of Jerison's (1973) extra neuron views (Holloway, 1966, 1974), and from the next sections on the empirical data base.

Since so much apparently relies on Shariff's (1953) work on primates in the analyses of my work by Jerison (1973), Passingham (1973), and Passingham and Ettlinger (1973), it is appropriate to look more closely at Shariff's results, and see how well the human values for various measures are predicted from its brain and body weights, as extrapolated from other primate data.

Shariff's (1953) Data

The hypothesis that many neural variables can be parsimoniously explained and predicted once one knows brain and body sizes has been suggested by Jerison (1973), Passingham (1973, p. 338), and Passingham and Ettlinger (1973), to mention but a few. In fact, Passingham has published a number of predictions of human neural parameters based on diverse data, for example, Shariff (1953), by using the formulas empirically derived from log–log regressions from nonhuman primates alone. For example, Passingham (1973, p. 339) shows that on the basis of the Stephan *et al.* (1970) data, the actual value of human neocortex is 3.2 times that expected for a nonhuman primate of human body weight, and 2.9 times the expected value if only simian (excluding prosimians) values are used. In the same article (p. 342), Passingham shows that Stephan's (1969) values for striate cortex, when placed in a regression analysis for nonhuman primates, show that the *Homo sapiens* value of striate cortex is that predicted for a primate of his body weight. In the Passingham and Ettlinger (1974, p. 242) article the same thing was done, *except* striate cortex was plotted against brain weight. In this case, the human value fell *well underneath* the line, as I pointed out previously (Holloway 1976, p. 334). Of more interest perhaps, is Passingham's (1973, pp. 346–347) attempt to plot Shariff's (1953) figures for $\log_{10}$ eulaminate cortex against $\log_{10}$ neocortex for nonhuman primates. The human value predicted is about the same as that actually found by Shariff (1953). In this case, however, the eulaminate cortex already accounts for 85% of total neocortex in *Homo sapiens*, so that the *two should* be highly intercorrelated! Further on (p. 355), we find Passingham regressing the number of nerve cells against neocortex (both in logs) from Shariff's data. Curiously, there is no regression for number of cells, for different cortical regions or density, against brain weight, which according to Jerison could be of such value to predicting other neural parameters.

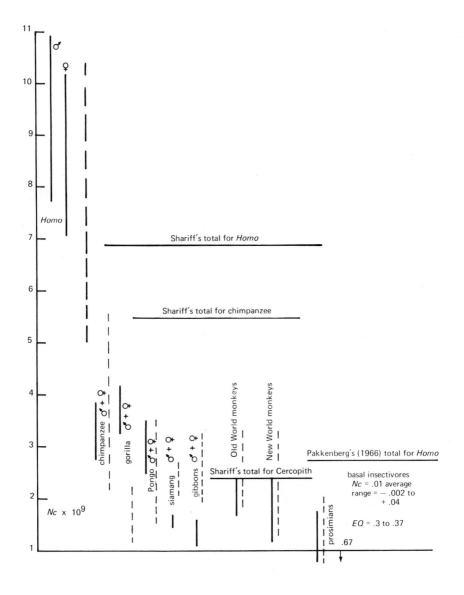

parameters. Passingham (1973, p. 356) then concludes that all of the *Homo sapiens* values can be related to increase in neocortex, body weight, or brain weight.

One of the criticisms of my previous works (1968) was that I did not perform regression analysis. I will now correct this lapse.

Regression analyses were performed on Shariff's (1953) data by plotting only the nonhuman values, finding the regression equation, and comparing the predicted (expected) with actual values. In my analyses, I selected three additional variables: (*a*) Shariff's (1953, p. 392) brain weights; (*b*) Bauchot and Stephan's (1969) *average* brain and body weights for each species; and, (*c*) a striate cortex figure for each species, found by multiplying Stephan's (1969) listed striate percentages by the total neocortex figures Shariff gave.

Tables IV.1 and IV.2 indicate the closeness of actual versus predicted values for all variables. Basically, these regressions show the following:

1. The average cell size for all cortex types (eulaminate, koniocortex, agranular) is *always more* than expected on basis of body size, brain size, Shariff's (1953) neocortex volume, or Stephan's (1969) volume.
2. The total numbers of cells in any cortical type is *less* than expected on the basis of size.
3. Densities for any cortical type are *less* than expected on basis of size, and *considerably* so.
4. a. The volume of eulaminate cortex is *more* than expected for a primate of that body size.

Figure IV.2. This shows the ranges of *Nc* and *EQ* values for various primates based on healthy adult values only (Jerison, 1973). The human data is from Pakkenberg and Voigt's 1964 study of Danish brain and body weights, kindly lent to this author for further statistical study. The remaining primate data (pongids) were taken from Bauchot and Stephan's (1969) compilations, choosing only those adult values which appeared reasonable. The remaining primate and insectivore data were taken from Stephan, Bauchot, and Andy (1970), and are average values for species. The solid vertical lines represent the *Nc's* and the dashed vertical lines the *EQ's* for each taxon. The horizontal lines represent the empirically determined total neuron numbers as published by Shariff (1953) and Pakkenberg (1966). The scale for *Nc's* and *EQ's* are the same except that the *Nc's* are in units of 10°. As can be seen, the *Nc's* from *Homo sapiens* are greatly above the empirical observations, the chimpanzee well below, and the Cercopithecoids also below but closer to Shariff's value for *Cercopithecus*. Note also the small degree of overlap in *EQ* values for *Homo sapiens* and chimpanzee, and the differences in degree of overlap between *Nc's* and *EQ's* for gorilla, the siamang, the gibbons. *Homo sapiens*, *N* = 667; chimp, *N* = 38; gorilla, *N* = 15; Pongo, *N* = 39; siamang, *N* = 5; gibbons, *N* = 44; *Old World monkeys*, *N* = 6; New World monkeys, *N* = 12; prosimians, *N* = 18; basal insectivores, *N* = 11. (*see facing page*.)

TABLE IV.1
Actual versus Estimated Values of Neural Variables from Log-Log Regressions.[a]

Depend. variable	Independ. variable	Exp. value	Actual val.	Abs. diff.	Percent diff.	A/E	Corr.	Signif.
Av. size eul. cells	Brain wt., 1450gm	1001	1621	620	38	1.6	.977	.011
	Body wt., 65,000gm	907	1621	714	44	1.8	.981	.009
	Tot. cort. × 2	950.8	1621	670	41	1.7	.961	.019
Av. size agr. cells	Brain wt.	1220	2468	1248	50	2.0	.996	.006
	Body wt.	1095	2468	1373	55	2.2	.992	.004
	Tot. Cort. × 2	1165	2468	1303	53	2.1	.999	.0002
Av. size konio. cells	Brain wt.	675	895	220	24	1.3	.952	.023
	Body wt.	647	895	247	28	1.4	.960	.019
	Tot. Cort. × 2	683	895	212	24	1.3	.925	.037
Tot. no. of cells	Brain wt.	29.6	13.8	15.8	115	.47	.978	.011
	Body wt.	16.3	13.8	2.5	18.3	.84	.978	.010
	Tot. cort. × 2	11.4	6.9	4.4	64.0	.62	.975	.012
No. of eul. cells	Brain wt.	27.7	11.4	16.3	143	.41	.977	.011
	Body wt.	13.6	11.4	2.2	19.2	.84	.978	.011
	Tot. cort. × 2	10.1	5.7	4.4	77	.56	.972	.014
No. of agr. cells	Brain wt.	2.93	1.02	1.91	187	.35	.995	.002
	Body wt.	1.55	1.02	.53	52	.66	.993	.003
	Tot. cort. × 2	.787	.51	.28	54	.65	.998	.001
No. of konio. cells	Brain wt.	2.65	1.4	1.25	89	.53	.878	.061
	Body wt.	1.90	1.4	.50	36	.74	.874	.063
	Tot. cort. × 2	1.18	.7	.48	69.	.59	.899	.050

[a]Eul., kinio., and agr. are eulaminate, koniocortex, and agranular cortex. Exp. value = the expected human value based on the regression from nonhuman primates. A/E is the ratio between actual and expected values. The correlation = the Pearson correlation coefficient based on the nonhuman sample alone, as is the significance (significance level). The significance figures in brackets are for the density variables are those when the total data is regressed (i.e., including the human values). Correspondingly, the correlations similarly increase. The total cortex × 2 is Shariff's total cortex (eulaminate, konio, agranular) multiplied by two to give a whole, rather than one-half brain figure. (Neocortex, Stephan) is Stephan's (1970) published values for total neocortex in those same primate species.

TABLE IV.2
Actual versus Estimated Values of Table IV.2 Neural Variables from Log–Log Regressions

Depend. variable	Independ. variable	Exp. value	Actual val.	Abs. diff.	Percent diff.	A/E	Corr.	Signif.
Density, eulaminate	Brain wt., 1450gm	46.57	29	17.57	60.6	.62	−.73	.134 (.03)
	Body wt. 65,000gm	58.17	29	29.17	100.6	.50	−.71	.14 (.04)
	Tot. cort. × 2	49.02	29	20.02	69	.59	−.71	.11 (.027)
Density, agranular	Brain wt.	35.23	18.2	17.03	93	.52	−.91	.043 (.008)
	Body wt.	42.84	18.2	24.64	135	.42	−.898	.05 (.022)
	Tot. cort. × 2	37.2	18.2	19	104	.49	−.949	.025 (.01)
Density, koniocortex	Brain wt.	121.3	97.2	24.1	24.7	.80	−.952	.023 (.002)
	Body wt.	153.85	97.2	56.65	58.2	.63	−.942	.028 (.007)
	Tot. cort. × 2	131.7	97.2	34.5	35.5	.74	−.974	.013 (.002)
Vol. eulam. × 2	Brain wt.	311,533	195,480	16,053	59	.63	.995	.002
	Body wt.	115,501	195,480	79,979	41	1.69	.988	.006
	Tot. cort. × 2	199,359	195,480	3879	2	.98	.999	.0001
Vol. agranular × 2	Brain wt.	34,448	27,700	6748	24	.80	.995	.002
	Body wt.	18,622	27,700	9078	33	1.48	.982	.008
	Tot. cort. × 2	30,938	27,700	3238	12	.89	.999	.0003
Vol. konio. × 2	Brain wt.	12,071	7220	4851	67	.60	.978	.001
	Body wt.	6162.5	7220	1057	15	1.17	.944	.028
	Tot. cort. × 2	8935	7220	1715	24	.81	.972	.014
Tot. vol. (E+A+K)	Brain wt.	352,201	230,400	121,801	53	.65	.997	.001
	Body wt.	138,318	230,400	92,082	40	1.66	.988	.005
	(Neocortex, Stephan)	295,704	230,400	65,304	28.3	.78	.988	.001

   b. The volume of eulaminate cortex is *less* than expected for either brain weights, and significantly so.

5. The same pattern as in *a* and *b* holds for koniocortex, and agranular cortex.

6. Shariff's values for striate cortex are less than expected for brain weight, body weight, and total cortex size, using either Shariff's raw figures or Stephan's 1.5% applied to Shariff's data.

7. While the volumes of eulaminate cortex (association) from Shariff's data are *always less* than expected on the basis of brain size, the volume for eulaminate is 1.69 more than expected on the basis of body weight. Since eulaminate cortex makes up 85% of the human cortex, the relationship to body weight is more indicative; on the other hand, the striate cortex makes up but 1.5–3.0% of the total cortex, and thus less with respect to brain size, and the in-built correlation is thus less severe.

The Stephan (1969) Data on Visual Striate Cortex

As mentioned earlier, Passingham and Ettlinger (1973) did not quantify the disparity between *actual* and *expected* human striate cortex values as related to brain weight. Using Stephan's (1969) percentage figures for striate cortex, and multiplying these by the neocortex values as in Stephan (1969), then plotting the resultant logs of visual striate cortex against the logs of brain and body weight, it is apparent (see Table IV.3) that the expected *Homo sapiens* value is on target for body weight as Passingham (1973) claims, *but is 95.1% off the mark where brain size is considered.* Here, the A/E ratio is .51, or one-half less than expected (based on *Pan troglodytes Cercopithecus ascanius, Callithrix jacchus, Galago senegalensis, Tarsius syrichta,* and the following percentages for striate cortex as a part of neocortex: *Homo* = 1.5%; *Pan* = 3.6%; *Cercopith* = 8.0%; *Callithrix* = 13.6%; *Galago* = 12.6%; *Tarsius* = 19.4%). The equation is, without *Homo sapiens*:

$$\text{striate cortex} = 113.12 \text{ brain weight}^{.77329}$$

In sum, the Stephan (1969) data support the results I obtained from reanalysis of Shariff's (1953) data.

The Solnitsky and Harman (1946) Data

Using brains of *Pongo, Cercocebus, Galago,* and *Homo sapiens*, Solnitsky and Harman attempted to quantify the striate and peristriate (areas 17, 18, and 19) volumes.

TABLE IV.3
Homo Sapiens Neocortical and Striate Cortex Volumes Predicted from Stephan's (1970) and Shariff's (1953) Data[a]

Depend. variable	Indep. var.	Expected	Actual	Abs. diff.	Percent diff.	A/E	Corr.	Signif.
Neocortex (Stephan)	Body weight	451,039	1,006,525	555,486	55	2.23	.995	.002
Neocortex (Shariff)	Body weight	138,318	230,400	92,082	40	1.66	.988	.005
Neocortex (Stephan)	Brain weight	1,195,731	1,006,525	189,206	19	.84	.996	.002
Striate cortex (Stephan)	Body weight	14,971	15,097.8	127.8	.85	1.008	.9796	—
Striate cortex (Stephan)	Brain weight	29,457	15,097.8	14,359	95.1	.51	.994	—

[a]Body weight $= 65{,}000$ gm; brain weight $= 1365$ gm; and neocortical and striate cortex units in mm^3

Table IV.4 shows the results when *Homo sapiens* is excluded, and the nonhuman primate regressions used to predict the human values. Again, the same patterns emerge as in the Shariff (1953) data base:

1. Relative to body weight, the expectations for striate and peristriate cortex are closer than when regressed against brain weight.
2. The various areas are more than expected when plotted against body weight, yet less (and relatively *much less so*) when plotted against brain size.

The Popoffs' (1929) and Filiminov's (1933) Data

The data from two early German publications (Popoff & Popoff, 1929; Filiminov, 1933) are of considerable interest since they are based on observations made on several brains for each species. Filiminov studied four Orang brains, three Macaca, and eight human, and recorded their brain weights, the surface areas of the total occipital lobe, and areas 17, 18, and 19.

Table IV.5 shows the results when *Homo sapiens* is excluded from the regressions and the actual values compared to those predicted. Again, the expected value for area 17, striate cortex, is considerably less than expected, whereas peristriate cortex, areas 18 and 19, are significantly more, yet the amount of occipital cortex en toto is almost exactly what would be expected, as the A/E ratio is 1.082.

The Popoffs' (1929; Popoff & Popoff, 1929) measured four hemispheres of three chimpanzee brains. Using their data, the average brain weight for this species was 390 gm, and the average surface area for area 17 was given as 1996 mm². Using the Filiminov data-based regressions on Orang and Macaca, the expected value for chimpanzee was 1966 mm². Using the regression for Macaca, Orang, and *Homo sapiens*, the expected chimpanzee value was 1726.8 mm², giving a percent difference of 12.1, and an A/E ratio of 1.14. In other words, the chimpanzee values, independently derived, match expectations very closely, but the *Homo sapiens* data does not.

Thus, from four separate independent sources, the results for expected versus actual values for *Homo sapiens* visual striate cortex are the same: *Homo sapiens* has less than expected for a primate of its brain weight. Perhaps I may be guilty of a premature judgment, but it appears that:

1. Brain weight is *not* necessarily a good predictor for "other interesting variables."
2. *Homo sapiens* shows definite signs of reorganization with regard to relative amounts of visual striate, koniocortex, peristriate, and as-

TABLE IV.4
Solnitsky and Harmon's Data[a]

Dependent variable	Independent variable	Expected[3] value mm³	Actual value mm³	Abs. diff. mm³	Percent diff.	A/E ratio	r corr.	Signif.
Total occip. cortex	Body[b]	7493.9	10,490	2996	28.6	1.4	.957	.09
Total occip. cortex	Brain[c]	17,605.8	10,490	7115.8	67.8	.59	.985	.05
Area 17	Body	2721.2	2613	108.2	4.1	.96	.962	.08
Area 17	Brain	5638.7	2613	3025.6	115.8	.46	.989	.04
Area 18	Body	2410.9	3948	2018	38.9	1.63	.9507	.10
Area 18	Brain	5966.5	3948	1143	51.1	1.66	.981	.06
Area 19	Body	2746.5	3890	1143.5	29.4	1.42	.981	.103
Area 19	Brain	8733.7	3890	4843.7	124.5	.44	.948	.063
Area 18 & 19	Body	5016.6	7838	2821.4	36.0	1.56	.98	.100
Area 18 & 19	Brain	13,595.1	7838	5757.1	73.5	.57	.95	.06

[a]Regressions based on Orang, Cercocebus, Galago.
[b]Body weight = 65,000 gm
[c]Brain weight = 1,330 gm

TABLE IV.5
Predicting *Homo sapiens* Values from Filiminov's (1933) and Popoff's (1929) Data

Dependent variable	Independent variable	Actual mm²	Expected mm²	Diff mm³	Percent diff.	A/E	r	Signif.
Regio Occipitalis	Brain wt. (1470) gm	10550	9747	802.8	.6	1.082	.984	.00003
Area 17	Brain wt. (1470) gm	2652.4	3858.5	12061.4		.69	.9687	.00016
Area 18	Brain wt. (1470) gm	3943.6	2752	1192	30.2	1.43	.9834	.00003
Area 19	Brain wt. (1470) gm	3946.4	3123.5	322.8	20.8	1.26	.94052	.0008
Peristriate	Brain wt. (1470) gm	7890	5867.9	2002	25.6	1.34	.96687	.00019
For Chimpanzee (Popoff, based on Macaca and Pongo Regression)								
Area 17	Brain wt. (390) gm	1964	1996	32	1.6	.98		
(Based on Macaca, Pongo, Homo)								
Area 17	Brain wt. (390) gm	1964	1726.8	237.2	12.1	1.14		

sociation cortex, which is in agreement with my earlier points on interpretation of visual cortex and certain of the fossil endocasts (Holloway 1975, 1976a).

Some warnings about these analyses are in order. The Filiminov and Popoff data were based on surface area extent of supposedly cytoarchitectonically distinct cortical moieties in the occipital lobe, a framework based on Brodmann's (1909) parcellations. On the other hand, the Shariff (1953), Solnitsky and Harman (1946), and Stephan (1969) data were based on volumes. Histological and mensuration techniques differed in each study. With the exception of Popoffs' and Filiminov's data, measurements were made on a single specimen for each species, so that variability is not taken into account with the later studies. Brain weights of the actual specimens (except for *Homo sapiens*) in Shariff's (1953) and Solnitsky and Harman's data were not available. Body weights for Popoffs' (1929) and Filiminov's (1933) specimens were not available. The analyses from Stephan's (1969) data are based on average body and brain weights for each species. Extrapolations from the Filiminov data to *Homo sapiens* are based on two groups, Macaca and Pongo, and will naturally give a straight line with almost perfect correlation since a straight line is defined by two points. The *Homo sapiens* brain used by Shariff (1953) has doubts surrounding its normality, which doubts incidentally, are attibuted to me by Passingham (1953, pp. 346–347) on the basis that its use gives unexpected values for relative amounts of association cortex. In fact, my hesitancy about that specimen was based on Sholl's (1956, pp. 32–33) comments, and the apparent lack of agreement between Shariff's figures and those previously found by earlier neuroanatomists.

In sum, I do not believe these analyses are in any sense free from a multiplicity of procedural and methodological problems, but they are the best we have at present, and if Passingham's (1973) methods are viewed as a valid attempt at objectivity (e. g., Jerison 1975, p. 43), then it can be seen that by using such methods, the picture takes an opposite cast when applied more fully.

For my part, I believe that one of the major issues requiring some thought and testing is whether or not one should use such approaches when in fact plotting something very small along with something very large. These will inevitably (particularly in $\log_{10}$ terms) give high correlations, and a straight line. When the sample sizes are small, the curved 95% confidence limits on either side of the regression line become extremely divergent at the extreme ends of the distribution. It is possible to be 200% wrong in a prediction of an expected value, and yet testing that result for significance will show the difference as nonsignificant.

With such low degrees of freedom, what else can be expected?[8] Are the regressions phyletically meaningful? What, precisely, does allometry explain at the genetic levels, and in terms thereof, of evolutionary changes at the species level (Holloway, 1974, 1976a, 1976b)?

Some Preliminary Multivariate Analyses of the Stephan, Bauchot, and Andy (1970) Primate Data

I must confess that when I first read Sacher's (1970) results from factor analyses on the data set from Stephan Bauchot, and Andy (1970), I was surprised that size accounted for so much of the total variance, and almost came to agree with his premise that I had "thrown out the baby with the bath water" in stressing reorganization and discounting size-related changes in neural components. What I wish to report here are only some *explorations* that have been made from that data base.

My assumption is as follows: If size accounts for almost all of the variance and is "taken out," either by a first factor in principle components or by allometric correction using linear regression, where the log of each structure is regressed against either or both total brain and body size, very little information should be left in the residuals, and *that information should be insufficient to classify the taxa correctly by discriminant analyses.* Or alternatively put, the hypothesis is that there is still sufficient information in the taxonomic patterning of residuals to permit a reasonably high percentage of correct classifications within taxonomic groups. I decided to limit these explorations to the Primate data base alone, deleting the Insectivora. Each neural structure, except the telencephalon, was regressed against brain and body weights for the Prosimians, New World Monkeys, Old World Monkeys, Pongids, and *Homo sapiens*, in $\log_{10}$ units. A multiple regression routine was also tried in which both brain *and* body weights were used, such that: Neural structure = k × brain weight$^\alpha$ × Bodyweight$^\beta$, which in log terms is:

$$\log_{10} \text{Structure} = \log_{10} k + \alpha \times \log_{10}$$
$$\text{Brain weight} + \beta \times \log_{10} \text{Body weight}$$

Each equation was then used to calculate a predicted structure size from the total primate data base. The predicted values were then subtracted

---

[8] I tried significance testing, which must be done on the log values, since the tests are linear for regressions. I soon gave up when I encountered values 100–200% off the actual values being *not* significantly different, and simply, claim that until the samples are larger, and d.f.s higher, significance testing of these values is pointless.

from the actual values for each species, and these residuals became the variables used in discriminant analyses. Each equation, of course, yielded correlations that were about .96 and often higher, and Table IV.6 shows, only as an example, the changes in multiple r from the multiple regression equations. The discriminant analyses were run using the "direct method," in which all variables are entered, rather than by a stepwise method, on the assumption that, after all, these were parts of the brain and should be entered! The question I was asking was *not* which structures were best in discriminating between the taxa, but whether there was sufficient information left in the residuals to correctly classify the taxa. Hence, all structures except telencephalon were entered, since its inclusion would be duplicative. In some runs, I left in the olfactory residuals, and in others I omitted the neocortex, simply to see if the subcortical residuals alone would give high classifications. *Homo sapiens* was sometimes left out, and sometimes placed in the Pongids, as the sample size of the latter is so small ($N = 2$).

Before discussing the results, I want to stress again the exploratory nature of these procedures. First, the sample sizes in each taxon are

TABLE IV.6

Changes in Multiple R When Combining Brain and Body Weights [Structure = A (Body Weight$^\alpha$ × Brain Weight$^\beta$)]

Medulla	Body	.972
	Brain	.990
Cerebellum	Body	.971
	Brain	.995
Mesencephalon	Body	.960
	Brain	.994
Dienephalon	Body	.964
	Brain	.995
Olfactory	Body	.436
	Brain	.635
Paleocortex	Body	.946
	Brain	.973
Septum	Body	.970
	Brain	.985
Striatum	Body	.955
	Brain	.994
Schizocortex	Body	.965
	Brain	.969
Hippocampus	Body	.972
	Brain	.977
Neocortex	Body	.94
	Brain	.999

highly disparate (18 Prosimians, 12 New World Monkeys, 6 Old World Monkeys, 2 Pongids, 1 *Homo sapiens*). Second, since there are only four groups, there can only be three discriminate functions. Third, there are more variables (10, if telencephalon and olfactory structures are omitted) than groups, and in the case of Old World Primates, more variables than specimens or cases.

The results are basically the same regardless of the combinations used: The percentage correctly classified into their taxonomic groups, broadly defined, runs about 80%.

Indeed, using factor analysis, and deleting the first factor upon which brain and body size are loaded so heavily, discriminate analyses on the remaining factor scores gave results of roughly 69–82 correct classifications. In these cases, the number of factor scores tends to match more closely the number of specimens within the taxonomic groups.

Another investigation recently tried was based on using the brain structures for the basal insectivores ($N = 11$), as provided by Stephan (1970). The reasoning behind this approach was as follows: the basal insectivores represent the best approximation to an ancestral group from which the Primates evolved, including most particularly the Prosimii. The regression equations, as shown in Table IV.7 are very interesting, in that almost all brain structures tend to have a slope of 1.0 when regressed against brain weight, and about .6 against body weight. This suggests an almost pure scaling of diverse brain components against size. These equations were then used as follows: The Primate values for these neural structures (from Stephan, 1970) were calculated as if they were basal insectivores of their respective brain and body weights. The actual brain structural values were then divided by the expected values based on the "basal insectivore" equations. This yielded the "progression indices" for each structure of each primate species. The logs of these indices were next regressed against brain weight, since the indices were clearly related to brain weight, as the correlations were all quite high ($r = .8–.9$) and highly significant. These equations were then used to calculate a second set of residuals after the original indices were corrected for brain size. These residuals were then used as the variables in a discriminant analysis. Again, the telencephalon variate was omitted. The percentage of groups correctly classified by this method was 87.18% (*Homo sapiens* was included in the Pongid group).

For a wide range of methodological reasons and my own sense of insecurity in venturing into the multivariate realm, I prefer not to push these studies until the data and techniques are more fully analyzed. Nevertheless, I believe that these preliminary results indicate that *both size and organization* are of taxonomic and functional significance, and that the residual 4 or 5% information remaining in the total variance not accounted for by brain and body weights needs careful consideration, and should not be the "new" baby that gets thrown out with the bath water!

Considerations of space forbid me to add and adequately discuss all

TABLE IV. 7

Regression Equations for "Basal Insectivores," $N = 11$, from Stephan (1970)

Constant		Exp.	Corr.
Medulla			
.0066	Body	.59050	.99149
.1224	Brain	.90680	.99356
Cerebellum			
.0040	Body	.67591	.98841
.1123	Brain	1.04175	.99412
Mesencephalon			
.0027	Body	.60202	.99157
.0535	Brain	.92387	.99299
Diencephalon			
.0031	Body	.62606	.98613
.0692	Brain	.96921	.99623
Telencephalon			
.0227	Body	.64632	.99137
.5536	Brain	.99848	.99943
Olfactory			
.0029	Body	.71499	.99353
.0993	Brain	1.09498	.99291
Paleocortex			
.0064	Body	.65961	.99232
.1670	Brain	1.01290	.99440
Septum			
.00084	Body	.58818	.99313
.0154	Brain	.90409	.99617
Striatum			
.00199	Body	.61154	.98583
.0480	Brain	.94511	.99485
Schizocortex			
.0013	Body	.62676	.96019
.0284	Brain	.97829	.97801
Hippocampus			
.0046	Body	.56540	.98216
.0747	Brain	.87870	.99607
Neocortex			
.0049	Body	.64319	.96151
.1194	Brain	1.00483	.98024

the data regarding the prediction accuracy of components based on brain and body weights. Table IV.8 is a more intuitive approach, and shows the percent deviations from expected *EQ* values for each structure, when the appropriate animal is deleted from the sample. In other words, I am comparing the predictive power for chimp and gorilla with *Homo* in the first top half of Table IV.8. To follow Passingham's (1973) technique, one would have to run the Stephan, Bauchot, and Andy (1970) primate data at least 39 times to do the same for each species. I thought limiting this approach to the *Hominoidea* would be sufficient.

TABLE IV.8

Percent Deviations from Expected *EQ* Values When Each Species in Turn Is Omitted from Regression of Log Structure versus Log Body weight

	Homo		Pan		Gorilla	
	−	+	−	+	−	+
Medulla	64.0		4.3			4.2
Cerebellum	.9			0.6		25.7
Mesencephalon	16.8		7.9		11.4	
Diencephalon	53.6		11.6		7.3	
Telencephalon	1.4		.2		5.6	
Paleocortex		10.6	41.6			9.7
Septum		27.8	.4			14.1
Striatum	68.9		20.2		24.5	
Schizocortex		22.4	7.1			6.6
Hippocampus		13.2	13.1		4.1	
Neocortex	10.3		1.7		9.4	

Ranges of Percentage Deviations of Expected from Actual EQ *Values*

	Prosimians		New World Monkeys		Old World Monkeys[a]	
	−	+	−	+	−	+
Medulla	47.2	28.9	36.6	21.8	12.4	10.2
Cerebellum	12.4	21.4	41.1	8.8	44.5	1.3
Mesencephalon	38.0	30.6	14.4	10.5	8.4	8.7
Diencephalon	29.4	24.0	11.1	6.1	13.6	2.7
Telencephalon	9.6	4.7	2.9	7.3	1.1	6.4
Paleocortex	68.3	44.2	57.9	5.5	23.9	8.6
Septum	46.3	32.7	64.9	9.8	32.9	9.4
Striatum	37.7	28.5	18.1	13.5	16.8	6.1
Schizocortex	23.1	56.9	77.1	14.3	71.5	19.0
Hippocampus	46.6	44.7	99.4	19.8	30.5	16.1
Neocortex	20.9	11.9	2.5	16.0	2.5	11.6

Based on non-human regressions of $\log_{10}$ structure versus $\log_{10}$ brain weight.

The bottom half of Table IV.8 shows the ranges of percent deviations for the broader taxa. Finally, Table IV.9 is included to show how accurate and in what directions the human predicted values are when using either the entire Primate order data, or just that for the *Anthropoidea*. A number of points should be made:

1. Certain structures are *not* well predicted in any given species, and these are most likely indicative of neural system specificity with respect to ecological zoning and behavioral (including locomotory) adaptation.

2. All of these figures are entirely relative to the width or diversity of the data base used, as one can see by the A/E reversals shown in Table IV.9, and thus different interpretations *could* be made regarding the combinations of neural structures which are so different in *Homo sapiens*.

TABLE IV.9
Prediction of *Homo sapiens* Structures Using Different Primate Samples

		Taxon 1[a]		Taxon 2[b]	
		Percentage deviation	A/E	Percentage deviation	A/E
Medulla	Body	64.4	.61	31.8	1.47
	Brain	48.7	.67	49.7	.7
Cerebellum	Body	.9	.99	62.0	2.63
	Brain	11.8	1.13	22.8	.81
Mesencephalon	Body	16.8	.85	50.2	2.0
	Brain	7.8	.93	3.5	.97
Diencephalon	Body	53.6	.65	44.7	1.91
	Brain	38.3	.72	35.3	.74
Paleocortex	Body	10.4	1.11	57	2.33
	Brain	18.9	1.23	6.4	1.07
Septum	Body	27.8	1.39	66.7	3.0
	Brain	35.3	1.55	25.5	1.34
Striatum	Body	68.9	.59	46.8	1.88
	Brain	51.1	.66	54.5	.65
Schizocortex	Body	22.4	1.29	63.0	2.71
	Brain	31.8	1.47	16.0	1.19
Hippocampus	Body	13.2	1.15	57.0	2.35
	Brain	23.0	1.30	11.3	1.13
Neocortex	Body	70.4	3.38	69.9	3.32
	Brain	10.3	.91	0.76	1.01
				---	

[a]Based on Prosimii, New World Monkeys, Old World Monkeys, Pongids
[b]Based on New World Monkeys, Old World Monkeys, Pongids (Both without *Homo sapiens*) Underlined values = reversal

3. It is inescapably true, as Sacher's (1970) analysis showed, that many neural structures can indeed be predicted if brain and body weights are known, as clearly many of the percent deviations are small, and the A/E ratios tend toward unity, or 1.0. Certain of them, however, are not so close, and it is their combinations that surely allow for relatively higher percentage-correct classifications by discriminant analysis. The obvious next steps are to create behavioral and adaptational variables which can be analyzed with the brain structure data to give a more interesting, and one expects, more provocative picture of neural size and organizational moieties, which will enrich our understanding of the evolution of the Primate brain. I sincerely doubt Primate evolution, or any single species within the order, can ever be explained as allometry pure and simple. It is my belief that allometry is but the first step in producing *theories* about brain evolution.

Conclusion

Given that the data base for quantitative measures of components in primate brains is incomplete, disparate, and built on different method-ologies, and that our statistical procedures are often ill-suited to the data (or visa versa), I think it is inescapable that size, reorganization, and hierarchy have been important in shaping our brains. I never believed size had been unimportant in human brain evolution, but freely admit that I did not in the past deal with the question in any depth. The data on visual striate cortex, as gleaned from the Popoff, Filiminov, Solnitsky and Harman, Shariff, and Stephan data, all point to the correctness of my concept of reorganization, using the very methods advocated by the criticisms of Jerison (1975, 1976), Passingham (1973), and Passingham and Ettlinger (1974). The only presently secure data base for neural statistics that can be predicted from knowing brain and body weights (see Jerison, 1973) is Shariff's study. Here, it should be clear, that *if* the data are correct, the human brain weight becomes a poor predictor for those variables, at least within the primate groups tested by Pas-singham's (1973) technique. If this were a singular result, it would per-haps be readily dismissed, but each study indicated the same result.

To the extent that the extra neuron, Nc, concept is tied into neuron density predictions for *Homo sapiens* from the rest of the Primate data, the Nc values surpass all other empirical findings for total neuron numbers.

Although size of brain and body are clearly of importance in account-ing for brain structual variation within the Primate order (and probably all orders), preliminary analyses of the residuals shown taxonomic patterns which are "information," suggesting broad aspects of reorganization that permit relatively high degrees of taxonomic classification, and thus one assumes, functional importance in terms of behavioral adaptations and past natural selection forces.

"Brain size" is not "the brain," and although I can easily appreciate the difficulty of adequately investigating the size, organizational, and hierarchical elements that make up the "brain" in so many of the genetic strain analyses reported in this volume, I believe we must realize that until we do, our analyses remain crude, and much in the way of potentially significant data literally goes out in the trash.

By cathecting on size alone, all evolutionary paradigms become reduced to natural or genetic selection operating on incremental size increases and behavioral efficiency, which always has the underlying implicit structual argument that "intelligence" equals "brain size." Thus, for example, all of hominid evolution becomes "scaling," "allometry," or quantitative increases, whereas these are only *distal* manifestations of something more complex and important. In other words, all of individual variation, the very stuff that evolution works on, is reduced to a single dimension of either small or large. In fact, it is likely that the selection events in any animal's life depend more on the timing of maturational events, epigenesis within the central nervous system (CNS), and everyday events—that is, the "nitty-gritty" life-death "selection walks"—are matters of hierarchical organization, differentiation, and development, of which the outcomes through time can only be measured (thus far) as size increments. We should and can demand richer explanations.

Acknowledgments

I wish to thank Mike Billig, Barry Cerf, and Tim Wolfe for their help in processing these data, and in particular David Post for his advice and caveats regarding the statistical analysis. Any errors therein are to be attributable solely to me.

References

Bauchot, R., & Stephan, H. Encéphalisation et niveau évolutif chez les simiens. *Mammalia* 1969, *33*, 225–275.
Bok, S. T. *Histonomy of the cerebral cortex.* New Jersey: Van Nostrand-Reinhold, 1959.

Brodmann, K. *Vergleichende Lokalisationslehre der Grosshirnrinde*. Leipzig, 1909.
Denenberg, V. A., Garbanati, J., Sherman, G., Yutzey, D. A., & Kaplan, R. Infantile stimulation induces brain lateralization in rats. *Science*, 1978, *201*, 1150–1152.
Dewson, J. H., III. Preliminary evidence of hemispheric asymmetry of auditory function in monkeys. In S. Harnard, R. W. Doty, L. Goldstein, I. Jaynes, & G. Krauthamer (Eds.), *Lateralization in the nervous system*. New York: Academic Press, 1976. Pp. 63–74.
Dubois, E. Sur le rapport du poids de l'encéphale avec le grandeur au corps chez les mammiferes. *Bulletin de Société Anthropologique*, 1897, *8*, 248–262.
Edinger, T. Paleoneurology versus comparative brain anatomy. *Confina Neurologica*, 1949, *11*, 5–24.
Filiminoff, I. N.: Über die Variabilität der Grosshirnrindenstruktur. *Journal für Psychologie und Neurologie*, 1933, *45*, 69–137.
Flechsig, P. Die *Leitungsbahnen im Gehirn und Rückenmark des Menschen auf Grundentwicklungsgeschichtlicher Untersuchungen*. Leipzig: Engelmann, 1876.
Goldman, P. S., Crawford, A. T., Stokes, L. P., Galkin, T. W., & Rosvold, A. E. Sexdependent behavioral effects of cerebral cortical lesions in the developing rhesus monkey. *Science*, 1974, *186*, 540–542.
Gould, S. J. Allometry in Primates, with emphasis on scaling and the evolution of the brain. In F. Szalay (Ed.), *Approaches to primate paleobiology: contributions to primatology*, Vol. 5. Basel: Karger, 1975. Pp. 244–292.
Harnard, S. R., Steklis, H. D., & Lancaster, J. Origins of language and speech. *Annals of the New York Academy of Science*, 1976, *280*, 1–914.
Harris, L. J. Sex differences in spatial ability: Possible environmental, genetic and neurological factors. In M. Kinsbourne (Ed.), *Hemispheric asymmetries of function*. New York: Cambridge University Press, 1976.
Holloway, R. L. Cranial Capacity, Neural Reorganization and Hominid Evolution: A Search for More Suitable Paramters. *American Anthropologist*, 1966, *68*, 103–121.
Holloway, R. L. The evolution of the primate brain: some aspects of quantitative relationships. *Brain Research*, 1968, *7*, 121–172.
Holloway, R. L. Some questions on parameters of neural evolution in primates. *Annals of the New York Academy of Science*, 1969, *167*, 332–340.
Holloway, R. L. Neural parameters, hunting and the evolution of the human brain. In C.R. Noback & W. Montagna (Eds.), *The primate brain*. New York: Appleton-Century-Crofts, 1970, Pp. 299–309.
Holloway, R. L. Australopithecine endocasts, brain evolution in the hominoidea and a model of hominid evolution. In R. Tuttle (Ed.), *The functional and evolutionary biology of primates*. Chicago: Chicago Aldine Press, 1972. Pp. 185–204.
Holloway, R. L. On the meaning of brain size. Book review of Jerison's 1973 *Evolution of the brain and intelligence*. *Science*, 1974, *184*, 677–679.
Holloway, R. L. 43rd James Arthur lecture at American Museum of Natural History, 1973. The role of human social behavior in the evolution of the brain. New York: American Museum of Natural History, 1975.
Holloway, R. L. Paleoneurological Evidence for Language Origins. In Origins and evolution of language and speech. *Annals of the New York Academy of Science*, 1976,In S. R. Harnard, H. D. Steklis, & L. Lancaster (Eds.), *280*, 330–348. (a)
Holloway, R. L. Some problems of Hominid brain endocast reconstruction, allometry and neural reorganization. Coloquium VI of the IX Congress of the U.I.S.P.P. Nice, 1976. (b)
Jerison, H. J. *Evolution of brain and intelligence*. New York: Academic Press, 1973.

Jerison, J. J. Fossil evidence of the evolution of the human brain. *American Review of Anthropology*, 1975, *4*, 27–58.

Jerison, H. J. Discussion paper: The paleoneurology of language. *Annals of the New York Academy of Science*, 1976, *280*, 370–382.

Molfese, D. L. Infant Cerebral Asymmetry. In S. J. Segalowitz & F. A. Gruber (Eds.), *Language development and neurological Theory*. New York: Academic Press, 1977. Pp. 22–37.

Mountcastle, V. B. An organizing principle for cerebral function: the unit module and the distributed system. In S. M. Edelman (Ed.), *The mindful brain*. Cambridge: M.I.T. Press, 1978. Pp. 7–50.

Oke, A., Keller, R., Mefford, I., & Adams, R. N. Lateralization of Norepinephrine in human thalamus. *Science*, 1978, *200*, 1411–1413.

Pakkenberg, H. The number of nerve cells in the cerebral cortex of man. *Journal of Comparative Neurology*, 1966, *128*, 17–19.

Pakkenberg, H. & Voigt, V. Brain weight of the Danes. *Acta Anatomica*, 1964, *56*, 297–307.

Passingham, R. F. Anatomical differences between the cortex of man and other primates. *Brain Behavior and Evolution*, 1973, *7*, 337–359.

Passingham, R. E., & Ettlinger, G. A comparison of cortical functions in man and other primates. *International Review of Neurobiology*, 1973, *16*, 233–299.

Popoff, I. Über einige Grössverhältnisse der Affenhirne. *Journal für Psychologie und Neurologie*, 1929, *38*, 82–90.

Popoff, I., Popoff, N. Beitrag zur Kenntnis der quantitativen Differenzen zwischen den Menschen-und Affenhirnen. *Journal für Psychologie und Neurologie*, 1929, *38*, 168–178.

Radinsky, L. The fossil evidence of anthropiod brain evolution. *American Journal of Physical Anthropology*, 1974, *41*, 15–28.

Radinsky, L. Viverrid neuroanatomy: Phylogenetic and behavioral implications. *Journal of Mammology*, 1975, *56*, 130–150.

Radinsky, L. Early primate brains: facts and fiction. *Journal of Human Evolution*, 1977, *6*, 79–86.

Sacher, G. A. Maturation and longevity in relation to cranial capacity in hominid evolution. In R. Tuttle (Ed.), *Primate functional morphology and evolution*. The Hague: Mouton Press, 1973.

Sacher, G. A. Allometric and factorial analysis of brain structure in insectivores and primates. In C. R. Noback & W. Montagna (Eds.), *The primate brain*. New York: Appleton-Century-Crofts, 1970. Pp. 245–287.

Sacher, G. A. & Staffeldt, E. F. Relation of gestation time to brainweight for placental mammals: Implications for the theory of vertebrate growth. *The American Naturalist*, 1974, *108*, 593–615.

Salamy, A. Commissural transmission: Maturational changes in humans. *Science*, 1978, *200*, 1409–1411.

Shariff, G. A. Cell counts in the primate cerebral cortex. *Journal of Comparative Neurology*, 1953, *98*, 381–400.

Sholl, D. A. *The organization of the cerebral cortex*. London: Methuen, 1956.

Snell, O. Die Abhängigkeit des Hirngewichtes von dem Korpergewicht und den geistigen Fahigkeiten. *Archiv für Psychiatrie*, 1892, *23*, 436–446.

Solnitsky, O. & Harmon, P. J. The regio occipitalis of the lorisoform lemuriod *Galago demmidovii*, *Journal of Comparative Nuerology*, 1946, *84*, 339–384.

Stephan, H. Quantitative investigations on visual structures in primate brains. Basel: Karger, *Proceedings of the Second International Congress on Primates*, 1969, *3*, 34–42.

Stephan, H., Bauchot, R., & Andy, O. J. Data on the size of the brain and of various brain parts in insectivores and primates. In C. R. Noback & W. Montagna (Eds.), *The primate brain*. New York: Appleton-Century-Crofts, 1970. Pp. 289–297.

Szentagothai, J. The "module concept" in cerebral cortex architecture. *Brain Research*, 1975, *95*, 475–496.

Tower, D. B. Structural and functional organizational of mammalian cerebral cortex: The correlation of neurone density with body size. *Journal of Comparative Neurology*, 1953, *101*, 19–52.

Welker, W. Brain evolution in mammals: A review of concepts, problems and methods. In R. B. Masterton, M. E. Bitterman, C. B. G. Campbell, & N. Hotton (Eds.), *Evolution of brain and behavior in vertebrates*. New Jersey: Lawrence Erlbaum Associates, 1976. Pp. 251–344.

Chapter V

Cerebral Indices and Behavioral Differences

WILLIAM I. RIDDELL

Intelligence: General Ability or Task Specific

During the last few years, renewed interest in the relationship between cerebral development and behavior has resulted in numerous
papers (e.g., Masterton & Skeen, 1972; Riddell & Corl, 1977) attesting
to the strong positive relationship across species between brain indices
and learning abilities. In recent work in our laboratory, we have tried
to dissociate species-specific abilities and learning scores in an attempt
to avoid confusing special abilities with other factors. This type of analysis is based on the assumption that each species possesses a separate
ability, that is, intelligence or general ability, which is different from
special abilities and thus independent of task. While this notion em-
bodies a classic view in psychology, it is out of phase with recent thinking in the area (e.g., Lockard, 1971) that views intelligence as the sum
of special abilities, or as the interaction between special purpose
systems.

The choice between these alternatives, intelligence versus task specific
abilities, is not straightforward. If it were possible to show similar performance on some measure among individuals of a species, regardless
of the task, then this would be unambiguous evidence of the general
ability model. However, species may differ considerably in the special

89

DEVELOPMENT AND EVOLUTION
OF BRAIN SIZE

abilities they possess. Thus for any given problems, the difficulty in finding a constant general ability is obvious.

If one assumes for a moment that the general ability, intelligence, exists, and that it has evolved in the same manner as other special abilities, several hypothesis may be posited concerning both its function and evolution. It is initially suggested that this general ability (intelligence) has the function of permitting changes in behavior ontogenetically. The critical term here is changes, and in this respect does not refer to those situations where organisms fit appropriate stimuli to preestablished templates. Language acquisition, mother–child recognition, and all cases where the appropriate stimulus for individual members of a species varies within a specific subset are modes of behavior where stimuli and preestablished templates are connected.

Alcock (1975) has called behaviors that change ontogentically, open innate releasing mechanisms IRMs. In Alcock's scheme open IRMs occur when the genetic template is not rigid, but allows for differential experience to modify both the releaser and the response. Templates for this type of IRM may be either restrictive, that is, allowing for a specific type of learning, or semirestricted, a condition that provides for more than one possibility, but restricts the range of behaviors available. While Alcock denies the notion of varying degrees of intelligence, he does specify the occurrence of open templates, that is, systems that provide the basis for behavior that is highly flexible and reversible and that is not tied to a given control mechanism. It is just such systems, differing in both complexity and size between species (morphological differences), which foster those behavioral differences that have been generally considered to denote varying degrees of intelligence.

Before dealing with the basic question of how one measures an ability called intelligence, or perhaps more interestingly, to denote both phyletic and morphological correlates of this ability, several other types of behaviors must be examined. These are in an obscure area between restricted or semirestricted templates and open templates. Many of these behaviors involve initial plasticity within the central nervous system, and thereby allow the individual to adjust physiological mechanisms to best fit its given environment. Receptive field development and the development of binocularity are perhaps two clear examples of this type of behavior. Although Grobstein and Chow, in a recent review (1975) suggest that maturational effects might have confused earlier dramatic reports concerning the effects of selective visual experience, there is still little doubt that, in the cat at least, early visual experience has a profound effect on the orientation selectivities. The evidence concerning binocular input matching also strongly suggests that appropriate individual experience is necessary for the establishment of cortical cell responsiveness to input from either eye in roughly the same visual place. Grobstein and Chow suggest what they call the "principle of restricted potential" as an explanatory device. This position suggests that, while the nervous system is sharply constrained by a genetic program, this program permits a realization of behavioral differences, which are governed by experience. This principle is, therefore, almost identical with Alcock's semirestricted templates. The distinguishing characteristic between these abilities and intelligence, however, lies in the fact that these abilities are tied to a particular system and do not represent a general ability, which transcends systems at least within a modality. Other perceptual abilities, however, such as adaptation to distorted visual input (prism compensation) might indeed reflect a general ability, since the effects are reversible and appropriate compensation certainly involves a total reorganization rather than alternate response to a given stimulus. In this respect, it is interesting to note that available evidence indicates a positive correlation between this ability and relative brain size (Taub, 1968).

Intelligence is therefore seen as having two basic characteristics; (1) It allows for behavioral changes to novel events (conditions which have not been specifically genetically coded); and (2) it is not tied to a sensory modality but operates within a modality and across modalities. This type of general ability is seen as essential for the survival of any species, since it allows individuals to deal with some fluctuations in their environment. Intelligence may operate in those situations in which there is no consistent environmental demand to warrant the development of a special ability.

Testing Various Hypotheses about Intelligence

In order to test the foregoing hypotheses concerning the function and physiological correlates of varying degrees of intelligence, several initial decisions were necessary concerning both the independent and dependent variables. Although many measures of brain size are available, for example, Nc ("extra neurons") Jerison (1973), absolute brain size (Rensch, 1956), endocranial cavity-foramen magnum ratio (Radinsky, 1967), prefrontal system (Masterton & Skeen, 1972), A–S ratio (Holloway, 1966), initial work in our laboratory used Sacher's (1970) Species Factor I. Sacher's index was employed because: It encompassed the species first tested (*Homo sapiens*, *Saimiri sciureus*, and *Tupania glis*); accounts for body weight (P); made no assumptions concerning relic forms;

and used as its basic data the most complete information available on brain components in insectivores and primates (Stephan & Andy, 1964). Recent work has employed Jerison's Nc or a modification of EQ (Jerison, 1973) as the independent variable. The change was mandated by the fact that Sacher's measure could not be computed on species other than those presented by Stephan and Andy (1964). The adoption of Nc for comparisons within mammals and EQ for cross-class comparisons was largely the result of the need for a measure that could be applied over a wide range of species, had considerable predictive validity, and could easily be derived in our laboratory.

The evolution of Jerison's extra neurons index (Nc) may be traced through several articles (Jerison, 1955, 1963), and is presented fully in his (1973) book. In general, this formulation is based on the following lines of reasoning: 1. For archaic mammals there is a general relation between E (brain weight) and P (body weight) given by the allometric equation $E = 0.03P^{2/3} \times 2$. E can be subdivided into two parts, E_v, the portion of E associated with primitive functioning, and E_c, the portion of E associated with intelligence; 3. in primitive mammals $E = E_v$; 4. the equation $E_v = 0.03P^{2/3}$ can be employed to calculate that portion of E in contemporary mammals allocated to primitive function; 5. E_c may then be calculated by subtracting E_v from E; and 6. E_c is then converted into total neurons available for other than primitive functioning, the resulting number of neurons being designated Nc. Nc thereby indicates the number of neurons in that portion of the brain defined as E_c, and is a numerical measure of progressiveness beyond that required for a given body size.

Although Jerison's measures, especially Nc, have been questioned by Holloway (1966, 1974), we have found that Nc correlates well with behavioral differences, Spearman ρ between this measure and learning set performance as shown in Figure V.1 being $+.98$ (Riddell & Corl, 1977). When we compared the predictive success of Nc to either (H), Herschel's (1972) body/brain ratio $B^{1/3}/b^{1/2}$ where B equals body weight and b equals brain weight, or gross brain weight (E), Nc was consistently superior to both measures, and brain size alone (E) was superior to H in predicting behavior over the limited range of species and tasks sampled. This finding can be easily interpreted as suggesting that the possible number of interneuronal connections, regardless of body weight may be more important than deviations from the general square–cube relationship between E and P. Since Nc is a measure of E after accounting for that part of E associated with P (E_v), under Jerison's model, the added predictive power of Nc is probably due to the ability to factor out the effect of P on E. It should also be the case that if Nc, or any other measure independent of P, could be used as an indicant of neuronal connections, an even more powerful measure might evolve. Although the predictive power of Sacher's Species Factor I, and a cortical–subcortical ratio are extremely high, $>.90$, the extremely limited sample sizes available limit the generality of these measures.

The criticisms of Nc can be largely classified as either questioning the

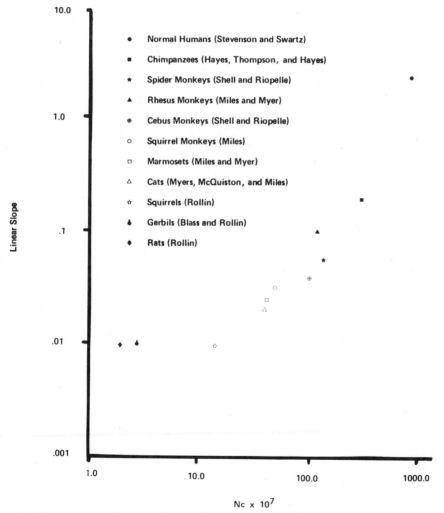

FIGURE V.1. Linear slope of learning set performance shown as a function of Nc. Adapted from Riddell and Corl (1977), by permission.

basic data, that is, the use of 2/3 as a constant slope in the allometric equation $E = P^{2/3}$, questioning the use of constant neural densities across species, or noting that the model does not take accout the possible differential organizational schemes across species. Athough Dr. Holloway will specifically address these questions in his chapter, the use of Nc as the major independent variable in our investigations demands that some of the problems raised be addressed here. Holloway's concern over "fictional numbers" (Holloway, 1974), and the possibility that the calculation of the number of extra neurons (Nc) might become a passion, is a shared concern. I do not believe that Jerison would argue that mean Nc values for a species are cut in stone. In this respect, all the extremely high correlations reported between Nc and behavior were rank order correlations. The criticism concerning the inability of the index to account for differential organization is side-stepped in this research; since the basic goal of the behavioral measure employed is to factor out species—specific special abilities, that is, those behaviors most likely to be linked with differential organization. Generally, however, although differential organization may well be attributed to behavioral differences, there is presently no way to quantify these differences across a wide range of species. As behavior, as shall be seen later, seems to be an exponential function of Nc it may well be the case that organizational differences, if correlated with Nc, are attributing to this result.

A possibly more telling problem with Nc involves the assumption that $E = E_v + E_c$. This formulation implies that primitive and advanced behavior are independent, and that new function is added with the addition of new or expanded structure. The notion of the pyramiding of structure and function has long been discarded in favor of the notion of greater differentiation of function with the addition of new structure. For example, this argument led Bitterman (1965) to ask "whether extensive cortical damage will produce in the rat the kinds of behavior which are characteristic of precortical animals, such as the fish, or animals with only very limited cortical development [p. 402]." While the results of testing these subjects on both visual and spatial, reversal and probability problems indicated that under some conditions the performance of decorticate rats was closer to fish than their whole brain peers, and in general was similar to turtles, there were no reports of egg laying or gill growing in this group. That is, I suggest that the removal of any given structure in one species will never short circuit millions of years of evolution. The total integration of different neuronal structures, and the spread of function across both phyletically old and new structures in more advanced species, precludes the compartmentalizing of function with the appearance of new structures. The present use of Nc or any other measure of relative brain development should therefore be seen as an attempt at an indicator of morphological differences, which reflects differences in the ability to handle and process information.

Attempts of Comparative Psychology to Study between Species Differences

The history of comparative learning could be simply classified as disappointing. Since Darwin initially laid the theoretical ground work in the area, few if any fundamental questions have been answered concerning the nature of species differences in regard to learning abilities. The comparative psychologist often appears to know little more than the grade school child who would rather have a pet dog than bird, or bird than fish, or fish than worm, simply because they make better friends, as they can be taught more. This state of affairs did not arise without considerable effort. Countless hours were spent testing numerous species on a variety of problems, in an attempt to find some measure that would yield consistent meaningful differences. Without exception however, any task that required members of species to learn a given problem either failed to yield such differences over a wide range of species, or the performance of species changed differentially as either the stimuli or procedural variables were manipulated. These failures are described presently as an inability on the part of comparative psychologists to control for species—specific special abilities, a problem that according to Lockard (1971) is insolvable. Lockard contends that learning abilities of a species are simply the sum of the special abilities, a position that is supported by these previous failures. The only class of problems that have been used with some limited success across species have required subjects to use previously learned information in one condition as a basis for future learning, that is, transfer designs. The most notable of these tasks is successive acquisition–extinction of an instrumental response (Voronin, 1962), successive discrimination reversals (Bitterman, 1965; Gossette, 1969), objects quality learning sets (Miles, 1957), and the reversal/acquisition ratio (Rumbaugh & Pournell, 1966).

Although each of these tasks has its problems (e.g., Devine, 1970, found on a series of learning set problems most if not all of the variance was due to procedural differences rather than species differences; Warren, 1967, indicated that the reversal index correlates with original learning, and the reversal/acquisition ration requires matching performance across species), they still manage to do a fair job in assessing behavior. The high correlation between learning set performance and Nc in Figure

V.1 attests to their usefulness. This correlation however, resulted from using the slope of the obtained curve from chance to asymptote as a dependent variable, since final asymptotic performance level is a function of a stimulus and task variables (Riddell, Corl, Bennett, & Reimers, 1974).

In choosing a specific task therefore, what is needed is a procedure in which special abilities are controlled, and that probably measures the ability of a species to transfer information from problem to problem. The inability to control for special abilities has been a major stumbling block in the study of comparative learning. An early solution to this problem was advanced by Bitterman (1960, 1965), when he suggested that one should look for functional differences between species, and employ the method of control by systematic variation. Although theoretically sound, the method of control by systematic variation is almost a procedural impossibility, and one would always seem to be in the position trying to prove the null hypothesis in those cases where functional differences are not initially evident. However, the problem raised by Bitterman remains unresolved, namely, that control by equation is an impossibility in comparative learning. If one cannot control by equation and control via systematic variation is too costly, the only possible solution seems to be to employ a within species control procedure similar in concept to the classic within subjects designs, which are used to control for individual differences. This is not a new thought and was the basis of the reversal index (RI) proposed by Rajalakshmi and Jeeves (1965), and serves as the basic proposition behind the reversal acquisition ratio suggested by Rumbaugh and Pournell (1966). As it became quickly apparent, however, that neither a simple ratio of original learning to reversal one performance, nor difference scores would control for differences between species (Gossette & Gossette, 1967; Warren, 1967), another technique was needed.

Removing Special Abilities from Performance Scores

As the only problems which have exhibited some success in eliciting reliable species differences have been problems which entail inhibition, and since the ability of subjects to shift responses from dimension to dimension might be the basis for the differences using learning sets, a series of extradimensional shifts were chosen for the present basic paradigm. In general, the procedure employed (a detailed procedure can be found in Riddell, *et al.*, 1974) the testing of two experimental groups on a series of three two-choice discrimination problems, where Problem

1 was identical to Problem 3. The two different discrimination tasks used in the initial series of experiments were Position, P (right = positive) and Brightness, B (on = positive). Within each species, one group received the sequence Position-Brightness-Position (P_1-B_2-P_3) for their three problem series, and the other received the sequence B_1-P_2-B_3. A daily session consisted of 30 noncorrection trials, during which time one of the two stimulus displays was illuminated for all problems (i.e., light was relevant for brightness problems and variable irrelevant for position problems). Testing continued on a given discrimination until a subject achieved at least 90% correct within a daily session. To date *Rattus norwegicus, Paca paca, Tupia glis, Samiri scireus, Cebus albifrons,* and *Homo sapiens* have been tested, using this procedure. As Problem 3 performance in each sequence was thought to be an index of inhibitory control, three control groups of rats were run to test this contention. The first two conditions merely involved omitting Problem 2 in each sequence and retesting the subjects on Problem 1 after waiting for the mean number of days it took subjects in the experimental groups to solve Problem 2. The third control condition involved removing the irrelevant dimension of brightness on Problem 3 in the Position-Brightness-Position sequence. For each of these groups, if the learning of Problem 3 was largely determined by the degree of inhibitory control, one would expect the error scores in these control groups to be small. As the mean number of errors (including criterion session) was less than 8 for all groups, we felt comfortable with this assumption.

We found there was no significant correlation between error scores and brain size, therefore if there was some general species factor involved in performance, it was obscured by species-specific special abilities. In order to attempt to remove the effects of these special abilities several initial assumptions (as stated earlier) had to be made. First it was assumed that there exists a general factor for every species that in part determines the observed performance; second, observed performance is a function of this general ability factor, plus the level of special ability for the given task; third, this general factor should be reliably related to brain size.

As an initial attempt to factor out these special abilities, the following functional relationship was suggested (Riddell, Corl, & Gravetter, 1976): Inhibition = K(relative difficulty)$^\alpha$. This particular function was chosen to relate relative difficulty to inhibition, since it makes no assumption concerning the value of the species factor (K) or α. It should be the case however, that K will be primarily influenced by species differences, since it controls the magnitude of inhibition, while α expresses the role of task difficulty. Relative task difficulty was initially defined as (P_2 −

$P_3)/(B_2 - B_3)$ or the inverse, that is, $(B_2 - B_3)/(P_2 - P_3)$. This measure was determined by assuming that errors on Problem 2 reflect the inhibition of Problem 1, the inhibition of any dimension in the subject's hierarchy between the dimension relevant in Problem 1 and the relevant dimension in Problem 2, and finally the learning of Problem 2. Similarly it may be assumed that Problem 3 requires the inhibition of Problem 2, the inhibition of dimensions between the relevant dimension for Problem 2 and the relevant dimension for Problem 3, plus any retention decrement. Since it can be assumed for the sake of simplicity that errors attributable to retention loss or inhibition of intervening dimensions are negligible or relatively consistent across problems, then Problem 2 minus Problem 3 should give a reliable estimate of problem difficulty for a species. From this discussion, it is therefore inferred that the errors on B_2 minus the errors on B_3 (B_2-B_3) provides a measure of the difficulty of the Brightness discrimination and similarly, $P_2 - P_3$ measures the difficulty of the Position problem. The ratio of these two values gives an indication of relative problem difficulty within each species. It further follows that the errors on the third problem in each sequence are primarily due to the difficulty of inhibiting responses learned during the previous problem.

These values give a set of two simultaneous equations for each of the species tested

$$P_3 = K[P_2 - P_3)/(B_2 - B_3)]^\alpha$$
$$B_3 = K[(B_2 - B_3)/(P_2 - P_3)]^\alpha.$$

These equations were solved for K and for α for each species. Figure V.2 indicates the results of this analysis for each species as a function of Nc. From Figure V.2, it is obvious that this formulation, which attempted to account for special abilities, orders the species very nicely along the Nc continuum ($P_1 - .94$). It can also be noted that K and Nc appropriately described the behavior of species from within the same subfamily, that is, Cebinae, and also made the unintuitive predication that a rodent, *Paca paca*, would perform in a manner more similar to the Primates than to its fellow rodent.

Although this demonstration of a nearly perfect relationship between K and cerebral development is certainly encouraging, it is only a partial test of the concept of general ability. If a single value of learning ability exists for each species and is measured by K, then the obtained values should not only provide a meaningful ordering of species, but also should be constant within species across tasks, procedures, motivational

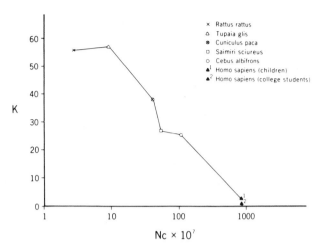

FIGURE V.2. *K* used as a function of *Nc* × 10⁷ for all species tested. Adapted from Riddell, Corl, and Gravetter (1976), by permission.

level, etc. As a partial test of the stability of *K*, rats, cebus monkeys, and college students were tested on a variety of problems designed to produce sizable variability in the raw data (Gravetter, Riddell, Hewitt, & Rogers, 1979). Using the same procedure as noted before, rats were tested on six different problems where either the saliency of brightness dimension was altered [20 foot-candles (fc) or 1.5 fc], trials per day (continuous running to criterion, or 30 trials, or 10 trials), or previous experience of the subjects (naive or sophisticated), was varied. The cebus monkeys were tested on a form versus size discrimination, using the standard procedure. The college students received four additional ex-tradimensional shift problems, which either entailed a form versus size discrimination, size versus position, color versus form, or position ver-sus alternation discrimination. As in the standard brightness versus position paradigm, the relevant dimension for one problem was a var-iable irrelevant for the other problem.

Initial analysis of error scores indicated that for each species the dif-ferent problems yielded significantly different error scores, and the pres-ence of significant interactions between Problems, Order, and Sequence indicated that the pattern of errors within each sequence was dependent on the particular experimental condition.

For this set of experiments the general formula to calculate *K* was slightly modified as follows.

$$\text{Learning Score} = K(\text{rel. diff})^{\alpha} \times (\text{abs. diff})$$

Where the value of K was theoretically determined by the species general ability, the relative difficulty of the two tasks is used as an index of special abilities, and α is expected to reflect the role of task difficulty. For each species and for each pair of problems, the values of K and α were found by solving two simultaneous equations in two unknowns.

$$A3 = K(\text{rel. diff. } A/B)^\alpha \times (\text{diff. } A)$$
$$B3 = K(\text{rel. diff. } B/A)^\alpha \times (\text{diff. } B)$$

Where,

1. $A3$ was defined as a number of errors on problem A when it was third in the series. Similarly, $B3$ was the learning score for problem B.
2. The difficulty of each problem was defined as the sum of the errors committed during the three presentations of that problem. For example, diff. $A = A1 + A2 + A3$.
3. Relative difficulty was defined as the ratio of the absolute difficulties.

Thus, although K and α are theoretical values, they are not free parameters but are completely determined by the data.

Although this formulation is consistent with the formula proposed earlier, the exact formula is modified with respect to two details. First, problem difficulty is now simply defined as the total number of errors committed on the problem, rather than the amount of savings from initial learning to relearning. The original definition may have been subject to confounding by group differences, since separate groups of subjects were being compared, and it led to occasional low Ks in situations where learning and relearning were both difficult, and the amount of savings was small. The second modification is the introduction of absolute task difficulty as a factor contributing to the learning score. It should be noted that while the new formulation reduces the magnitude of the obtained general learning scores (K-values), the ordering of species is the same as produced by the original formula.

The means and standard errors for each of the species tested, along with the single points obtained previously are shown in Figure V.3. An analysis of variance on the obtained K values for the three species tested yielded a significant difference between groups, $F(2, 10) = 7.94; p < .01$. As is clear from Figure V.3 the correlation between Nc and K is again high, this time yielding a Spearman correlation of $+.90$. The data for the *Pacas* were omitted from this analysis because of the change in the formula for K, since the data were not derived from two independent groups of subjects (Riddell *et al.* 1976).

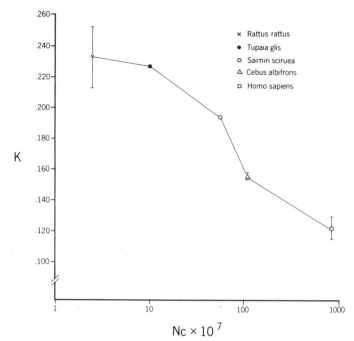

FIGURE V.3. Mean K values and standard errors shown as a function of $Nc \times 10^7$.

This demonstration of consistency within species lends support to the concept of a single value for species learning ability. It should also be made clear however, that this set of results leaves many problems and unanswered questions. In particular, there is some overlap in the K values of diverse species, for example, the lowest K for rats (.143) is less than the highest K for humans (.150). If we are correct in assuming that differential brain development should be reflected in differential general learning ability, then this result is unacceptable. However, the results presented demonstrate enough consistency within species and proper differentiation between species to indicate that some underlying general ability is being measured.

As these results yielded considerable support for the basic premise that relative brain size differentiated species in respect to general learning ability, it was decided to extend the model on both the independent and dependent variables. This was attempted by testing fish, that is, the class of vertebrates with the smallest relative brain size, on the extradimensional shift paradigm. The testing procedure for the fish involved shock avoidance in a symmetrical Y-maze. This apparatus was also used to reevaluate the learning scores for rats, therefore providing a test for the stability of K between the two-choice appetitive situation and the Y-maze shock avoidance situation, in rats.

The apparatus and procedure used were almost identical to those described by Caul and Barrett (1973) for rats, with the exception of the addition of a top grid and water for the fish. Thirty trials were given each day and subjects were tested until the 90% criterion level was obtained. The standard Position–Brightness shift sequences were used. The shock levels were set at the minimal level possible to obtain an escape response. Although bullheads, brown trout, rainbow trout, chubs, and goldfish have successfully completed the three problem sequences, only the data for the chubs are presented, because of the small number of subjects in each of the other groups. The data for the chubs was obtained on 10 subjects (5 per condition). The data for the other species is not dramatically different from that obtained from chubs, and would lead to the same conclusions.

In order to compare fish with the mammals tested earlier, it is necessary to use a different index of brain development, since Nc is obviously restricted to species with neocortex. The index chosen was EQ. There have been many variations of this measure, which is simply the ratio of the observed brain weight of a species to the expected brain weight. The differences between measures are a result of either expressing the ratio as a percentage, or differences in the calculation of expected brain weight. As the purpose of the measure was to compare performance across vertebrates, the use of the expected brain weight of the standard average mammal (i.e., the expected weight used by Jerison), did not seem appropriate. Instead, it was decided to employ as an expected weight the brain weight of the vertebrate with the smallest brain size. The log–log plot of brain and body weights for fish, is shown in Figure V.4, from which it is apparent that the lamprey possesses the smallest relative brain size, $E = .007P^{2/3}$. Our measure of EQ was therefore defined as EQ_L—observed brain weight/expected brain weight, where expected brain weight equalled $.007P^{2/3}$. The slope of two-thirds was chosen, since it was not only conventional but closely approximated the slope between the adult and transformer lamprey points.

The actual performance of the fish was superior to that expected. Figure V.5 shows the total number of errors for this species, and the mammals previously tested on the standard sequence. As is clear from Figure V.5, fish made approximately the same number of errors as tree shrews, and considerably less than the cebus. The K value (using the newer formulation) was considerably less than expected, and in fact suggests that the chub ($K = .183$) and squirrel monkey ($K = .194$) are approximately equivalent in terms of general learning ability as shown in Figure V.6. This result is obviously unreasonable, if one wishes to maintain that *K* is measuring anything at all. Although trial by trial data were not collected on any species, the pattern of errors was distinctly different for fish both within and between sessions. In particular, although one could predict fairly accurately the performance of the mammals from trial to trial and session to session, this orderliness was absent in the fish. They seemed to respond, on Problems 2 and 3, in an all or nothing matter. That is, there would be frequent runs on the early session on Problem 3 or the late sessions of Problem 2 of seven or more correct responses followed by seven or more incorrect responses, and

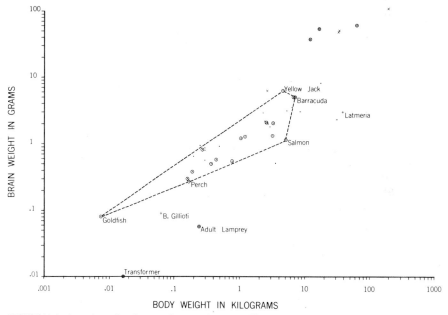

BODY WEIGHT IN KILOGRAMS

FIGURE V.4. Log–log plot shown of mean brain and body weights of fish. The teleost data was obtained from Crile and Quiring (1940) and has been expressed within a minimum convex polygon after Jerison (1973). The points outside the polygon represent either sharks (brain weights in excess of 10 gm) or relict forms (*B. gillioti, Latermia,* or *Lamprey*). The shark data was obtained from Ebbesson and Northcutt (1976). The data for lampreys (adult and transformers) was obtained in our laboratory. Although it is clear that the "standard" slope of two-thirds fits the teleost data, the value of the intercept is approximately .028 rather than the .007 reported by Jerison. This discrepancy resulted from using mean weights and not including either reptiles or relict forms. The intercept for the relict forms is approximately .007, that is, the value used to compute EQ_{L}. It is interesting to note that the shark data is clearly different from either the relict forms or present teleost data, suggesting that within fish one might find the same differences between groups as found in mammals.

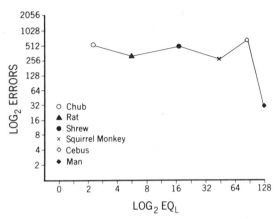

FIGURE V.5. Total errors, shown on both sequences for the standard Position/Brightness sequences as a function of EQ_L.

it seemed that it was just a matter of chance whether or not criterion was reached. The mammals, on the other hand, responded consistently both within and between sessions. The behavior of the fish here is reminiscent of the performance of fish on probability problems, reversal learning, and ID versus ED shifts (Tennant & Bitterman, 1973). On each of these problems, fish do not show the typical pattern of performance exhibited by mammals, and Sutherland and Mackintosh (1971) have described the difference as an attentional deficit in fish relative to mammals. As the present paradigm deals directly with the inhibition of observing or attentional responses, and as fish might well be qualitatively different from mammals in this respect, it is not surprising that the result did not fit the expected pattern. This interpretation is strengthened by the relationship between the number of errors made on a given

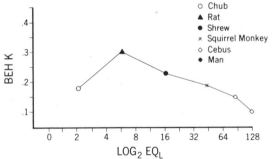

FIGURE V.6. K shown as a function of EQ_L for the mammals tested and a representative fish.

discrimination when presented as Problem 1 (original learning), or as Problem 2 (ED shift). Although 10 of the 12 possible such comparisons for mammals (considering only Position or Brightness problems) indicated Problem 2 was more difficult than Problem 1, of the 7 possible comparisons for fish, only 3 indicated the typical interference effect.

The performance of the rats was consonant with the prediction that K should be consistent within a species across tasks and methodologies. The observed K value for these subjects was .237, a value which is close to the mean K value of .222 observed in the two-choice appetitive situations. Although one additional positive result does not a measure make, the fact that this K value falls within the standard error computed from other data certainly would be difficult to predict if each K value is assumed to represent a distinct special ability.

In any discussion of comparative learning the question as to qualitative versus quantitative differences between species or within species across different tasks becomes paramount. Since the goal of the present formulation was to factor out special abilities, the question of qualitative differences within species may become moot to the extent that the formulation is effective. The question as to whether the different K values between species reflect different processes or simply a greater processing ability in some species, I do not know the answer. Two recent papers from Bitterman's lab (Bitterman, 1976; Bitterman & Woodard, 1976) directly address the issue, and attest to the inherent difficulties in this area: "Quantitative differences in process may produce qualitative differences in performance, and "Qualtitative differences in performance do not necessarily mean there are qualitative differences in process [p. 218]." The weight of the evidence presented here however, suggests quantitative differences in K between species. This conclusion is most parsimonious as there is a smooth orderly relationship between Nc and K and it can be argued that Nc reflects quantitative differences in processing ability within mammals.

Given what appears to be a reliable relationship between indexes of brain development and learning abilities, questions can at least be asked concerning the nature of this relationship. Although I have a general mistrust of trying to reduce complex behavioral phenomena to rigid mathematical formulations, the orderliness of the data warrants this type of speculation. Figure V.7 shows the basic learning set slope data and K values presented earlier as a function of Nc, to which two theoretical lines have been added. One line represents the best fit to the data if the behavior is considered to be a linear function of Nc, and the second line represents the relationship if behavior is considered an exponential function of Nc. From Figure V.7, it is obvious that the expo-

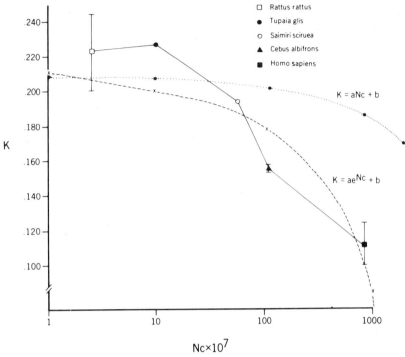

FIGURE V.7. Best fit linear and exponential curves of learning set slope plotted as a function of Nc.

nential curve best fit the data. In general the data indicate that while large changes in relative brain size are necessary for behavioral differences at "low" Nc values, the same relative or even absolute change at "higher" Nc values would produce much greater changes in behavior, or, as grandma used to say, "the rich get richer." The most obvious causal mechanism for this type of relationship is the number of neuronal connections. As suggested by Rensch (1956), increases in brain size lead to a geometric increase in the number of possible interneuronal connections, a condition which Rensch described as the necessary condition for greater behavioral flexibility. Dr. Holloway's suggestion that differential organization must be taken into account also fits neatly with this result, as one would expect that the complexity of possible neuronal patterns might well increase at a greater than linear rate as relative brain size increases. In this respect, although it is not suggested that e^N is an indicant of the actual number of connections, it should be directly related to the actual number by some geometric or exponential function. The theoretical exponential curves could also explain the inability to find any within species differences as a function of relative brain size. In studies done in our laboratory with fish, rats, or gerbils, and in other studies conducted by colleagues that entailed some learning tasks, we have tested for the presence of a within species correlation between brain size and performance. In the more than 20 such tests performed to date, the average correlations is $-.01$. Given the degree of variability in brain index values within a species (about 10%), and the flattening of the curve at low Nc values, this lack of correlation would be expected. It is also interesting to speculate on the relationship between brain size and behavior from an evolutionary perspective. Given the condition that small changes in brain size in large brained species have a greater behavioral effect than equivalent changes in small brained species, the evolutionary increase in brain size in such groups would proceed in a much more orderly and consistent fashion, assuming, of course, that this increase was advantageous.

Conclusion

In conclusion, the present data indicate that the use of relative brain size as an independent variable seems to allow for the systematic study of species along an orderly and appropriate continuum. While the present set of studies was concerned with learning abilities, there is no a priori reason why this type of continua could not be employed in studying many other types of behavior.

Acknowledgments

The author is indebted to Frederick Gravetter, who has collaborated on much of the work presented, and to Stanley Wechkin for his advice and criticisms of the paper and constant intellectual support. A special thank you is also given to all those students who have tested subjects over the years, expecially Gerald Dewey, whose help in the preparation of this paper has proven invaluable.

References

Alcock, J. *Animal behavior: An evolutionary approach.* Sunderland, Mass.: Sinauer Associates, 1975.
Bitterman, M. E. Towards a comparative psychology of learning. *American Psychologist,* 1960, *15,* 704–712.

Bitterman, M. E. Phyletic differences in learning. *American Psychologist*, 1965, *20*, 396–410.

Bitterman, M. E. Issues in the comparative psychology of learning. In R. B. Masterson, M. E. Bitterman, C. B. G. Campbell, & N. Hotton (Eds.), *Evolution of brain and behavior in vertebrates*. New York: Erlbaum–Wiley, 1976.

Bitterman, M. E., & Woodard, W. T. Vertebrate learning: Common processes. In R. B. Masterson, M. E. Bitterman, C. B. G. Campbell, & N. Hotton (Eds.), *Evolution of brain and behavior in vertebrates*. New York: Erlbaum–Wiley, 1976.

Caul, W. F., & Barrett, R. J. Shuttlebox versus Y-maze avoidance: value of multiple response measures in interpreting active-avoidance performance of rats. *Journal of Comparative and Physiological Psychology*, 1973, *84*(3), 572–578.

Crile, G., & Ouiring, D. P. A record of the body weight and certain organ and gland weights of 3690 animals. *Ohio Journal of Science*, 1940, *40*, 219–259.

Devine, J. V. Stimulus attributes and training procedures in learning-set formation of Rhesus and Cebus monkey. *Journal of Comparative and Physiological Psychology*, 1970, *73*, 62–67.

Gossette, R. L. Variation in magnitude of negative transfer on successive discrimination reversal (SDR) tasks across species. *Perceptual and Motor Skills*, 1969, *29*, 803–811.

Gossette, R. L., & Gossette, M. F. Examination of the reversal indices (RI) across fifteen different mammalian and avian species. *Perceptual and Motor Skills*, 1967, *24*, 987–990.

Gravetter, F. J., Riddell, W. I., Hewitt, W., & Rogers, W. Towards a valid measure of species differences. In preparation. 1979.

Grobstein, P. & Chow, K. L. Receptive field development and individual experience. *Science*, 1975, *190*, 352–358.

Holloway, R. L. Cranial capacity, neural reorganization, and hominid evolution: A search for more suitable parameters. *American Journal of Physical Anthropology*, 1966, *25*, 305.

Holloway, R. L. On the meaning of brain size. *Science*, 1974, *184*, 677–679.

Jerison, H. J. Brain to body ratios and the evolution of intelligence. *Science*, 1955, *121*, 447–449.

Jerison, H. J. Interpreting the evolution of the brain. *Human Biology*, 1963, *35*, 263–291.

Jerison, H. J. *Evolution of the brain and intelligence*. New York: Academic Press, 1973.

Lockard, R. Reflections on the fall of comparative psychology. *American Psychologist*, 1971, *26*, 168–179.

Masterson, B., & Skeen, L. Origins of anthropoid intelligence: Prefrontal system and delayed alternation in hedge hog, tree shrew, and bush baby. *Journal of Comparative and Physiological Psychology*, 1972, *81*, 423–433.

Miles, R. Learning-set formation in the squirrel monkey, *Journal of Comparative and Physiological Psychology*, 1957, *50*, 356–357.

Radinsky, L. Relative brain size: A new measure. *Science*, 1967, *155*, 836–838.

Rajalakshmi, R. & Jeeves, M. A. The relative difficulty of reversal learning (Reversal Index) as a basis of behavioral comparisons. *Animal Behavior*, 1965, *13*, 203–211.

Rensch, B. Increase in learning capability with increase in brain size. *American Naturalist*, 1956, *90*, 81–85.

Riddell, W. I., & Corl, K. G. Comparative investigation of the relationship between cerebral indices and learning abilities. *Brain, Behavior and Evolution*, 1977, *14*, 305–308.

Riddell, W. I., Corl, K. G., Bennett, V. D., & Reimers, R. Discrimination learning differences and similarities as a function of brain index. *Phsyiology and Behavior*, 1974, *13*, 201–205.

Riddell, W. I., Corl, K. G., & Gravetter, F. J. Cross order comparisons using indexes of cerebral development, *Bulletin of the Psychonomic Society*, 1976, *8*, 578–580.

Rumbaugh, D. M., & Pournell, M. B. Discrimination-reversal skills of primates: The reversal/acquisition ratio as a function of phyletic standing, *Psychonomic Science,* 1966, *4,* 45–46.

Sacher, G. A. Allometric and factor analysis of brain structure in insectivores and primates. In C. R. Noback & W. Montagna (eds.), *The primate brain: Advances in primatology,* New York: Appleton-Century-Croft, 1970.

Stephan, M., & Andy, O. J. Quantitative comparisons of brain structures from insectivores to primates. *American Zoologist,* 1964, *4,* 59–74.

Sutherland, N. S., & Mackintosh, N. J. *Mechanisms of animal discrimination learning.* New York: Academic Press, 1971.

Suen, O. E. Ebesson & R. C. Northcutt. Neurology of anamniotic vertebrates. In. R. B. Masterson, M. E. Bitterman, C. B. G. Campbell, & N. Hotton (eds.), *Evolution of brain and behavior in vertebrates.* New York: Erlbaum–Wiley, 1976.

Taub, E. Prism Compensation as a learning phenomenon: A phylogentic perspective. In S. J. Freedman (Ed.), *The neuropsychology of spatially oriented behavior.* Homewood, Ill.; Dorsey Press, 1968.

Tennant, W. A., & Bitterman, M. E. Some comparisons of intradimensional and extradimensional transfer in discrimination learning of goldfish. *Journal of Comparative and Physiological Psychology,* 1973, *83,* 134–139.

Voronin, L. Some results of comparative-physiological investigations of higher nervous activity. *Psychological Bulletin,* 1962, *59,* 161–195.

Warren, J. N. An assessment of the reversal index, *Animal Behavior,* 1967, *15,* 493–498.

Chapter VI

Correlated Brain and Intelligence Development in Humans[1]

HERMAN T. EPSTEIN

All correct reasoning is a grand system of tautologies, but only God can make direct use of that fact. The rest of us must painstakingly and fallibly tease out the consequences of our assumptions.

> H. A. Simon [*The Sciences of the Artificial*, Cambridge, Mass., MIT Press, 1969]

This report is mainly a selective summary of what is in the literature—selective not in the sense that I have knowingly excluded evidence counter to the propositions to be put forth, but selective in that it is impossible, in any such brief presentation, to include all the relevant studies.

I shall be looking at correlations between brain and intelligence in two different biological contexts. The first context is that of developmental biology, leading to the question, "Is there any connection or correlation between brain development measured biophysically and intelligence development measured psychologically?" The second context is that of neuroanatomy, leading to the question, "Is there any correlation between the properties of any brain region measured neuroanatomically and intelligence measured psychologically?" The answer I shall give to the first question is that there appears to be very solid scientific evidence

[1]This research was supported by the Ruth Newton Fund and by Biomedical Research Support Fund Grant RR07044.

DEVELOPMENT AND EVOLUTION
OF BRAIN SIZE

showing such a correlation. The answer to the second question is that there is already a basis for a working hypothesis about a locale for some significant aspects of human intelligent functioning.

My approach was to ask what can be learned about what appear to be the strategies and tactics of brain growth and development through studies of the ontogenic aspects. It is not important to this approach whether or not ontogeny might recapitulate phylogeny. What is important is that by learning *when* major brain changes take place, we can ask what functional changes appear at those ages. In turn, those discovered functional changes permit inferences about the "reasons" for those particular anatomical changes, so that we can establish working hypotheses about what kinds of reasons are important to nature in the development of brains. Such hypotheses always suggest looking at additional details of the actual brain growth, thereby modifying the details of the behavioral studies to be examined. In this way, my study has gone back and forth from brain to behavior to brain, trying always to sharpen both of the emerging pictures of development.

At first sight it was, admittedly, unlikely that anything of much significance could be learned by ascertaining the facts about the overall growth of the brain. There was a widespread reaction to the presenting of the data showing the average brain weight as a function of age from birth to brain maturity at around age 18 years; this reaction was "so what?" At most, so I was told, I could stop writers of textbooks from telling medical students that the human brain reaches essentially adult size by about age 2 years or 4 years—as if the remaining respective increases of 30% or 15% were unlikely to be of immense significance for a species so very dependent on the extent and complexity of its neural networks.

The major self-imposed restriction on what I shall tell you is that I will confine my discussion to cognitive and sensory aspects of behavior. Brain functions include psychiatrically and psychologically interesting aspects, which have been studied, but which will not be discussed here.

General Features of Organ Development

The growth of the brain should have aspects in common with the growth of other organs, as well as aspects specific to the requirements for efficient development of the brain. The normal growth patterns of a number of human organs are illustrated in Figure VI.1, which is a collection of data from several independent sources as put together by Clatworthy, and Anderson (1944). It shows the ratio of organ volume

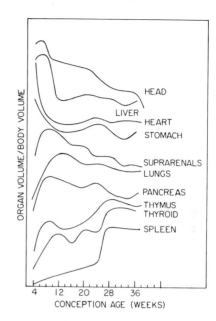

FIGURE VI.1. Organ volume/body volume of various human organs shown from shortly after conception until birth. [Data from Clatworthy & Anderson, 1944.]

to body volume from a few weeks after conception until birth. The overall changes in this ratio range from a sharp relative increase for some organs to a relative decrease for other organs, with most organs showing an intermediate pattern, resulting in little overall change in the ratio during gestation. In addition to the overall change, there are some readily seen temporary variations. The spleen, for example, drifts along in a very slow increase in the ratio until about 5 months, at which age a tripling of the ratio takes place in a very few weeks. Similar, though less dramatic, changes may be seen in all organs. The head shows three such change periods: about 6 weeks after conception, 16–20 weeks after conception, and about 6–8 weeks before birth. We will later discuss the significance of the fact that the latter two head growth periods are paralleled by readily measured bursts of synthesis of DNA in the brain (Dobbing & Sands, 1970).

Embryologists tell us that, as organs develop, they all experience at various stages a cellular differentiation leading to a new function, (e.g., secretion of a new hormone or enzyme). The newly differentiated cell type then multiplies rapidly so as to be able to supply an amount of the new function suited to the needs of the growing organism. This process is generally termed functional differentiation, and is signalled by the rapid increase in mass of the organ, which contrasts with the overall growth pattern of that organ. Presumably then, the various short-term increases in organ/body volume ratio are signals for the appearance of important new functions.

Not all significant changes in organ functioning take place through cell differentiation. For example, thymus cells can apparently be recruited to new functions by factors elaborated by the first cells that interact with incoming antigens; no significant cell replication seems to be necessary (Dutton, *et al.*, 1971). Further, not all such changes occur prenatally. Growth stages are evident in organ weights at various postnatal ages, as shown by the data of Coppoletta and Wolbach (1933). Significant brain changes will be shown to be examples of both points made in this paragraph.

Human Brain Growth

Examination of the data on postnatal growth of the brain reveals significant changes in the brain/body weight ratio at various ages. These changes might be ascribed to the usual fluctuations in any set of measurements, were it not for the fact that all four collections of autopsy data that I have found, which cover the entire birth to brain-maturity period, show the changes at the same ages (Epstein, 1974a). Since that publication, additional data have been located covering less than the entire 0–18 year span, but still yielding significant information about brain growth over these more restricted periods. Currently, brain growth data show stages at 3–10 months, and 2–4, 6–8, 10–12 +, and 14–16 + years.

The data can be substantially augmented by recent work that shows that human brain weight is proportional to the cube of the head circumference (Burns, Birkbeck, & Roberts, 1975; Cooke, Lucas, Yudkin, & Pryse-Davies, 1977; Epstein & Epstein, 1978; Rosso, Hormazabal, & Winick, 1970; Winick & Rosso, 1969). This relation holds for brain weights of 15–1500 g.

The largest collection of head circumference data is that of Nellhaus (1975), which is shown in biennial increment form in Figure VI.2. Growth peaks may be seen around ages 3–4, 7, 11–12, and 15–16 years. These are similar to those given earlier for brain weight growth peaks. The quality of the data in Figure VI.2 is indicated by the fact that the standard errors are smaller than the data points. Another indication of data quality is that peaks and troughs are evident in head circumference growth, despite the fact that the data are from a dozen different countries (presumably using a variety of instruments and methods), and obtained with varying age ranges. The inability of these sources of variation to "wash out" the peaks and troughs bespeaks a thoroughly synchronized

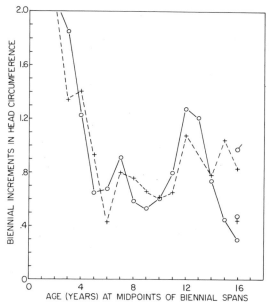

FIGURE VI.2. Biennial increments in human head circumference given at various ages. [Data from Nellhaus, 1975.]

brain growth pattern. An illustration of longitudinal data is given in Figure VI.3, which is taken from the Berkeley Growth Study (Eichorn & Bayley, 1962). It shows sharp peaks and troughs at the same ages as given in Figure VI.2. Not evident in Figure VI.3 is the finding that all 35 boys and girls have zero head growth between ages 8 and 9 years, indicating an extraordinary degree of synchronization. I have discussed elsewhere (Epstein, 1978) the possible significance of the substantial sexual dimorphism shown at ages 11 and 15 years.

The increments in brain weight are each 5–10% over the 2 year periods, so that these brain growth stages account totally for an increase of 30% in brain weight after age 1½ years. Since there is little or no net increase in brain DNA after that age (Dobbing & Sands, 1973), the 30% growth takes place with no net increase in cell number. Because of their relatively small size, growth of the more numerous glial cells should not account for a major portion of the weight increase that is, therefore, ascribable to the growth of neurons. This implies that growth would have to be composed of elongation and branching of axons and dendrites along with myelination of the axons. Thus, during the last four brain growth stages, there is a major increase in the complexity of the neural networks.

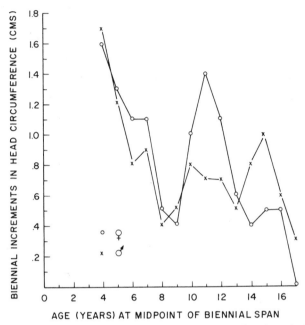

FIGURE VI.3. Biennial increments in human head circumference taken from the longitudinal Berkeley Growth Study. [Data from Eichorn & Bayley, 1962.]

Such an increase in neural network complexity is obviously likely to be reflected in a markedly increased complexity of brain functions, so that the growth stages are presumably instances of functional differentiation of the kind that occurs in the absence of cell replication. As an example of such functions, we can take the literature data described elsewhere (Epstein, 1978), which show that the brain is being programmed for binocular vision, language, and hearing during the 2–4 year brain growth stage. The evidence is that earlier-occurring defects in those functions can be remedied only during the growth stage.

The three properties just mentioned as having special remedial periods are frequently encountered in discussions of critical periods. Whatever critical periods may be, they are definitely not the equivalents of the growth stages. My analysis concerns the normal growth and development of brains, apart from any questions about the results of insults during that growth. It is true that one can ask about the different consequences of insults during and apart from growth stages, but these are an aid to the discovery of normal developmental stages. Critical periods are discovered through insults only, and therefore constitute parts of aberrant growth rather than of normal growth. To give this point the emphasis I believe it both deserves and requires, I am labeling it with a word that has been derived from the Greek *phrenoblysis*, meaning correlated brain and mind growth stages found in normal development. The correlation aspect appears in this definition in order to separate body growth related brain growth from that associated with mental growth, as will be discussed later. The subjects of critical periods and mental growth stages will both appear in subsequent aspects of our discussion.

Animal Brain Growth

From the point of view presented thus far, it should follow that all mammals will be found to have organ growth stages, including brain growth stages, and that these will be associated with the appearance of new behavioral competencies. The evidence for rats and mice that appeared recently (Gottlieb, Keydar, Epstein, 1977) shows brain growth stages at ages 0–6, 8–12, and 17–23 days after birth. The analysis will not be repeated here; instead some additional aspects of rodent brain development will be presented later.

Data for primates are not yet extensive enough to give a reliable picture of brain growth from birth to maturity, even for the most frequently studied primate, the rhesus monkey. However, through the cooperation of several of the primate research centers in the U. S. A., we have obtained some data concerning brain weights and monkey ages. There seem to be enough animals studied to give a preliminary drawing of the growth curve during the first 500 days of life. Both brain and behavior data have been analyzed (Horr & Epstein, manuscript in preparation), and the brain data are in the bottom part of Figure VI.4. The numbers near the bottom of the figure are the number of animals at each age point, using four as the minimum number to be included in the analysis. A brain growth plateau occurs between about 120 days and 270 days, and a second plateau is apparently being started around 400 days of age. Thus, in the rhesus monkeys there are two brain growth stages as shown in Figure VI.4: 0–120 days and 270–400 days. The top portion of the figure will be discussed later.

Data for cats are even more sparse than those for monkeys, as is evident from Figure VI.5. Most of the data appear in the form of brain–body weight ratios. If these were ample data, I would interpret them as showing a brain growth stage at ages 1–10, 20–30 +, and probably

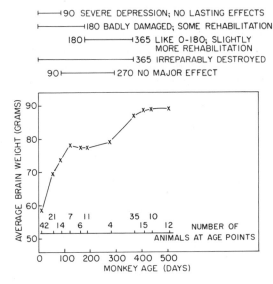

FIGURE VI.4. Average rhesus macaque brain weight seen as a function of age from birth to 500 days—data are from the New England, Oregon, and Wisconsin Primate Research Centers. The information at the top is discussed in the text. [Data from Sackett, 1968.]

after 90 days. It may be of significance that the 20–30 + days brain growth stage is quite close to the critical period for vision studied so extensively by Wiesel and Hubel (1965).

We can now take a first look at comparative brain growth since we have preliminary data for humans and for three nonhuman animals. We can ask about similarities and differences between the main events taking place in the brain growth stages in the various species. If similar events are found in individual growth stages in different species, the similarities could be explained in at least two ways. The first is that nature used, or was compelled to use (because of the kinds of problems and solutions available to her), similar developmental strategies and tactics. Alternatively, we could suppose the similarity to be a result of evolutionary selection, as follows: Consider the common ancestor of humans and rodents. Presumably that organism had one or more brain growth stages. If more than one existed, its origin would then be imagined to have been the result of a mutation in the system regulating brain growth. If the resultant larger brain led to an increased survival, then the mutant organism would eventually have replaced the smaller-brained organism. After the divergence of the lines leading to the present species of humans and rodents, the species had separate evolutionary histories. But, it is unlikely that the original growth stages were altered in their main features. Therefore, by examining the brain growth

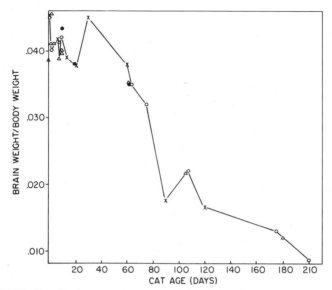

FIGURE VI.5. Brain/body weight ratios of cats shown from birth to age seven months: [Data from Blinkov & Glezer, 1968 (●); Agrawal, Davis, and Himwich, 1968 (X), Kobayashi, 1963 (○); and Count, 1947 (△).]

stages in humans and rodents, we may expect to find that a particular stage in mice has the same main features as one of the stages in humans (e.g., both would manifest peak DNA synthesis in the cerebellum). Elsewhere, we (Epstein & Miller, 1977), have outlined evidence leading to the equating of the 8–12 day brain growth stage of rodents with the 3–10 month stage in humans. A similar correspondence was noted between the main events in the next brain growth stages in those species (17–23 days in rodents and 2–4 years in humans). This double set of parallelisms supports the descriptive notions that preceded, and if it is assumed that the analysis is correct, it affords a rather substantial improvement in our ability to extrapolate events from one species to another.

Manifestations of Brain Growth Stages in Properties Other Than Weight

One of the most frequently encountered erroneous inferences about the existence of brain growth stages is that all brain properties must show highly correlated growth stages. The weight increases during plateau periods are, of course, much lower than during growth stages, but that does not mean that no brain properties change appreciably during the plateau periods. Indeed, we can learn about developmental strategies from discovering which properties do in fact show correlated and unrelated growth stages. However, the growth stages must be manifested in specific details, including regionalization and the expression of weight changes in physical, chemical, physiological, and anatomical terms. In addition, there are quite clear predictions that follow from the inference that the stages are manifestations of sharp increases in neural network complexity.

It has already been mentioned that the last two prenatal brain growth stages in humans are paralled by sharp rises in DNA. Dobbing and Sands (1973) studied both protein and DNA in whole brain and separately in brain stem, cerebellum, and cerebrum. The protein/DNA ratio affords an estimate of the size and complexity of cells, and the ratio shows sharp rises at the stages just mentioned, as well as during the first postnatal stage at about 3–10 months. These parallels were already obtainable from the earlier but much less abundant data of Winick (1968), who found a rough tripling of the protein/DNA ratio between about 17 and 21 weeks after conception, as well as a very appreciable increase starting at about 3–4 months after birth.

Winick also measured RNA in his study, and the RNA/DNA ratio affords an estimate of the level of biosynthetic activity in general. This ratio doubles between 17 and 21 weeks, paralleling the protein/DNA ration. But, instead of staying up at the new level (RNA/DNA = 1.3), it drops sharply back down to about .7 by about 26 weeks. On the other hand, the protein/DNA ratio remains at its higher level, which is as expected of a parameter that reflects amounts rather than activities. These two measurements permit us to infer that the level of biosynthetic activity actually drops, which is evidence for an effective regulation of activity. The RNA/DNA ratio stays at the lower level until a sharp rise appears starting at about the postnatal age 2.5 months, shortly before the rise in protein/DNA, and reaches a plateau at about 10–12 months.

The biophysically-based electroencephalogram (EEG) also provides evidence of the stagewise development of the brain. Petersen and co-workers (Matousek & Petersen, 1973; Hagne, Persson, Magnueson & Petersen, 1973) studied EEG developmentally from birth to age 20 years. John (1977) transformed the Petersen group's data into energy form (they were originally given as amplitudes), so that it is possible to compute the energy associated with each of the standard frequency ranges of the EEG. It turns out that the fraction of the total EEG energy that appears in the alpha frequency range increases from about 8% at age

1 year to about 70% in the adult. This major shift in energy distribution occurs in stages as shown in Figure VI.6, which gives the biennial increments in alpha frequency energy as a function of age. There are four alpha energy growth stages at precisely the ages of the brain weight growth stages. Thus, without knowing the meaning of the alpha, it is possible to know that extremely sharp and significant brain network changes are occurring at specific ages. In addition, the Petersen group's study of EEG changes during the first year of life reveals a substantial spurt in higher frequency components covering the middle of the first year, just as would be expected for concordance with the first postnatal brain growth stage. Thus, all postnatal brain growth stages are signalled by very marked changes in the EEG.

The EEG changes found in the cat (Meier & Peeler, 1960) correlate well with the tentative stages of brain growth given earlier based on brain weight growth spurts. Brain growth stages also correlate in ages with changes in a number of other electrical aspects of rodent brain functioning: (a) Development of steady electric potential (Sobotka, Seminovsky, & Springler, 1968); (b) visual evoked potential (Rose, 1968; (c) Auditory evoked potential (Hassamanova, Rokyta, Zahlava, & Myslivecek, 1968); and (d) the results of electroshock (Millichap, 1957). In this volume, Fuller shows that the audiogenically primed convulsions of mice appear in the 17–23 day brain growth stage. Millichap also studied the guinea pig, and the absence of postnatal brain growth stages in that species correlates with the absence of postnatal functional stages in that species.

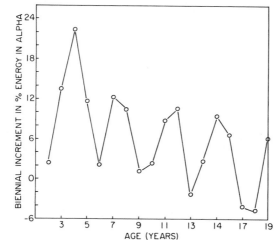

FIGURE VI.6. Biennial increment in the percentage of EEG energy found in the alpha frequency range. [Data from John, 1977.]

There is an enormous amount of data on many different aspects of rodent brain growth. We will give a partial listing of aspects that relate to the expectations based on the presumptive increase in neural network complexity, and which shows onsets, changes, and plateaus, which parallel in ages those already given for brain weight growth stages. These include aspects such as: oxygen utilization and death due to oxygen deprivation (Fazekas, Alexander, & Himwich, 1941): sodium channel appearance as measured by tetrodotoxin binding (Unsworth & Hafeman, 1975); axon density in sensorimotor cortex (Eayrs & Goodhead, 1959); granule and stellate cell replication (Altman, 1970); arborization of Purkinje cells (Berry & Bradley, 1976); cell migration and mitotic activity (Del Cerro & Snider, 1968); dendritic spine density in pyramidal cells of the visual cortex (Shapiro & Vukovich, 1970); myelination in many brain regions (Chase, Dorsey & McKann, 1967; Jacobson, 1963; Suzuki, 1965); acetylcholinesterase activity (Adlard & Dobbing, 1971); synapse number in molecular layer of parietal cortex (Aghajanian & Bloom, 1967); cell density and blood vessels in rat cerebral cortex (Caley & Maxwell, 1970); degeneration in ventrobasal complex after unilateral aspiration of somatosensory cortex (Matthews, Narayanan, Narayanan, & St. Onge 1977); a number of vesicle-containing profiles in lateral geniculate nucleus (Karlsson, 1967); and concentration of beta-adrenergic receptors (Harden, Wolfe, Sporn, Perkins, & Molinoff, 1977). Almost no data on topics similar to those just listed can be found for humans. One of the rare corresponding studies is by Sobotka and May (1977), who measured visual evoked potentials and reaction times in children, finding that in the parietal region there were sharp changes in reaction time and in latency of the first negative wave starting around age 11 years.

A final way in which we can look into age-related aspects of brain growth is to ask if perturbations of biophysical aspects of brain function bear any relationship in their effectiveness to the ages of the brain growth stages. An obvious perturbation seems to be the changes associated with epilepsy. It turns out (Gibbs & Gibbs, 1952) that there is no concordance in ages of appearance of grand mal or petit mal, but the onset of the petit mal variant is appreciably more likely at the onset of each of the brain growth stages. The formation of substantial numbers of new interconnections among neurons could well be associated with the creation of new connections aberrant enough to produce the known changes in brain waves and behavior.

There are still other possible perturbations of brain growth that could be the consequences of malnutrition, oxygen deprivation, etc., and that could occur at various ages. As far as I have been able to determine, other than the undernutrition studies already cited, there have not been age-limited human catastrophes that have yielded interpretable results related to this question. However, it is possible to create such catastrophes in experimental animals, and some of these kinds of experimental results were listed before as revealing correlations with brain growth stages.

Regionalization of Brain Growth Stages

The studies of Yakovlev (1962) give indications of the kinds of regionalization that can be detected. His study of progressive myelination during the first postnatal year of humans in five areas of the cerebral cortex shows the major change between 3 and 12 months is in the inferior parietal lobule. In agreement with the well known Flechsig picture of primary, secondary and tertiary stages of myelination of various areas that are parallel to their increasingly complex functions, this area is one of the last to myelinate. There are hints of an evolutionary devlopment that drops the slope of the Sylvian fissure from being somewhat more vertical in monkeys to being more nearly horizontal in humans. The later growth and myelination of the region at the end of the fissure are in correspondence with this inference. This is the region which Geschwind (1968) has characterized as being "the association area of association areas," on the basis of its anatomical connections and its location. A ready hypothesis is that the cross-modal connections permit cross-modal analysis to be located importantly in the inferior parietal lobule. The functional data relating to this proposition will be discussed later.

The data of Dobbing and Sands (1973) show clearly that the cerebellum has its major and virtually its final growth during the first postnatal year. This covers the 3–10 month brain growth stage. The data of Winick, Rosso, and Waterlow (1970) show an approximately threefold increase in cerebellar DNA compared to cerebral DNA during the first postnatal year. Paralleling the rapid replication of cells in the cerebellum is a tripling of the protein/DNA ratio in the cerebrum, bespeaking a striking increase in size and complexity of those cells.

At this point, it might be useful to return to the EEG results presented earlier to point out that the data in Figure VI.6 are for the P-O (parietal-occipital) electrodes. An entirely similar set of data is obtained for the T-T (temporal) electrodes, but not for electrodes over the frontal and central regions. Thus, the stages depicted in the figure are for a region which may be described as P-O-T, which corresponds reasonably to the inferior parietal lobule. There seems to be a general concordance of growth stages in all cortical areas through about age 7 or 8 years, after which only P-O-T peaks agree well with the brain growth stages. The later peaks of the other regions are thus at ages of virtually no brain growth, so they would seem to be related to maturation of earlier brain growth rather than to the appearance of significant new brain growth. The correlation of the development of the inferior parietal lobule EEG with brain growth stages suggests a relationship between the new cognitive competencies and the development and functions of that special region. This will be discussed subsequently.

The Functional Significance of the Brain Growth Stages

The evidence for functionally-related brain growth stages includes the implication that their major anatomical expression is in the very much increased complexity of neural networks, due to increased elongation and branching of axons and dendrites. Of the three main brain functions (cognitive, sensory, and emotional), the sensory functions have already been indicated as developing rapidly and rather exclusively at the time of the second postnatal human brain growth stage. We now turn to other functions to see if there is evidence for or against the proposition that they, too, show stagewise growth and growth stages correlated with those of the brain.

It needs no emphasis from me that measures of intelligence or of learning capacity are at best rough estimates of not-yet-well-defined properties of human beings. Yet, properties such as mental age and general intelligence factors have been used so extensively that we know rather more about their developmental aspects than about what they represent. To the extent to which they are related to intelligent functioning, their developmental aspects will be relevant for us.

It turns out that mental age shows developmental stages at ages that agree, within experimental error, with those found for the brain. The first collection of such correlations is in an earlier report (Epstein, 1974b), and will not be recapitulated here. These correlated brain and mind growth stages *(phrenoblysis)* are but a particular instance of the functional differentiation discussed at the beginning of this report.

It is of greater use to note that the first four brain growth stages coincide with the classically given ages of onset of the four main stages of intelligence development found by Piaget and his associates (Piaget, 1969). I have discussed elsewhere (Epstein, 1978) the question of age-relatedness, versus stage-relatedness, of the Piagetian stages. What will be discussed here is the fact that the brain has five postnatal growth stages, and one of them (the fifth, 14–16 + years) has no Piagetian counterpart. Therefore, the identification of the brain growth stages with the Piagetian stages leads to a critical test of the phrenoblysis concept: A fifth Piagetian stage should be found, and it should have its onset in the 14–16 year period. Since that prediction was made, Arlin (1975) has given the first evidence for the existence of a fifth stage, and her more recent work has narrowed down its appearance to precisely the predicted period.

The concordance of the brain and Piagetian stages allows us to take over the entire body of results of 4 decades of work by the Piagetians to give detailed indications of what is happening functionally during those growth stages. This may permit a relatively detailed characterization and localization of those stages as follows. Consider the Piagetian stage of concrete operations. As we discover the main features of brain growth during the 6–8 year period, we thereby acquire an initial working hypothesis about the nature and location of those concrete operations. A similar statement can, of course, be made about the other growth periods. As a further check on our inferences, we can use a finding by Webb (1974), which is the counterpart of the Piagetian concept of decalage. When a new stage of intelligence appears, it is first manifest in rudimentary form, and then undergoes a maturation process which generally lasts a year or two. What Webb discovered was that the time for maturation of the new stage is inversely related to the IQ of the children. Maturation of the age 11 year stage took only a very few months in the 160 IQ children he studied, contrasted with the 1 or 2 years needed by average IQ children. The study of brain changes in high and average IQ children should serve as a sensitive check on the inferences drawn from the correlative data. This IQ-linked maturation difference could already be tested by searching out differences in EEG and blood flow, apart from any information available by chance in autopsy material.

Do brain growth stages manifest themselves in still other functional ways? A case can be made for using the phrenoblysis concept to explain the massive failure of Head Start programs to improve cognitive competence of children from deprived situations. Such programs have dealt with children very close to the 4–6 year age—a span of minimum brain growth. The few programs that started by age 2 years (Hunt, 1975) all produced large and lasting increases in IQ and in school performance. Of the thousands of programs using 4- to 6-year-old children, only that by Sprigle (Van De Riet & Resnick, 1973) seems to have produced lasting positive consequences. His strategies and tactics illuminate significant aspects of phrenoblysis beyond the scope of this discussion.

Another brain growth plateau on which we have done some analysis, as well as starting field work, is that between 12 and 14 years. This covers the middle school or junior high school, and the hypothesis being tested is that novel intellectual challenges are not readily accepted by those nongrowing brains. The apparent slow cognitive growth of such children is generally ascribed to biological and personal distractions associated with sexual maturation. I would not deny the existence of those distractions, but our work would indicate that, though the main problem is actually biological, it is located at the other end of the body.

The next set of questions bears on the possibility that the inferior parietal lobule is developmentally correlated with intelligence. I do not intend to minimize the involvement of the frontal lobes of higher primates and man. The emphasis on that lobule relates only to its correlation with a number of aspects of intelligence development that are common to humans and rodents.

Is there evidence that cross-sensory functioning has a stagewise nature? Birch and Belmont (1965) studied equivalence judgments of auditory and visual patterns, finding a spurt between ages 5.8 and 7.7 years, followed by a virtual plateau from 7.7 to 9.7 years, followed in turn by another substantial increase, the extent of which was not clear because the study included children only up to age 12 years.

Is there evidence that intelligent functioning (already shown to be correlated in a stagewise fashion with brain growth stages) has a degree of localization in the inferior parietal lobule? Two studies indicate the nature of the evidence on this question. Ingvar (1976) has measured blood flow in the brains of humans engaged in a variety of activities. For example, motor activities show an increased blood flow in motor regions of the brain. What is important for us is his study of reasoning. The only nonfrontal region showing increased blood flow is the region of the inferior parietal lobule, an increase that also shows up as part of the pattern found during talking.

The second study related to this point is that by Weinstein and Teuber (1957). They studied Korean War veterans who had survived penetrating brain wounds in other than frontal regions. These men were retested for IQ many years after they had been given their first such test on induction into the army as 18-year-olds. There was no effect of the injury on IQ unless the injury was in the inferior parietal lobule, in which case there was more than a 25-point difference between such men and those who had either sustained no injury or else had been injured in other parts of the nonfrontal brain. Only about one-half of those injured in this region were aphasic, so that barring subtle dysphasic situations, the intellectual deficits cannot be attributed only to language difficulties.

There is, then, evidence that cross-sensory functioning grows stagewise and in correlation with the phrenoblytic stages and that the presumptive locale of this functioning has a direct connection with intelligent functioning. Is there any evidence for the rather obvious proposition that cross-sensory functioning is related directly to intelligence? There is little direct study on this proposition, but two papers by Reitan and his group may be relevant. In the first study (Reitan, 1970) they compared two groups of minimally brain damaged children, one with and the other without impaired cross-sensory (sensorimotor) functions. Those showing impaired cross-sensory functioning also did much more poorly on such intelligence tests as the Wechsler-Bellvue, the Halstead and the Minnesota Multiphasic Personality Inventory. In another study, Finlayson and Reitan (1976) compared two groups of children on the basis of the number of errors made on tactile-perceptual tests. The poorly performing group made an average of 8–9 errors per test, while the better performing group made about .3 errors per test. This thirty-fold increase in error rate of the poorer group paralleled a decrease in average IQ of about 8 points. The authors considered the results as "further support for a relationship between sensorimotor impairment and higher-level cognitive functioning."

Two Examples of Brain–Behavior Stage Correlation in Animals

Animal data on the functional manifestations of brain development are exceedingly rare. For rodents this is because of the great difficulty in measuring behavior of animals whose eyes are not open until about 2 weeks after birth. One of the few developmental studies (for others see the article by Nagy in this volume) is that of Riccio and Schulenberg (1969) who measured the performance of rodents placed on an insulated disc sitting on an electrified table. One hundred-day-old animals learned in one trial to remain on the disc. Thirty-day-old animals also learned in one trial. Twenty-day-old animals learned in one to two trials, while ten-day-old animals learned in an average of five trials. But, fifteen-day-old animals never learned, stepping off the disc on an average of every fifty seconds. The ten- and twenty-day-old animals are in brain growth stages, while the fifteen-day-old animal is in the middle of a long plateau. Our interpretation would be that the latter animal is incapable of readily learning new behaviors.

The extensive monkey studies by the Harlow laboratory at Wisconsin have yielded data relevant to the brain–behavior correlation. In the top part of Figure VI.4 there are results summarized by Sackett (1968). Monkeys placed in total social isolation from birth to ages 3, 6 and 12 months, may be seen to exhibit increasingly serious damage to their eventual social competence, with only the 0–3 month animals being entirely rehabilitabable. It may also be seen that total social isolation from 6 to 12 months is hardly less devastating than is 0–6 months. Yet, isolation from 3 to 9 months has virtually no effect at all. It can be seen by comparison with the brain growth data in the bottom part of that figure that the 3–9 month animals are in a brain growth plateau, while the others all cover one or more growth stages entirely, except the 0–3 month animals, which have about another month to go before the end of the brain growth period during which they are isolated.

Summary

Evidence is presented that human brain weight and head circumference manifest growth stages at about 3–10 months, 2–4, 6–8, 10–12 +, and 14–16 + years. Since net DNA synthesis in the brain ceases around age 1½, the last four stages must be expressed mainly in elongation and branching of axons and dendrites, and in myelination of axons. Evidence for that expression is shown to occur in correlated stages of (a) energy needs, (b) synapse formation, (c) synthesis of synaptic enzymes, (d) neurotransmitter syntheses, and (e) changing functions of neural networks. Corresponding evidence is presented for the existence of a similar situation in rodents, along with indications of a perhaps similar situation in cats and monkeys.

Functional correlates of the stages are found in human mental age stages and in the Piagetian stages of intelligence development. Examples of what may be similar correlations in animals are also given.

Some evidence is presented indicating that the correlated human brain and mind growth stages have a primary localization in the anatomical and functional aspects of the inferior parietal lobule.

Acknowledgments

Many individuals gave generously of their time trying to make sure that I understood what I was trying to think about. For this I am especially grateful to Norman Geschwind, Thomas Kemper, Simeon Locke, Sanford Miller, and Alberto Monroy, who, of course, are not responsible for my failures to understand.

For access to monkey brain weight data I am indebted to W. McNulty of the Oregon Primate Research Center, K. Schiltz of the Wisconsin Primate Research Center, and R. Garcia of the New England Primate Research Center, as well as to my colleague, David Horr, who made those contacts.

References

Adlard, B. P. F., & Dobbing, J. Vulnerability of developing brain. III. Development of four enzymes in the brains of normal and undernourished rats. *Brain Research*, 1971, *28*, 97–107.

Aghajanian, G. K., & Bloom, F. E. The formation of synaptic junctions in developing rat brain: A quantitative electron microscopic study. *Brain Research*, 1967, *6*, 716–727.

Agrawal, H. C., Davis, J. M., & Himwich, W. A. Developmental changes in mouse brain: Weight, water content and free amino acids. *Journal of Neurochemistry*, 1968, *15*, 917–923.

Altman, J. Postnatal neurogenesis and the problem of neural plasticity. In W. A. Himwich (Ed.), *Developmental neurobiology*. Springfield, Ill.: C. C. Thomas, 1970. Pp. 197–237.

Arlin, P. K. Cognitive development in adulthood: A fifth stage? *Developmental Psychology*, 1975, *11*, 602–606.

Berry, M., & Bradley, P. The growth of the dendritic trees of Purkinje cells in the cerebellum of the rat. *Brain Research*, 1976, *112*, 1–35.

Birch, H. G., & Belmont, L. Auditory-visual integration, intelligence and reading ability in school children. *Perceptual and Motor Skills*, 1965, *20*, 295–305.

Blinkov, S. M., & Glezer, I. I. *The human brain in figures and tables*. New York: Basic Books, 1968.

Burns, J., Birkbeck, J. A., & Roberts, D. F. Early fetal brain growth. *Human Biology*, 1975, *47*, 511–522.

Caley, D. W., & Maxwell, D. S. Development of the blood vessels and extracellular spaces during postnatal maturation of rat cerebral cortex. *Journal of Comparative Neurology*, 1970, *138*, 31–48.

Chase, H. P., Dorsey, J., & McKhan, G. M. The effect of malnutrition on the synthesis of a myelin lipid. *Pediatrics*, 1967, *40*, 551–559.

Clatworthy, H. W., & Anderson, R. G. Development and growth of the human embryo and fetus. *American Journal of Diseases of Children*, 1944, *67*, 167–175.

Cooke, R. W. I., Lucas, A., Yudkin, P. L. N., & Pryse-Davies, J. Head circumference as an index of brain weight the fetus and newborn. *Early Human Development*, 1977, *1(2)*, 145–149.

Coppoletta, J. M., & Wolbach, S. B. Body lengths and organ weights of infants and children. *American Journal of Pathology*, 1933, *9*, 55–70.

Count, E. W. Brain and body weight in man: Their antecedents in growth and evolution. *Annals of the New York Academy of Science*, 1947, *46*, 993–1122.

Del Cerro, M. P., & Snider, R. S. Studies on the developing cerebellum. *Journal of Comparative Neurology*, 1968, *133*, 341–362.

Dobbing, J., & Sands, J. Timing of neuroblast multiplication in developing human brain. *Nature*, 1970, *226*, 639–640.

Dobbing, J., & Sands, J. Quantitative growth and development of human brain. *Archives of Diseases in Childhood*, 1973, *48*, 757–767.

Dutton, R. W., Flakow, R., Hirst, J. A., Hoffman, M., Kappler, J. W., Kettman, J. R., & Vann, D. Is there evidence for a non-antigen specific diffusible chemical mediator from thymus-derived cell in the initiation of the immune response? In B. Amos (Ed.), *Progress in Immunology*. New York: Academic Press, 1971. Pp. 355–368.

Eayrs, J. T., & Goodhead, B. Postnatal development of the cerebral cortex in the rat. *Journal of Anatomy*, 1959, *92*, 385–402.

Eichorn, D., & Bayley, N. Growth in head circumference from birth through early adulthood. *Child Development*, 1962, *33*, 257–271.

Epstein, H. T. Phrenoblysis: Special brain and mind growth periods. I. Human brain and skull development. *Development Psychobiology*, 1974, *7*, 207–216.(a)

Epstein, H. T. Phrenoblysis: Special brain and mind growth periods. II. Human mental development. *Developmental Psychobiology*, 1974, *7*, 217–224.(b)

Epstein, H. T. Growth spurts during brain development: Implications for educational policy and practice. In J. S. Chall & A. F. Mirsky (Eds.), *Education and the Brain*. (Yearbook of the N.S.S.E.). Chicago: University of Chicago Press, 1978. Pp. 343–370.

Epstein, H. T., & Epstein, E. B. The relationship between brain weight and head circumference from birth to age 18 years. *American Journal of Physical Anthropology*, 1978, *48*, 471–474.

Epstein, H. T., & Miller, S. A. The developing brain: A suggestion for making more critical interspecies extrapolation. *Nutrition Reports International*, 1977, *16*, 363–366.

Fazekas, J. F., Alexander, F. A. D., & Himwich, H. E. Tolerance of the new born to anoxia. *American Journal of Physiology*, 1941, *134*, 281–287.

Finlayson, M. A. J., & Reitan, R. Tactile-perceptual functioning in relation to intellectual, cognitive and reading skills in younger and older normal children. *Developmental Medicine and Child Neurology*, 1976, *18*, 442–446.

Geschwind, N. Disconnection syndromes in animals and man. *Brain*, 1968, *88*, 237–294; 585–644.

Gibbs, F. A., & Gibbs, E. L. *Atlas of electroencephalography*, Vol. 2, Epilepsy. Reading, Mass.: Addison Wesley Press, 1952.

Gottlieb, A., Keydar, I., & Epstein, H. T. Rodent brain growth stages: An analytical review. *Biology of the Neonate*, 1977, *32*, 166–176.

Hagne, I., Persson, J., Magnusson, R., & Petersen, I. Spectral analysis via fast Fourier transform of waking EEG in normal infants. In P. Kellaway & I. Petersen (Eds.), *Automation of clinical electroencephalography*. New York: Raven Press, 1973. Pp. 103–109.

Harden, T. K., Wolfe, B. B., Sporn, J. R., Perkins, J. R., & Molinoff, P. B. Ontogeny of beta-adrenergic receptors in rat cerebral cortex. *Brain Research*, 1977, *125*, 99–108.

Hassmannova, J., Rokyta, R., Zahlava, J., & Myslivecek, J. Intercentral relationships in the auditory system during ontogeny. In *Ontogenesis of the Brain*. Prague: Charles University Press, 1968. Pp. 319–326.

Horr, David E., & Epstein, H. T. Manuscript in preparation.

Hunt, J. M. Reflections on a decade of early education. *Journal of Abnormal Child Psychology*, 1975, *3*, 275–336.

Ingvar, D. H. Functional landscapes of the dominant hemisphere. *Brain Research*, 1976, *107*, 181–197.

Jacobson, S. Sequence of myelinization in the brain of the albino rat. *Journal of Comparative Neurology*, 1963, *121*, 5–29.

John, E. R. *Functional neuroscience* Vol. 2. Hillsdale, N.J.: Lawrence Erlbaum Associates, 1977.

Karlsson, U. Observations on the postnatal development of neuronal structures in the lateral geniculate nucleus of the rat by electron microscopy. *Journal of Ultrastructure Research*, 1967, *17*, 158–175.

Matousek, M., & Petersen, I. Frequency analysis of the EEG in normal children and adolescents. In P. Kellaway & I. Petersen (Eds.), *Automation of clinical electroencephalography*. New York: Raven Press, 1973. Pp. 75–102.

Matthews, M., Narayanan, C. H., Narayanan, Y. & St. Onge, M. Neuronal maturation and synaptogenesis in the rat ventrobasal complex: Alignment with developmental changes in rate and severity of axon reaction. *Journal of Comparative Neurology*, 1977, *173*, 745–772.

Meier, G.W., & Peeler, Jr., D. F. Development of behavioral and electroencephalographic patterns in the kitten. *Psychological Reports*, 1960, *6*, 307–314.

Millichap, J. G. Development of seizure patterns in newborn animals. Significance of brain carbonic anhydrase. *Proceedings of the Society for Experimental Biology and Medicine*, 1957, *96*, 125–129.

Nellhaus, G. Personal Communication. 1975.

Piaget, J. *Psychology of intelligence*. New Jersey: Littlefield, Adams, 1969.

Reitan, R. M. Sensorimotor functions, intelligence and cognition, emotional status in subjects with cerebral lesions. *Perceptual and Motor Skills*, 1970, *31*, 275–284.

Riccio, D. C., & Schulenberg, C. J. Age-related deficits in acquisition of a passive avoidance response. *Canadian Journal of Psychology*, 1969, *23*, 429–437.

Rose, G. H., The comparative ontogenesis of visually evoked responses in rat and cat. *Ontogenesis of the brain*. Prague: Charles University Press, 1968 Pp. 347–358.

Rosso, P., Hormazabal, J., & Winick, M. Changes in brain weight, cholesterol, phospholipid and DNA content in marasmic children. *American Journal of Clinical Nutrition*, 1970, *23*, 1275–1279.

Sackett, G. P. Abnormal behavior in laboratory-reared rhesus monkeys. In M. W. Fox (Ed.), *Abnormal behavior in animals*. Philadelphia: W. B. Saunders, 1968. Pp. 293–331.

Shapiro, S., & Vukovich, K. Early experience effects upon cortical dendrites: a proposed model for development. *Science*, 1970, *167*, 292–294.

Sobotka, K. R., & May, J. G. Visual evoked potentials and reaction time in normal and dyslexic children. *Psychophysiology*, 1977, *14*, 18–24.

Sobotka, P., Semiginovsky, B., & Springler, V. Correlations of some biochemical and electrical properties in the developing brain. In *Ontogenesis of the brain*. Prague: Charles University Press, 1968. Pp. 299–302.

Suzuki, K. The pattern of mammalian brain gangliosides. III. Regional and developmental differences. *Journal of Neurochemistry*, 1965, *12*, 969–979.

Unsworth, B. R., & Hafeman, D. R. Tetrodotoxin binding as a marker for functional differentiation of various brain regions during chick and mouse development. *Journal of Neurochemistry*, 1975, *24*, 261–270.

Van De Riet, V., & Resnick, M. B. *Learning to learn*. Gainsville: University of Florida, 1973.

Webb, R. A. Concrete and formal operations in very bright six to eleven year olds. *Human Development*, 1974, *17*, 292–300.

Weinstein, S., & Teuber, H. L. Effects of penetrating brain injury on intelligence test scores. *Science*, 1957, *125*, 1036–1037.

Wiesel, T. N., & Hubel, D. H. Comparison of the effects of unilateral and bilateral eye closure on cortical unit responses in kittens. *Journal of Neurophysiology* (London), 1965, *28*, 1029–1040.

Winick, M. Changes in nucleic acid and protein content of the human brain during growth. *Pediatric Research*, 1968, *2*, 352–355.

Winick, M., & Rosso, P. Head circumference and cellular growth of the brain in normal and marasmic children. *Journal of Pediatrics*, 1969, *74*, 774–778.

Winick, M., Rosso, P., & Waterlow, J. Cellular growth of cerebrum, cerebellum and brain stem in normal and marasmic children. *Experimental Neurology*, 1970, *26*, 393–400.

Yakovlev, P. I. Morphological criteria of growth and maturation of the nervous system in man. *Mental Retardation*, 1962, *39*, 3–46.

Chapter VII

Genetic Techniques as Tools for Analysis of Brain—Behavior Relationships

THOMAS H. RODERICK

Rationale for Using Genetic Techniques

The term "analysis" implies a search for and understanding of caus-ative pathways. This discussion will be confined to paths in the direction of brain-to-behavior, although analyses of causes in the opposite direc-tion are proving most worthwhile (Rosenzweig, this volume). I shall, for the most part, be considering normal variation in the brain and normal variation in behavior in contrast to gross anomalies of the brain and behavior where relationships are more obvious.

There are many characteristics of the brain and its components which intrigue us as to their influences on behavior. These include differences in size, relative size, patterns, microanatomy, biochemistry, develop-ment, and other attributes. If sufficient or consistent differences between animals exist for any of these traits, then there is a possibility of finding behavioral differences as correlates. A major problem then is to find large obvious differences, or possibly small differences, where the ex-perimental design permits an analysis.

Consider the dilemma of the investigator in Figure VII.1. It is his problem to determine how to find these differences in the brain so that the black box between brain and behavior can be explored. One way of producing observable differences in the brain is to manipulate the genes that produce differences in brain characteristics. Genetic manip-

133

DEVELOPMENT AND EVOLUTION
OF BRAIN SIZE

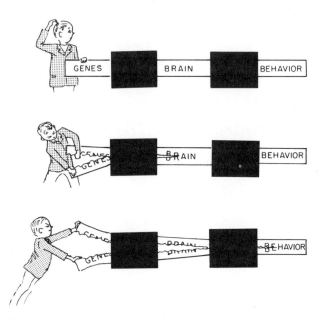

FIGURE VII.1. Genetic manipulation used as a tool to bring out differences in characteristics of the brain for studies of behavior correlates.

ulation by the experimenter can be of two main kinds. He can manipulate the genes in such a way to exaggerate the characteristics of the brain, for example as is done when selection is applied to a brain trait. Or he can take the given manipulation of genes, for example such as the development of independent inbred strains has provided, producing less obvious differences in brain characteristics, but producing them in a consistent and repeatable manner so that analyses of smaller differences in brain and behavior are feasible. Each of the genetic techniques available to the investigator is a means of controlling genetic variation in a prescribed way.

The nature of the relationship between genes and behavior could be simple in that one or perhaps two genes might cause great variability in a brain character. Or it might be complex in that the variation of a brain trait is under the influence of many genes. It does not necessarily matter for the investigator's purposes what the nature is of the black box between genes and brain, as long as the manipulation produces the desired differences in the brain. Genetic manipulation in this sense is a tool only, although it is the ultimate dream of many to understand more about the various pathways between genes and the brain.

The Genetic Tools

Selection

   Brains and behaviors have both evolved in time. One of the major interests of individuals in this volume is whether relationships between particular brain characteristics and certain attributes or behaviors can be elucidated by interspecies comparisons. An approach to the study of these associations is the use of artificial selection applied to laboratory mammals over a few generations, in an attempt to simulate eons of evolutionary changes. The fact that selection is applied over a very brief period without time for other genetic adjustments, which long term natural selection provides, is probably a major reason why artificial selection does not truly simulate natural selection. Furthermore, the associations between brain and behaviors that interspecies comparisons reveal do not necessarily tell us what traits have been selected. Clearly brain size in primate evolution, for example, was not the selected trait per se, although we are greatly interested in this trait and its associations with behavior. Thus, since different processess have taken place, we should not be surprised if interspecies associations between traits are not necessarily the same as the associations found within species between individuals.

   During the course of selection experiments, there are usually obvious changes in traits other than the selected trait. These correlated responses or correlated traits have long intrigued animal and plant breeders, particularly the responses having to do with viability and reproductive performance (Lerner & Donald, 1966). In the selection experiments concerning the brain, our search will be for correlated responses that are relevant to brain–behavior relationships. We should expect to find correlated responses in fitness traits, as well as a whole host of rather "uninteresting" traits from our viewpoint.

   Nevertheless, artificial selection as a tool can tell us some things about genetic associations between traits within species. Figure VII.2 shows four different possible interpretations of associations produced by selection. Model number one represents the common conception of the relationship between a selected trait and a correlated trait. In this case the selected trait itself is in the direct causative pathway of the correlated trait and is the main influence itself on the correlated trait. Such a simplistic model might be assumed for a study of selection for a brain characteristic and the correlated responses in behavior. Model number two may simplistically represent selection where one is using a behavioral trait as the selected trait and examining correlated responses in brain traits as potential intermediary mechanisms in producing behav-

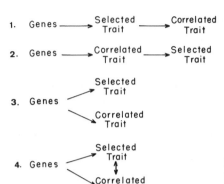

FIGURE VII.2. These four models describe the causative relationships between a selected trait and a correlated trait.

ioral differences. In both models one and two, the traits are directly conjoined, lying in a common causative pathway. Model number three, on the other hand, describes a situation where a correlated trait occurs not because it is in anyway directly causing or caused by the selected trait, but is altered through an independent causative pathway by the genes or a portion of them that cause the variation in the selected trait. We have called model number three an example of indirectly conjoined traits, not to burden us with more jargon, but rather to better depict the essence of the model (Roderick, Wimer, & Wimer, 1976). This model describes the commonly held view of the mechanism of pleiotropy, although actually all four models could represent pleiotropic effects. Model number four is a combination of the three previous models, all more of less playing a role simultaneously. Probably this complex model describes the majority of causative relationships when we use selection or other genetic techniques.

Selection has one major advantage. In selection experiments it is not uncommon for the response to equal between 10 and 20 times the phenotypic standard deviation of the foundation population (Falconer, 1960). Selection is therefore a means of greatly exaggerating a trait with the possible consequence of providing insight into traits otherwise only subtly associated. Selection is therefore a good initial step to providing clues to causative pathways, and it is a device to see how severely a particular phenotype can be altered and still be compatible with life. It thus is a way to test hypotheses of causative relationships as well as to generate new hypotheses by seeing what happens.

Selection may be a better instrument for determining what traits are *not* in the causative pathway of the selected trait, for if a suspected correlated trait does not respond appropriately at any time during selection, then that trait is probably of little if any importance in the mechanisms of variation of the selected trait.

There are several objections to using information on correlated traits to elucidate mechanisms of causation. One usually held assumption is that genetic correlations are valid throughout the range of phenotypic variation. But this may not necessarily be so. To move the phenotype of a population far from the norm is to make those individuals bizarre outwardly and probably to make them anatomically, physiologically, and biochemically bizarre as well. Other traits that must be altered to accommodate these bizarre attributes might not be traits necessarily important to the selected trait within one or two phenotypic standard deviations of the norm. So correlated traits may be qualitatively different, depending on the distance from the phenotypic mean.

Another problem is inferring the nature or extent of a biological association between traits, based on the results of one selected high line and one selected low line. Genetic drift of a nonselected trait may produce a spurious association, particularly when the breeding population is small, as is the case in almost all selection experiments in the laboratory. Even if a correlated response is due to common genetic variation for the two traits, one must be cautious in generalizing from the response of only two lines. If the correlated response is based on only a very few genes, then the association found after selection will depend on whether genetic variation exists at those loci in the particular foundation population. Also close linkage of a few genes controlling the selected trait and correlated trait could produce a correlated response of no interest in our search for causative relationships.

The same problems hold for two selected lines and a control line. Far better for generalizing are two sets of high, low, and control lines, with each set derived from a genetically independent foundation population. Genetic independence in practical terms means a population derived from sets of strains, each of which was derived independently from feral populations from different geographical locations. Genetically independent inbred strains are known and are available (Roderick, Ruddle, Chapman, & Shows, 1971). This design using two sets of lines is feasible for rodent selection experiments in most laboratories. It provides simultaneous replication with an attempt to control for genetic differences in base populations.

A control line is used to represent a nonselected population and to control for effects of inbreeding depression if it is propagated in the same way as are the selected lines. Two independent control lines should be included in any case if there is significant interest in asymmetry of response between high and low lines. One could be misled by the response of a single control line because it can, as any small closed population, be affected by genetic drift for many traits, including the selected trait.

One could make an inference about the genetic association of a correlated trait if that trait changed consistently across generations with the responses of the selected trait. The trouble with this approach is that, although we may have some idea at the outset what correlated responses may be of interest, we are often asking selection to tell us what associations may be important. We may discover the interesting associations only after the selected trait has diverged significantly, and the animals of the earlier generations are long gone. One possible solution is to freeze representative embryos of the foundation stocks and of each of the ensuing generations. The embryos from all the lines and all generations could be thawed at a specific time and samples of animals of all generations could be examined for the selected trait and any potential correlated traits, not only to verify the concomitant response of the correlated traits with the selected trait, but also to observe all traits without the consequences of between-generation environmental effects. Reliable techniques for freezing embryos are now used in many laboratories (Lyon, Whittingham, & Glenister, 1977). Superovulation in a female will provide about 25 eggs, which can be fertilized in the natural fashion. Embryos are collected about 3 days after mating. Using certain cryoprotective agents, the embryos are cooled at a rate of .6° centigrade (C) per minute down to $-80°C$, and then transferred to liquid nitrogen. They can be stored apparently indefinitely in that condition. When thawed, they are cultured for 24 hours and transferred to pseudopregnant females. About 50% of the embryos survive the freezing and thawing, and about another 50% survive the transfer and development in a foster mother, so a total yield of viable offspring is approximately 25% of those embryos originally frozen. The extent of our belief in recovery of animals from the frozen embryo state is evidenced by the fact that some experimentally important strains and stocks of mice now exist *only* in the frozen state.

One can go further and verify the importance of a correlated response by crossing the high and low lines and examining individuals in the F_2 for both traits. Similarly, such verification could be done in a replication of the foundation population or better, in a genetically independent and genetically heterogeneous population (Roderick *et al.*, 1976; Wimer, Wimer, & Roderick, 1969). Here the differences between individuals in the selected and correlated traits will not be as great as between the high and low selected lines, but in an analysis of a genetically heterogeneous population each individual will be the statistical equivalent of a single selected line. Thus smaller differences and smaller genetic associations should be borne out if they are real.

If a correlated response occurs in the selected lines from one base population and not in the lines from the other, one might wish to explore the reasons for the difference. Such an outcome might imply that a very few genes are involved in the correlated response, and thus there would be an opportunity to locate those genes and study them further. In addition to using an F_2 from the cross of the high and low lines, there may be a need to replicate the foundation population. If a foundation population is the F_2 from two inbred strains, then the genetic distribution of the F_2 can essentially be reconstituted because all of the individuals of the F_1 are genetically identical and thus repeatable. The same holds for a foundation population based on the third generation of systematic crosses of four inbred strains (see Roderick *et al.*, 1976 for examples of these breeding schemes). Here, even though the two F_1 populations are genetically different, they contain genetically identical individuals respectively and are thus repeatable respectively. A cross of repeatable but different genotypes will provide an opportunity to repeat the genetic distribution of the foundation population. An eight way cross (see Roderick *et al.*, 1976) is valuable in providing enormous genetic variability in the foundation population and in turn providing a better opportunity for a response to selection. But the genetic distribution of this population cannot be replicated, because each of the parents of this generation is genetically unique. If one were to anticipate the need to replicate an eight way cross, one could freeze embryos from later litters of the same parents of the foundation population.

Our experiments in selection for brain weight and other neuroanatomical traits were recently reviewed (Roderick *et al.*, 1976; Wimer, this volume). The lines are now being maintained without selection and are being further characterized for alleles at "isozyme" loci, which can be detected electrophoretically. This is an attempt to ascertain any correlated response in specific alleles, which might suggest close linkage with a major gene in determining brain weight. Further characterization of brain weights of these lines in the absence of selection should be interesting but will probably not help to shed further light on the behavioral implications. One correlated response, body weight, deserves mention. Although the results are preliminary, it appears that the correlated response in the body weight under selection for brain weight, was greater than had we selected for body weight per se. Such a result is theoretically possible when the selected trait has a very high heritability (in this case about .70), the correlated trait has a low heritability (about .25), and there exists a very high genetic correlation between the traits, that is, genes for the selected trait play a major role in the control of the variation of the correlated trait.

The response in visual impairment also deserves mention. Part way through our initial selection experiment for brain weight, we found that animals from both low lines could not learn a simple maze task that depended on visual cues. One hypothesis for this finding was that animals with low brain weight were incapable of this particular task. This simplistic hypothesis was disrupted by the fact that one of the high lines and the control lines also had animals that behaved as if they could not learn the task. Fortunately at this same time, the recessive gene retinal degeneration (rd) was discovered in many of the commonly used inbred strains of mice (Sidman & Green, 1965). Three of the eight strains making up our foundation population were rd, so we could expect about three-eighths of our lines to be fixed for rd sooner or later, if no selection were applied to visual acuity or any other trait affected by rd. We found that all the inability to learn our visual task could be explained by the degenerate retinas of mice. Thus the correlation of maze learning and brain weight was in this case spurious, although we considered the possibility that one way to reduce brain size could be to reduce visual sensation. The concept was that any genes reducing visual sensory input might be selected for as an intermediate trait leading to lowered brain weight (an example of model number two).

Inbred Strains

An inbred strain, to those dealing with mice and rats, is a strain which has reached 20 generations or its equivalent of brother–sister matings. This amount of inbreeding theoretically eliminates over 99% of the heterozygosity which was present at the outset, that is, the animals in the strain have an inbreeding coefficient exceeding .99. Genetic characterization of animals within these strains, particularly at histocompatibility and isozyme loci, has shown that in reality these animals are indeed homozygous at all identifiable loci and are as alike as identical twins except for the necessary sex dimorphism. Furthermore, although subline differentiation does occur after 20 generations or more of inbreeding, it does so at very low rates, implying genetic constancy of an inbred line over many generations (Bailey, 1978; Roderick, 1978). The important point is that variation within an inbred strain can be ascribed nearly totally to environmental causes and variation between inbred strains to both environmental and genetic causes. Inbred strains offer an enormous advantage for behavior testing in that animals of the same genotype can be exposed to various treatments where naivety of the treatments is important. The same advantage holds for any two tests where, because of practical procedures, one animal cannot be tested, examined, or characterized for all pertinent tests. Each strain then represents the genotype of an individual, and strain comparisons can be used to study associations between brain and behavioral traits. One might object to the fact that these animals, because of their complete homozygosity, are themselves bizarre genotypes upon which we should not generalize. My experience has been that this is not so generally, but the problem can be overcome by similar comparisons between a set of F_1 hybrids.

Again it is important to choose strains that are genetically independent, that is, which have their origins in different feral populations, if that can be ascertained. Our experience suggests that many of the commonly used laboratory strains of mice have a somewhat similar origin, probably in western Europe. One piece of evidence is the high frequency of *rd* already mentioned, a gene one would not expect to be advantageous in nature, and we have not found it in feral populations we have examined. So the presence of *rd* implies at least some common genetic heritage of the strains possessing it. It is also possible that the high frequency of *rd* in long established inbred strains represents not common ancestry, but rather selection for mutations that reduce sensitivity in a laboratory environment. Tameness is a strongly selected trait in the animal room, mostly because nontame animals escape. Any gene which can produce greater tameness perhaps through greater insensitivity may be advantageous in the laboratory. This long-term adaptibility to laboratory environments may be another good reason for considering newly developed inbred strains.

It is therefore important to consider new strains of mice, for example SK/Cam from the island of Skokholm off Wales, SF/Cam from San Francisco, IS/Cam from Israel, and a strain now nearly completely inbred from Peru. There are also strains now inbred from interfertile subspecies of the laboratory mouse, that is, *Mus musculus castaneus* and *Mus musculus molossinus*. One should also include those inbred strains that are characterized by unique alleles at one or more isozyme loci, because uniqueness suggests at least a unique segment of the genome and possibly independence of origin (Roderick *et al.*, 1971).

In two studies we used several different inbred strains of mice to examine brain characteristics (Roderick *et al.*, 1973, Wimer *et al.*, 1969). In the latter study the *molossinus* stock was examined along with 25 other inbred strains commonly available. *Molossinus* as a stock and now a strain had the lowest brain weight (14% below the next lowest), the lowest spinal cord weight (26% below the next lowest), and the highest ratio of brain to spinal cord weight (5% above the next highest). The stock also differs from laboratory strains in several behavioral traits, according to an unpublished study by Karen Winteringham. This strain, originally trapped in Japan, has a normal karyotype and is fully interfertile with laboratory strains. Obviously it is an example of the importance of new strains for study of genetic variation of brain and behavior.

Sublines of Inbred Strains

Sublines of fully inbred lines are being maintained in several laboratories. Basically they are a nuisance, because one can presume the allelic characterization of one will represent the other, but one can never be certain. But sublines do have one advantage; if mutational differences do appear between them, then mutation and its effects can be studied alone without the complication of other genetic background variability. If such a gene were to cause an effect in the brain, it would offer an opportunity to study its physiological and developmental effects. If its linkage could be determined it would afford an opportunity for tracking carriers with closely linked markers. So-called sublines exist not only for inbred strains, but for strains which were bifurcated before 20 generations of inbreeding (Bailey, 1978). In these cases one could still make possible use of the few genes that might differentiate two sublines because of residual heterozygosity at the time of separation. The general concept is that if sublines differ with respect to a particular trait, then one can presume the difference is due to relatively few genes.

Recombinant Inbred Lines

Recombinant inbred lines are separate lines inbred brother–sister from an F_2 of genetically independent inbred strains (Figure VII.3). Inbreeding proceeds quickly enough to freeze large segments of genes together in homozygous state before they can recombine. The resulting lines then provide an opportunity to study linkage relationships between any genes that have allelic differences between the original parental inbred lines. Since polymorphisms are very common and are being described at a great rate, the development and use of recombinant inbred (RI) lines has blossomed. A further, most important advantage of such lines is that preliminary estimates can be made on the number of genes controlling the variation of quantitative traits. The approach is to determine how many of the RI lines of a single set represent single quantum classes of the phenotype. If all fall into two classes, for example, one might assume only one gene is having a major effect on the phenotype. This may be important to the study of brain variation, as well as behavior variation and their relationships. Bailey (1971) and Taylor (1980) provide further discussion of the advantages, uses, and availability of RI lines.

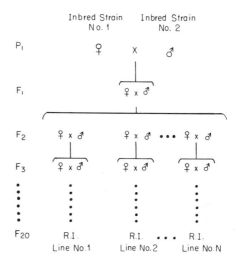

FIGURE VII.3. The mating scheme that produces recombinant inbred (R. I.) lines.

Inversions

Newly developed techniques have permitted the rapid induction and description of paracentric inversions in mice (Roderick & Hawes, 1974). Now over 30 of them are available and distributed among the chromosomes of the mouse. Those about 40 cM in length or less do not permit double crossing over. Thus, any linkage of specific genes within the inverted segment will remain linked indefinitely. We have induced most of these inversions on a specific inbred strain (DBA/2J) and are placing many of them on another strain background (C57BL/6J). After several generations of backcrossing, these lines are essentially congenic lines where the only genetic differences that exist between the inversion carriers and the host line occur within the inverted segment. The inversions are easily mapped because of the many markers available in the mouse (Davisson & Roderick, 1979), and thus the specific area of genes that might have effects on brain or behavior could be defined. If particular segments of chromosome are found to be important in behavioral or brain variation, overlapping inversions studied independently may help to define more precise map locations of important genes.

Mutations

Mutations exist for both the rat and the mouse affecting neuromuscular, brain, and behavioral functions. They are best known in the mouse (Green, 1980) and have been utilized effectively, for example by R. L.

Sidman and his colleagues, in studying the development of brain. These mutants produce a variety of behavioral effects that can be traced to a specific portion of the brain. Up to this point, we have made the distinction between normal brain and behavioral variation, and abnormal brain and behavioral variation, the latter class manifested by these single gene mutants with gross effects. Probably the distinction of variation is good, but there is considerable gray area in between them (pun intended). Thus, this vast mutational resource should be examined for its possible use in conjunction with studies of normal variation.

Mosaics

Finally, mention must be made of an exciting use of genetic mosaics of the mouse to elucidate the cellular or organismal origins of various behaviors (Nesbitt, Butler, & Spence, 1979). Mouse chimeras can be produced by fusing early embryos followed by implantation and normal uterine development. Strains A/J and C57BL/6J differ in many developmental and behavioral traits. Among these, of interest to Nesbitt and her colleagues, were activity, alcohol preference, cricket killing, and rope climbing, which differ dramatically between the strains. Chimeras from the fusion of embryos of both strains will contain aggregates and clones of both genotypes. But each chimeric mouse, because of developmental idiosyncrasies, will be characterized by its own unique proportion of cells of each parental genotype. Furthermore, the proportion of parental cells in the various clones and organs of the body will differ between animals. In this initial study they found that there were no correlations among behaviors of all the animals tested, thus indicating separate organ or cellular etiology of the behaviors.

This approach could be extended to study many behavioral differences between different strains and ultimately to classify behaviors as to the extent of their common genetic origins. Once this is done, then the search for the cellular or organ origins could begin. This will be the difficult part, and will necessitate the use of the anatomical and physiological investigation of the chimeric mice themselves, as well as the parental strains. It will require the ability to distinguish the genotypes of cells or aggregates of cells. This may be feasible because already pure clones of cells of different genotypes can be distinguished on the basis of chromosomal and isozyme characteristics, and it is even possible in some cases to estimate the proportion of each parental cell types where the two are mixed. The brain will not necessarily be the cellular seat of all these behaviors, but to make this approach feasible, we will look to advances in genotypic characterization of cells of the brain.

Comment

Two notions seem to emerge. The first is that there is no dearth in approaches to studying the genetic etiology of brain and behavioral traits and for studying the associations between these traits. Indeed, for experiments with mammals this seems to be a particularly exciting time for developing new genetic techniques and for embellishing old ones. The second is that each experimental approach offers certain advantages and disadvantages with respect to the problems to be solved. Each technique probes the intractable black boxes between genetics, brain, and behavior in somewhat distinct ways, distinct enough that each of us can no longer be expected to be satisfied with only one approach.

Acknowledgments

I am grateful for many valuable discussions with E. R. Dempster, R. E. Wimer, C. C. Wimer, R. L. Sprott and R. L. Collins.

References

Bailey, D. W. Recombinant-inbred strains. *Transplantation*, 1971, *11*, 325–327.

Bailey, D. W. Sources of subline divergence and their relative importance for sublines of six major inbred strains of mice. In H. C. Morse, III (Ed.), *Origins of inbred strains of mice*. New York: Academic Press, 1978. Pp. 197–215.

Davisson, M. T., & Roderick, T. H. Status of the linkage map of the mouse. *Cytogenetics and Cell Genetics*, 1978, *22*, 552–557.

Falconer, D. S. *Introduction to quantitative genetics*. New York: Ronald Press, 1960.

Green, M. C. Catalog of mutant genes and polymorphic loci. In M. C. Green (Ed.), *Genetic variants of the laboratory mouse*. Stuttgart, Germany: Gustav Fischer, 1980, in press.

Lerner, I. M., & Donald, H. P. *Modern developments in animal breeding*. New York, N. Y.: Academic Press, 1966.

Lyon, M. F., Whittingham, D. G., & Glenister, P. Long-term storage of frozen mouse embryos under increased background irradiation. In *The freezing of mammalian embryos*. Ciba Foundation Symposium 52 (new series). New York: Elsevier-Excerpta Medica, 1977. Pp. 273–290.

Morse, H. C., III. (Ed.) *Origins of inbred strains of mice*. New York: Academic Press, 1978.

Nesbitt, M. N., Butler, K., & Spence, M. A. Behavior studies in chimeras derived from differently behaving mouse strains. *Proceedings of the National Academy of Sciences*, 1979, in press.

Roderick, T. H. Further information on subline differences. In H. C. Morse, III (Ed.), *Origins of inbred strains of mice*. New York: Academic Press, 1978, Pp. 485–494.

Roderick, T. H., & Hawes, N. L. Nineteen paracentric chromosomal inversions in mice. *Genetics*, 1974, *76*, 109–117.

Roderick, T. H., Ruddle, F. H., Chapman, V. C., & Shows, T. B. Biochemical polymorphisms in feral and inbred mice (*Mus musculus*). *Biochemical Genetics*, 1971, *5*, 457–466.

Roderick, T. H., Wimer, R. E., & Wimer, C. C. Genetic manipulation of neuroanatomical traits. In L. Petrinovich & J. L. McGaugh (Eds.). *Knowing, thinking and believing.* New York: Plenum Publ. Corp., 1976. Pp. 143–178.

Roderick, T. H., Wimer, R. E., Wimer, C. C. & Schartzkroin, P. A. Genetic and phenotypic variation in weight of brain and spinal cord between inbred strains of mice. *Brain Research,* 1973, *64,* 345–353.

Sidman, R. L., & Green, M. C. Retinal degeneration in the mouse. *Journal of Heredity,* 1965, *56,* 23–29.

Taylor, B. A. Recombinant inbred strains. In M. C. Green (Ed.), *Genetic variants and strains of the laboratory mouse.* Stuttgart, Germany: Gustav Fischer, 1980, in press.

Wimer, R. E., Wimer, C. C., & Roderick, T. H. Genetic variability in forebrain structures between inbred strains of mice. *Brain Research,* 1969, *16,* 257–264.

Chapter VIII

Correlates of Mouse Brain Weight: A Search for Component Morphological Traits[1]

CYNTHIA WIMER

The Roderick-Wimer brain weight selection study (see Chapter VII, this volume and Roderick, Wimer, & Wimer, 1976) was planned as a first step in a series of experiments designed to investigate genetic aspects of brain morphology and associated behavioral traits. It had been shown (Roderick, Wimer, Wimer & Schwartzkroin, 1973) that brain weight has a substantial coefficient of genetic determination (about .65) among inbred strains of mice. The selection experiment was designed to determine whether the genetic variability in mouse brain weight was additive, and therefore usable, in selective breeding. If it were possible to select for high and low brain weight, the resultant stocks could then be used to detect both morphological and behavioral differences associated with variability in brain weight. Hopefully, the results would lead to increasingly more specific questions about finer aspects of brain morphology and their relationship to behavior.

Two concurrent replications of the selection experiment were carried out, each consisting of a high and low brain weight line and an unselected control. After the first few generations of selection, it was clear that there *is* considerable usable genetic variation in brain weight, for

[1]This work was supported in part by USPHS Grants NS 10284 from the National Institute for Neurological Diseases and Stroke and HD 02491 from the National Institute of Child Health and Human Development.

147

DEVELOPMENT AND EVOLUTION
OF BRAIN SIZE

the difference between the mean brain weights of the high and low selection lines steadily increased with each generation in both replications (called Sel 6 and Sel 7).

Behavior Correlates of Genetic Selection for Brain Weight

The behavior of mice genetically selected for brain weight was studied at several generations during the course of selection. Table VIII.I summarizes the results obtained (for a more detailed summary of behavioral results, see Roderick, Wimer, & Wimer, 1976). In early generations, the high brain weight mice were more active than the lows, and they were generally better learners—especially in tasks that required them to learn an active response. As selection progressed and more behavioral studies were carried out, however, it became apparent that behavioral differences were not entirely consistent from generation to generation. In addition, behavioral results varied somewhat between the Roderick-Wimer lines and another set of lines subsequently selected for brain weight by Fuller (Fuller, Chapter X, this volume; Fuller & Herman, 1974; Hahn, Haber, & Fuller, 1973). In a comparison of several brain weight selection lines on the same behaviors, Jensen (1977, and Chapter XI, this volume) found *no* consistent relationships.

The variability of the results obtained in the behavioral studies could be due to several factors, for selected lines of mice differing in brain weight may differ in a number of other characters that also affect behavior. In the comparison of lines selected for brain weight, one must be concerned with characters that have a consistent relationship with brain weight within one generation of a particular set of selected lines, but may relate differently to brain weight in independently selected lines and sometimes from generation to generation in the same line. Basically, there are two types of characters that are cause for concern. The first type includes all of those traits that are *not* genetically correlated with brain weight and affect behavior independently. Such characters may become associated with brain weight in selected lines due to genetic drift, that is, because by chance they were associated in the original mating pairs, or because some alleles were lost in the course of selection in a small population. Replicated lines selected from the same foundation stock may, particularly in later generations, differ markedly with respect to this type of character; lines from independent selection studies, using different foundation stocks, are even more likely to differ. (In the Roderick–Wimer brain weight selection study, for example, the

TABLE VIII.I
Behavioral Results for the Roderick–Wimer Brain Weight Selection Study[a]

Behavioral task	Reference	Generation of selection	Results
Open field activity	Wimer and Prater, 1966	3	High brain weight mice significantly more active than lows in two 5-minute trials. Lines did not differ in frequency of elimination or latency of response.
Brightness discrimination learning, water maze	Wimer and Prater, 1966	3	Highs reached the learning criterion in significantly fewer trials than lows.
Response to novelty and complexity	Wimer and Prater, 1966	3	Lines did not differ in amount of time spent exploring a complex or novel environment; both lines spent more time in such environments than in familiar or simple ones, when given a choice.
Open field activity	Wimer, Roderick, and Wimer, 1969	10	High brain weight line significantly more active than control lines over a three-day period.
Brightness discrimination learning, water maze	Wimer, Roderick, and Wimer, 1969	10	Highs reached criterion significantly faster than controls.
Active escape learning	Wimer, Roderick, and Wimer, 1969	10	High line escaped shock significantly faster than controls.
Passive avoidance learning	Wimer, Roderick, and Wimer, 1969	10	Lines did not differ significantly in learning to avoid shock by remaining passive, although the highs were *slower* to learn than the controls.
Reversal learning	Wimer, Roderick, and Wimer, 1969	10	Highs were significantly better than controls in switching from the passive-avoidance to the active-escape task, and significantly *poorer* at switching from active to passive.

[a]By generation 6, the low brain weight lines were fixed for retinal degeneration. Thus, most behavioral studies on later generations compared highs and controls only. Before generation 11, there were two replications each of the high, control, and low lines. In generation 11, each of these pairs of lines was crossed and selection was continued in the hybrid populations, so that subsequent comparisons were made among three lines rather than six.

(continued)

TABLE VIII.I (continued)
Behavioral Results for the Roderick–Wimer Brain Weight Selection Study[o]

Behavioral task	Reference	Generation of selection	Results
Spatial discrimination, learning and reversal, water maze	Elias, 1969	14	Lines did not differ in original learning, but high brain weight line was superior to controls on the discrimination reversal task.
Spatial discrimination learning and reversal, water maze	Collins, 1970a	15	Control line was poorer than *either* highs or lows on both original learning and reversal. Highs completed significantly more reversals than lows.
Aggressiveness	Collins, 1970b	15	When housed in large enrichment cages (lines separately), low brain weight mice showed significantly more scarring than controls. Highs were the least aggressive.
Spatial discrimination learning and reversal, water maze	Elias, 1970	17	No differences in original learning. High line mice learned first reversal in fewer trials and with fewer errors than controls, and were able to complete significantly more successive reversals. Controls escaped from the maze faster than highs.

gene for retinal degeneration was present in three of the eight strains that made up the foundation population, and this gene became fixed in both low lines and in one of the high lines in the course of selection.)

The second type of trait that can change during the course of selection comprises characters that *are* genetically correlated with brain weight and may also be in the causative pathway between genes and behavior. Correlated characters will always (unless fixed early by drift) change with the selected trait in repeated selection experiments, but *not* always to the same extent. Their response to selection will be a function of their variability in the foundation stock, drift during selection, and the degree of their correlation with the selected trait. If some of the genes that determine total brain weight also affect, for example, the size of a particular structure within the brain, producing a moderate correlation between the two characters in the foundation stock, the between-lines correlation between the two variables will approach unity as selection progresses, because in selecting for brain weight we are also selecting for *some* of the genes that determine the size of the correlated structure. (In the Roderick–Wimer study, body weight—which was moderately related to brain weight in the foundation stock—was a positively correlated character in both replications of the selected lines, although its correlated response to selection for brain weight occurred later and was less extreme in Sel 7 than in Sel 6.)

In any line selected for brain weight, there will be a number of traits that affect behavior, whether or not they are true genetically correlated characters. The search for some of these characters is the topic of several chapters in this book; Dudek and Berman, and Zamenhof and van Marthens, for example, have been concerned with biochemical differences in mice selected for brain weight. The focus of the present chapter is on component morphological variables, characters that are an intrinsic part of the complex trait operationally defined by the weight of the brain.

Volumes of Forebrain Regions in Mice Selected for Brain Weight

Several component structures of the forebrain were investigated in the brains of mice from the Roderick–Wimer selection study. Since the volumes of the brains of the selected lines were found to be almost perfectly correlated with brain weight (Hagerich, 1968; Tobey, 1965), volumes of component structures were compared to determine whether the structures had changed disproportionately. Table VIII.2 shows the

TABLE VIII. 2
Brain Weight and Volumes of Forebrain Structures in Mice from the Seventh Generation of Selection for Brain Weight

	Line					
Variable	Sel 6[a]			Sel 7[a]		
	High	control	Low	High	control	Low
Brain weight (g)	.5262	.4710	.4332	.5257	.5030	.4446
Volumes (cc)						
Total forebrain	.1533	.1348	.1133	.1472	.1358	.1214
Neocortex	.0482	.0424	.0370	.0478	.0425	.0392
Hippocampus	.0125	.0118	.0098	.0129	.0116	.0106
Caudate nucleus	.0110	.0098	.0068	.0104	.0098	.0088
Relative volumes[b]						
Neocortex	.3138	.3155	.3268	.3245	.3127	.3237
Hippocampus	.0811	.0879	.0862	.0874	.0855	.0876
Caudate nucleus	.0717	.0729	.0600	.0705	.0723	.0727

[a]Sel 6 and Sel 7 were two concurrent replications of the selection experiment.

[b]Relative volume was obtained by dividing the volume of total forebrain into the volumes of each of the three component structures.

results of a study of forebrain volume and the volumes of three regions within the forebrain (Gould, 1966). This study was carried out on the brains of mice from generation 7 of selection; by this generation, the brain weights of the three lines were already well separated in both replications (Sel 6 and Sel 7). To obtain the measures of volume, the forebrain was cut sequentially in 10 μm sections; in every twentieth section, the outlines of the neocortex, hippocampus, caudate nucleus and total forebrain were traced using a projecting microscope; areas were measured with a compensating polar planimeter and were integrated over the entire extent of each structure. The resulting volume estimates for the three component structures were divided by the estimate of forebrain volume to obtain measures of relative volume. Both absolute and relative volume estimates were averaged separately for each replication. As Table VIII.2 shows, the three selection lines differed in total volumes of the forebrain and of all structures measured, but *not* in the *relative* proportions of any of the substructures. The results of analyses of variance indicated that the highs and lows in both replications were significantly different in absolute volume of *all* of the structures measured; there were some significant differences in relative volume in Sel 6 (for hippocampus and caudate), but these were not replicated in Sel 7.

The lack of variability in relative substructure volume seemed inconsistent with the fact that there is a great deal of variability in the relative size of neocortex and hippocampus among inbred strains of mice, and, furthermore, that in inbred strains the total volume of the forebrain is highly correlated with neocortical volume but *not* with hippocampal volume (Wimer, Wimer, & Roderick, 1969). The search for the origin of the discrepancy between the results for the brain weight selection lines and for inbred strains is the primary topic to be considered in the remainder of this chapter.

Relationships between Brain Regions in Other Mammalian Species

In order to look for changes in component morphological traits, it is first necessary to define the traits to be examined. Morphological traits should consist of sets of substructures that tend to covary in size, independently of other sets. Several studies (e.g., Stephan, Bauchot, & Andy, 1970) have investigated normal variability in the relative size of brain regions in a variety of mammalian species. Analysis of species differences in statistical relationships among these regions of the brain might help to define some morphological traits that may have changed during the course of selection in the Roderick-Wimer brain weight selection study.

There are several structural relationships that hold across the whole range of mammalian brains. One of the strongest of these relationships is that between brain weight and cortical volume, which are nearly perfectly correlated (Elias & Schwartz, 1969; Jerison, 1973). Examination of this relationship, and of other correlations with brain weight, has led several authors (e.g., Sacher, 1970; Jerison, 1973) to the conclusion that— although there is some disproportionality in the size of major brain regions across species—a *general size factor* can account for over 90% of the between-species variability in the size of individual regions. One of the major analyses that led to this conclusion was Sacher's (1970) principal components factor analysis of data from Stephan, *et al.* (1970), on 63 insectivore and primate species. Table VIII.3 shows rotated factor loadings obtained by Sacher for the variables and structures measured in the Stephan, *et al.* study—brain weight, body weight, and the volumes of major divisions of the central nervous system and of substructures within the telencephalon. The factor loadings indicate a general size factor (I), which has very high loadings for all structures except olfactory bulbs, and a second factor that is clearly an olfactory one. Together the two factors account for 99% of the common variance of the 13 measures of the 63 species.

TABLE VIII.3
Varimax Factor Loadings for Body Weight, Brain
Weight, and the Volumes of 11 Brain
Structures in 63 Insectivore and Primate Species[a]

	Factors	
Variable	I	II
Body weight	.89	.38
Brain weight	.98	.19
Telencephalon		
Neocortex	.99	.10
Hippocampus	.93	.33
Schizocortex	.92	.36
Corpus Striatum	.98	.19
Septum	.94	.34
Paleocortex	.86	.46
Olfactory bulbs	.18	.91
Diencephalon	.98	.20
Mesencephalon	.96	.26
Cerebellum	.97	.24
Medulla	.94	.30

[a]Data adapted from Sacher (1970).

The Sacher (1970) analysis was not in the most useful form for comparison with the brain weight selection study. For such a comparison,
it was desirable to examine the residual covariance patterns when the
general size factor was removed. The general size factor is not just a
brain size factor; it is also a *body* size factor. And although for several
authors (see Jerison, Chapter III, this volume) the brain–body weight
relationship is a crucial one, it could be masking some of the brain
size–substructure correlations that are independent of body size. In
order to clarify these relationships, Sacher's correlation matrix was modified to eliminate the body weight variable. This was accomplished by
computing the partial correlation between each pair of variables with
the covariance due to their correlation with body weight statistically
removed. The resultant partial-correlation matrix is shown in Table
VIII.4, together with the original Sacher correlations (in parentheses).
While all of the correlations in the original matrix, with the exception
of those for olfactory bulbs, were .9 or greater, the partialed matrix
shows much more variability. The correlations of olfactory bulbs with
all the other variables are negative, the paleocortex correlations are considerably lower and many others are below .9. A new principal components factor analysis (Harman, 1967) with varimax rotation (Kaiser,
1959) was carried out on the partialed matrix, and the resulting three

TABLE VIII.4
Correlations between Brain Measures for Insectivores and Primates, with Body Weight Partialed Out[a]

Variable		2	3	4	5	6	7	8	9	10	11	12
Brain Weight	1	.95(.99)	.77(.98)	.73(.97)	.96(.99)	.84(.98)	.45(.94)	−.44(.35)	.96(.99)	.86(.98)	.96(.99)	.78(.98)
Neocortex	2		.72(.96)	.70(.95)	.96(.99)	.75(.96)	.26(.90)	−.51(.28)	.96(.99)	.84(.97)	.93(.98)	.69(.95)
Hippocampus	3			.90(.99)	.77(.97)	.72(.98)	.52(.95)	−.02(.47)	.82(.98)	.82(.98)	.82(.98)	.76(.98)
Schizocortex	4				.74(.97)	.86(.99)	.52(.95)	.08(.50)	.80(.98)	.78(.98)	.79(.98)	.74(.98)
Telencephalon												
Corpus striatum	5					.82(.98)	.43(.93)	−.39(.35)	.97(.99)	.83(.98)	.94(.99)	.76(.97)
Septum	6						.67(.97)	−.03(.48)	.84(.98)	.83(.98)	.87(.99)	.81(.99)
Paleocortex	7							.36(.58)	.41(.93)	.51(.95)	.44(.94)	.54(.96)
Olfactory bulbs	8								−.36(.37)	−.21(.42)	−.32(.39)	−.18(.44)
Diencephalon	9									.91(.99)	.95(.99)	.79(.98)
Mesencephalon	10										.87(.99)	.85(.98)
Cerebellum	11											.79(.98)
Medulla	12											

[a]Values in parentheses are the original correlation coefficients before the effects of body weight were removed. The original coefficients, which were computed on logarithmically transformed data, are from Sacher (1970).

significant factors are shown in Table VIII.5. The first factor is defined by the volumes of hippocampus and schizocortex (with substantial loadings for diencephalon, mesencephalon, and cerebellum). The second is an olfactory bulb factor and is negatively related to several other variables. The third has its highest loadings for paleocortex and septum.

There are, undoubtedly, a number of functional implications that can be derived from this analysis in terms of structures that load on the same factor. What is of particular interest in the present context, however, is that the covariance of brain weight is split between the three factors, with almost equal apportionment to Factors I and II. Cortical volume is also equally split between I and II, but does *not* load on Factor III. These results imply that—when common relationships with body weight are removed—the so-called size factor can be further broken down by region: that is, a large brain in one species may have an especially large hippocampus—schizocortex region, while in another species it may be characterized by particularly small olfactory bulbs, and so on.

Relationships between Brain Regions in Inbred Strains of Mice

The factor analysis of brain measures in 63 mammalian species reveals a hippocampus–schizocortex size factor that is only partially related to

TABLE VIII. 5

Factor Loadings for Brain Measures in Insectivores and Primates, with the Effects of Body Weight Removed

Variable	Factor		
	I	II	III
Brain weight	.66	.61	.42
Telencephalon			
Neocortex	.69	.67	.22
Hippocampus	.92	.07	.25
Schizocortex	.93	−.02	.30
Corpus striatum	.68	.57	.39
Septum	.66	.22	.66
Paleocortex	.31	−.20	.82
Olfactory bulbs	.01	−.88	.23
Diencephalon	.76	.52	.34
Mesencephalon	.74	.35	.43
Cerebellum	.75	.49	.39
Medulla	.65	.28	.49

brain weight and cortical volume—at least between insectivore and primate species. In order to relate this finding to the brain weight selection study, it was necessary to determine whether the same kind of relationship also appears within the species *Mus musculus*. As described above, some relationships among forebrain structures had already been determined in inbred strains of mice (Wimer, *et al.* 1969). Examination of these relationships via the factor-analytic approach would help to determine whether the morphological traits revealed in the between species analyses also describe the variability of component structures in the brains of mice.

Data were available for several relevant variables—body weight, brain weight, and volumes of total forebrain, neocortex and hippocampus—for 11 inbred strains of mice from The Jackson Laboratory (Wimer *et al.*, 1969; Roderick *et al.*, 1973; additional unpublished data). Strain mean values for these five measures are shown in Table VIII.6, together

TABLE VIII.6
Body Weight, Brain Weight, and Brain Volume Measures for Inbred Strains of Mice, and Correlations between the Measures

Strain	Body weight (gm)	Brain weight (gm)	Neocortical volume (cc)	Hippocampal volume (cc)	Remaining forebrain volume[a] (cc)
BABL/cJ	31.2	.540	.043	.012	.119
CBA/J	39.2	.496	.044	.011	.118
C57BL/6J	33.0	.489	.039	.010	.104
DBA/2J	32.6	.421	.031	.010	.093
LG/J	51.5	.549	.042	.010	.100
LP/J	33.1	.466	.033	.009	.091
MA/J	34.0	.484	.036	.012	.102
RF/J	36.4	.513	.045	.011	.111
SM/J	28.2	.486	.036	.011	.105
SWR/J	30.7	.477	.036	.010	.099
129/J	27.2	.445	.033	.011	.097
		Correlations			
Body weight		.57	.54	−.10	.15
Brain weight			.87	.40	.66
Neocortical volume				.40	.86
Hippocampal volume					.68

[a]Remaining forebrain volume was calculated by subtracting the values for neocortical and hippocampal volume from that for total forebrain volume. This was done to insure the experimental independence of the three volume measures. The Pearson product-moment correlation coefficients were computed on the logarithms of the mean values, to be consistent with the procedure followed in between-species analyses.

with the correlations between them. The correlations of body weight with the other measures are low compared to those obtained between species; the brain weight-neocortex volume correlation is high, as expected; forebrain volume has reasonably high correlations with the other three brain measures; and hippocampal volume has only low correlations with brain weight and neocortical volume.

Although a factor analysis with only 11 strains and five variables cannot really be definitive, an exploratory principal components analysis was performed on this correlation matrix, and the varimax-rotated factor loadings are shown in Table VIII.7. The two factors that emerged from the analysis appear to be consistent with the between-species studies. The first factor is defined by hippocampal volume and remaining forebrain (including schizocortex, which loaded with hippocampus in the modification of Sacher's 1970 analysis); the second factor has high and equal loadings for body weight, brain weight and neocortical volume. But brain weight and cortical volume *also* have reasonably high loadings on the hippocampal factor, just as they did in the between-species analysis.

The tentative conclusion to be drawn from the factor analysis—of an admittedly limited amount of data—is that the covariance of brain structures among inbred strains of mice consists of a general size factor involving body weight, brain weight, and cortical volume, and a second factor involving the volumes of the hippocampus and other forebrain structures. (If the forebrain were further subdivided, the factor structure would very likely change; the general size factor might be further broken down, and other specific forebrain factors might emerge.)

TABLE VIII.7
Factor Loadings for Brain Measures in Inbred Strains

	Factor	
Variable	I	II
Body weight	−.12	.80
Brain weight	.47	.77
Neocortical volume	.60	.78
Hippocampal volume	.81	−.04
Remaining forebrain volume	.90	.35

Relationships between Brain Regions in Mice Genetically Selected for Brain Weight

The lack of variability in relative structure volume among high, low and control line brains in the Roderick-Wimer brain weight selection study can be examined in the light of the factors accounting for variability among inbred strains of mice. For this purpose, factor scores[2] were computed for the six selected lines, for the hippocampal volume (I) and general size (II) factors from the inbred strains analysis. The factor scores should provide insight into the question of what aspects of the brain changed during the course of selection for brain weight: If the changes had involved only one of the two factors, the factor scores would "sort out" for the high, control and low lines for one factor, but not the other; the array of factor scores might also be different for the two replications, or for the high brain weight lines as opposed to the lows. Table VIII.8 shows the obtained factor scores, which indicate that the lines sort out on *both* factors, that is, both high brain weight lines are high on both factors and both low lines are low. There appear to be some differences between the lines and the replications: For the high lines, Sel 6 is higher on Factor I, while Sel 7 is higher on Factor II, and equal to the controls on Factor I; for the low lines, Sel 6 is lower on *both* factors than is Sel 7, and both replications are lower on Factor II than on Factor I. Conclusive statements cannot be made about these specific differences on

TABLE VIII.8
Factor Scores for Brain Weight Selection Lines

Line	Factor I	Factor II
Highs		
Sel 6	2.18	1.57
Sel 7	1.32	2.39
Controls		
Sel 6	.34	− .76
Sel 7	1.32	− .19
Lows		
Sel 6	− 1.77	− 2.56
Sel 7	− 1.11	− 1.79

[2]Factor scores characterize individuals, or groups of individuals, with respect to the obtained common factors, and can be calculated for any individual or group for which measures of the appropriate variables are available. The scores resemble standard scores, and are computed by combining the measures, weighting them according to their relative factor loadings. In this case, measures of all the variables in Table VIII.7 were available for brains from generation seven of the selection study.

the basis of these limited data, but the overall differences between the high and low lines on both factors are large enough to conclude that selection for brain weight involved both the hippocampal and the general size factor.

It appears that selection for brain weight produced a change in the volumes of all component structures that had even moderate correlations with brain weight, even though some of these might normally vary independently of each other. As a result, the correlations between the volumes of these structures, which are shown in Table VIII.9, were inflated so that they were *all* higher than those among the same variables for inbred strains. Particularly striking in this table are the correlations greater than .9 between hippocampal volume and both brain weight and neocortical volume, compared to values of only .4 for the inbred strains (see Table VIII.6). All the correlations with body weight are also higher than for the inbred strains. Even with body weight partialed out, as was done for the between-species study (Table VIII.4), the correlation coefficients are still all greater than .9.

TABLE VIII.9
Correlations between Body Weight and Brain Measures in Brain Weight Selection Lines

	Brain weight	Neocortical volume	Hippocampal volume	Remaining forebrain volume
Body weight	.76	.68	.58	.77
Brain weight		.96	.94	.96
Neocortical volume			.97	.97
Hippocampal volume				.96
Remaining forebrain volume				

Implications

These results have two implications for brain weight selection studies in general, and particularly for the study of behavior in stocks selected for brain size. First, when comparing behavioral studies on different selected lines (or even at different generations of selection in the same study), it would be wise to also compare the factor structure of the brain phenotype itself, since different studies may have selected for different aspects of brain size, and since the relative importance of these aspects may change over the course of selection.

The second implication is that in using *any* selected stocks to draw conclusions about the relationship between brain size and behavior, we run the risk of engineering a large or small brain that is not a "normally" large or small brain. That is, it is not only different in size from the "standard" mouse brain, but its substructures are in different proportions to each other, so that quantitative relationships between structures are changed, and functional networks may be distorted. In other words, artificial selection does not necessarily recapitulate natural selection.

Aside from the cautions that they suggest for the use of selected lines, the analyses carried out above represent some positive steps toward the structural analysis of the mammalian brain. First, they suggest some specific relationships between structures that define a set of morphological traits, and these traits appear to be consistent not only across a wide range of species, but also within a single species. And second, they illustrate that some real insights into structural relationships can be provided by the application of not-very-complicated statistical techniques to rather simple measurements of gross neuroanatomical variables.

Multivariate analysis has considerable potential for the study of brain–behavior relationships. Starting with the kinds of analyses presented above, there are several directions that could be taken. One possible direction would be to use the kinds of gross volumetric variables described here to define orthogonal morphological traits, and to attempt to link them to orthogonal *behavioral* traits defined by similar analyses of behavioral batteries (see Chapter XVII, this volume). Another direction is toward a finer analysis of gross structural traits, which could be accomplished by relating the statistically defined traits to increasingly more precise measures of the size and composition of substructures and the relationships between them.

References

Collins, R. A. Experimental modification of brain weight and behavior in mice: An enrichment study. *Developmental Psychobiology*, 1970, 3, 145–155.(a)

Collins, R. A. Aggression in mice selectively bred for brain weight. *Behavior Genetics*, 1970, 1, 169–171.(b)

Elias, H., & Schwartz, D. Surface areas of the cerebral cortex of mammals determined by stereological methods. *Science*, 1969, 166, 111–113.

Elias, M. F. Differences in spatial discrimination reversal learning for mice genetically selected for high brain weight and unselected controls. *Perceptual and Motor Skills*, 1969, 28, 707–712.

Elias, M. F. Spatial discrimination reversal learning for mice genetically selected for differing brain size: A supplementary report. *Perceptual and Motor Skills*, 1970, 30, 239–245.

Fuller, J. L. & Herman, B. H. Effect of genotype and practice upon behavioral development in mice. *Developmental Psychobiology*, 1974, 7, 21–30.

Gould, J. Effects of changes in total brain size on specific brain structures in mice. Unpublished student paper, The Jackson Laboratory, Bar Harbor, Maine, 1966.

Hagerich, J. A. Investigation of the causes of brain weight variation in mice. Unpublished student paper, The Jackson Laboratory, Bar Harbor, Maine, 1968.

Hahn, M. E., Haber, S. B., & Fuller, J. L. Differential agonistic behavior in mice selected for brain weight. *Physiology and Behavior*, 1973, *10*, 759–762.

Harman, H. J. *Modern factor analysis* (2nd ed.). Chicago: University of Chicago Press, 1967.

Jensen, C. Generality of learning differences in brain-weight-selected mice. *Journal of Comparative and Physiological Psychology*, 1977, *91*, 629–641.

Jerison, H. J. *Evolution of the brain and intelligence*. New York: Academic Press, 1973.

Kaiser, H. F. Computer program for varimax rotation in factor analysis. *Educational and Psychological Measurement*, 1959, *19*, 413–420.

Roderick, T. H., Wimer, R. E., & Wimer, C. C. Genetic manipulation of neuroanatomical traits. In L. Petrinovich & J. L. McGaugh (Eds.), *Knowing, thinking and believing*. New York: Plenum, 1976. Pp. 143–178.

Roderick, T. H., Wimer, R. E., Wimer, C. C., & Schwartzkroin, P. A. Genetic and phenotypic variation in weight of brain and spinal cord between inbred strains of mice. *Brain Research*, 1973, *64*, 345–353.

Sacher, G. A. Allometric and factorial analysis of brain structure in insectivores and primates. In C. R. Noback & W. Montagna (Eds.), *The primate brain. Advances in primatology*, Vol. 1. New York: Appleton-Century-Crofts, 1970. Pp. 245–287.

Stephan, H., Bauchot, R., & Andy, O. J. Data on size of the brain and of various brain parts in insectivores and primates. In C. R. Noback & W. Montagna (Eds.), *The primate brain. Advances in primatology*, Vol. 1. New York: Appleton-Century-Crofts, 1970. Pp. 289–297.

Tobey, W. R. Neuroanatomical differences in mice selectively bred for high and low brain weight. Unpublished student paper, The Jackson Laboratory, Bar Harbor, Maine, 1965.

Wimer, C., & Prater, L. Some behavioral differences in mice genetically selected for high and low brain weight. *Psychological Reports*, 1966, *19*, 675–681.

Wimer, C., Roderick, T. H., & Wimer, R. E. Supplementary report: Behavioral differences in mice genetically selected for brain weight. *Psychological Reports*, 1969, *25*, 363–368.

Wimer, R. E., Wimer, C. C., & Roderick, T. H. Genetic variability in forebrain structures between inbred strains of mice. *Brain Research*, 1969, *16*, 257–264.

Chapter IX

Brain Weight, Brain Chemical Content, and Their Early Manipulation[1]

STEPHEN ZAMENHOF
EDITH VAN MARTHENS

The main topics of this volume, brain size and its behavioral implications, have been discussed from various points of view. In our chapter, we would like to present first *our* interpretation of this problem.

To be entirely on the side of logic, the question, "How does the brain size affect brain functioning?" should be preceded by the question "How does the brain function?" We do not know. Perhaps it is too early to ask. After all, it is only the twentieth century. But we can compile a list of factors that (logically) should contribute to brain functioning:

1. Anatomical complexity of brain cells, especially neurons (dendritic and axonal arborization, spines, synaptic junctions), which allows for interactions with a multitude of other neurons
2. Neuronal circuitry ("wiring diagram"), which preprograms these interactions
3. Biochemical complexities that determine speed and efficiency of nerve conduction and of synapses
4. Integrity and nutritional status of cell bodies, which determine proper development and functioning

[1]The author's work has been supported by Grants HD-05615, HD-08927, and AG-00162 from the National Institutes of Health, U. S. Public Health Service, and EY-76-S-03-0034 from the U. S. Department of Energy.

163

5. Number of neurons (and glial cells that service them): obviously, this number, together with (and related to) the number of synapses, determines the richness of cell interactions in the brain. As discussed elsewhere in this volume, this number also increases steadily in the evolution from lower species to man.[2]

As we know, brain volume and brain weight are complex final outcomes of many of these factors. These two parameters obviously should depend on (a) anatomical complexity, because a well developed dendritic tree necessitates adequate distance between individual neurons; (b) nutritional status of cell bodies, which determines cell volume and development of the dendritic tree; and (c) above all, number of neurons and glial cells. Thus, it appears useful to study first the correlations between brain weight and other brain parameters. These correlations are discussed below.

Brain Weight: Correlations with Other Brain Parameters

The time when neuronal proliferation ends offers a unique opportunity for study of the correlations between brain cell number, which is then mostly full neuron complement, and brain weight or even body weight; later in life these weights change in a less predictable manner. The moment of cessation of neuron proliferation is, of course, different for different species. In humans, it is most inconveniently situated at around the eighteenth week of pregnancy (Dobbing & Sands, 1973). In the rat and rabbit, on the other hand, this moment is most conveniently situated at birth. At this time, cerebral cell proliferation (or DNA) in rats reaches a temporary plateau (Figure IX.1); what proliferates after birth are mostly (with few exceptions) just glial cells and nonneural elements. Taking advantage of this situation, we have studied several correlations in newborn rats and rabbits.

As mentioned before, neonatal brain cell number is a characteristic index of prenatal brain development. But the actual cell count on histological slides is a procedure that is both very laborious and subject to considerable error, especially since the count on each section has to be multiplied by the volume of the section and integrated through all sec-

---

[2]From an evolutionary point of view, one may surmise that this huge number of cells (brain), which is very expensive to nourish and to oxygenate (in humans approximately one-third of the total body oxygen consumption), would not be there if it were not needed: The economy of natural selection would never allow it to come into existence during the gradual evolution.

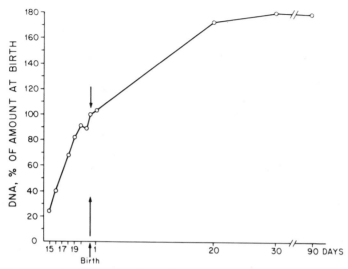

FIGURE IX.1. DNA synthesis in cerebral hemispheres of developing rat brain. Abscissa-embryonal (fetal) age before birth and age after birth. Ordinate-DNA, cited in percentage of the amount at birth. Before birth, both sexes measured together, after birth, only females.

tions to obtain the total count per brain. The *cell density* can be measured on histological slides, but the interpretation of this parameter is often misleading. Lower density may mean poor cell multiplication, but it may also mean a later stage in development (migration of cells away from each other). In general, *total* brain cell number appears to be a more meaningful parameter than cell density. One should also add that the number of cells and the cell densities change dramatically from one brain region to another: Whenever possible one should attempt to analyze various brain regions separately.

The most often used method for cell enumeration is determination of the DNA content of the brain. Normal neuron and glial cells *at birth* are esentially diploid, and the amount of DNA per diploid cell of a given species is constant. Only after birth do some specialized cells become polyploid (cerebellar Purkinje cells, Betz cells of the motor cortex or large pyramidal cells in the hippocampus; for a review, see Zamenhof & van Marthens, 1978). For all practical purposes, determination of neonatal brain DNA is a convenient and objective quantitative method for determination of total neonatal brain cell number (Zamenhof, Bursztyn, Rich, & Zamenhof, 1964; Zamenhof, Grauel, van Marthens, & Stillinger, 1972). From the DNA values per brain, the actual total number of brain cells can be calculated by dividing by a constant, DNA content per cell (6×10^{-6} µg for the rat; see Zamenhof et al., 1964).

Bearing the preceding in mind, one can look for correlations among parameters in neonatal animals. Although for any one individual a heavier brain weight does not necessarily mean more brain cells, for large numbers of animals the correlation between the two is very good (see Table IX.1) (Zamenhof, Guthrie, & Clarkson, 1974). In fact, for a sample of 250 neonatal animals, brain weight is also well correlated with brain protein, with cell size (illustrated by the ratio cerebral protein/cerebral DNA or cerebral weight/cerebral DNA), and even well correlated with neonatal body weight. The latter correlation is of particular practical importance for a sample of this size, because it allows us to predict brain weights without sacrificing the animals, and the animals can thus be studied postnatally.

Brain weight at birth, that is, at the end of a neuron proliferation, is not only well correlated with the cerebral cell number, which is mostly neuron number, but also shows other interesting correlations. It is, for instance, well correlated with cortical thicknesses as measured in rostral sections in several locations (Clark & Zamenhof, 1973). Curiously enough, it is also well correlated with the weight of the *placenta*, the organ responsible for supplying the nutrients for prenatal brain growth (Zamenhof, Grauel, & van Marthens, 1971). Thus, again, the neonates can be spared, for with a sample of this size, brain weights can be predicted from the weights of placentas.

Many of the correlations based on neonatal animals are not valid for adult animals. In adults cerebral cells are no longer predominantly neurons, but also include all glial cells and nonneural elements. For adult animals, body weight is no longer correlated with brain weight, and brain weight no longer with cell size, although brain weight is still well

TABLE IX. 1
Correlations between Cerebral Parameters in Neonatal Rats

Parameters correlated	r	p
Body weight—cerebral weight	.668	<.0005
Body weight—cerebral DNA	.426	<.0005
Body weight—cerebral protein	.214	<.0005
Cerebral weight—cerebral DNA	.537	<.0005
Cerebral weight—cerebral protein	.299	<.0005
Cerebral DNA—cerebral protein	.314	<.0005
Cerebral weight/cerebral DNA—cerebral weight	.572	<.0005
Cerebral protein/cerebral DNA—cerebral weight	.691	<.0005
Cerebral weight/cerebral DNA—cerebral DNA	.380	<.0005
Cerebral weight/cerebral DNA—cerebral protein	.754	<.0005
Cerebral protein/cerebral DNA—cerebral protein	.902	<.0005

correlated with brain cell number (DNA) and brain protein (Zamenhof *et al.*, 1974). Also, for adult animals, cerebral weight is no longer correlated with cortex thicknesses in rostral sections (Clark & Zamenhof, 1973).

The correlations for the most interesting brain, the human brain, have not been well studied. Data on neonatal normal brain weight with relation to neonatal brain DNA are not readily available. But in humans one can make a harmless measurement of neonatal head circumference. Winick and Rosso (1969) established a linear relation between head circumference and brain DNA of essentially normal infants during the first year of life. In our study on 91 normal infants born at the UCLA Hospital (Zamenhof & Holzman, 1973), we could establish a good correlation ($p<.001$) between neonatal head circumference and neonatal body weight, as well as placental weight. As in the rat, it would be more meaningful to study the brain at the end of neuron proliferation, which is around the eighteenth week of pregnancy, but the material is not available. One may add that neonatal head circumference cannot be used on rats because of the inconvenient geometry of the rat's head.

Natural Cell Death during Early Brain Development

Until a few years ago, the picture of the process of neuron multiplication resulting in a certain final number of neurons (and, therefore, later certain definite brain size) was somewhat like this: The neurons, or rather neuroblasts, in the ependymal layer, close to the ventricle, multiply quickly at first, then more slowly until they come to a plateau, as shown in Figure IX.1. How far the neuroblast proliferation will go, that is, how high the plateau, should be determined by both genetic and environmental factors. However, this picture does not represent what is really happening. We know now that neurons (neuroblasts) *are produced in excess*, and then a certain portion undergo *natural death*. The final number will, therefore, be a composite of *two* processes—neuronal proliferation and neuronal natural death. Neuronal death has been studied in the past in many different locations in the central nervous system, *excepting* the cerebral hemispheres (Cowan, 1973). The purpose and mechanism of this death of excess neurons is largely unknown. The most popular theory is that the purpose of the excess is to facilitate connections with other neurons, the "target cells." The excess, which are unable to find connections, die out, and are quickly phagocytized.

In the past there was no direct information on cell death in cerebral hemispheres. Hyndman has just finished studies of natural neuronal death in the cerebral hemispheres of the chick embryo (Hyndman & Zamenhof, 1978). The DNA of early neuroblasts was labeled with tritiated thymidine. If there were no cell death and cells proliferated in the presence of tritiated thymidine, more and more neuronal DNA would become labeled. The actual situation is represented in Figure IX.2. It can be seen that instead of steady increase, the amount of labeled cerebral DNA undergoes a sharp decline on days 10–14 and then again after day 16. This decline can be attributed only to destruction of already existing labeled DNA, that is, to cell death. The first decline is in neuronal (neuroblast) cells; the second is either in a second population of neuronal cells (the ones that originated later) or in glial cells. The loss of label in each case is considerable: our estimate is at least on the order of 20–30%. Further study reveals that this phenomenon of natural cell death is intricately coordinated with cell proliferation and maturation, as well as with the levels of relevant enzyme activities in the embryonal brain: In the period of embryonal cell death, the DNA degradative enzyme (thymidine phosphorylase) is on the increase, and the DNA synthesizing enzymes (thymidine kinase, thymidylate synthetase [Hyndman & Zamenhof, 1978] and DNA-dependent, DNA-polymerase [Margolis, 1969] are decreasing.

What determines the extent of natural cell death: heredity or environment? Since we do not know the mechanism, or the extent of hy-

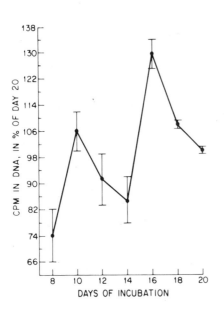

FIGURE IX.2. Radioactivity of labeled DNA of cerebral hemispheres of a chick embryo plotted as a function of age, following the introduction of 5 μci of tritiated thymidine onto chorio-allantoic membrane at 7 days of incubation. Data are shown in counts per minute (CPM) of total DNA function, expressed as percent of day 20 value. [From Hyndman & Zamenhof, 1978.]

pothetical "target cells," at present it is safest to suggest that both may be involved.

Variability of Brain Parameters

From the foregoing it appears that the study of brain parameters close to the end of neuron proliferation and at the conclusion of the natural cell death, will be more informative than the study of those parameters in adult animals. How constant and species-characteristic are these parameters?

The subject of genetic selection for brain size will be discussed further in the next section of our chapter. The subject and changing brain parameters by environmental manipulation will be the last section in our chapter. Here, we would like to discuss *natural variability* of brain parameters within species, independent of laboratory genetic or environmental *manipulation*.

In our sample of 91 human newborns, the body weight varied considerably ($\pm 20\%$, expressed as percentage of standard deviation). On the other hand, variability of neonatal head circumference was only $\pm 3.5\%$, suggesting that this parameter is very conservative indeed. In a sample of 720 newborn rats we could also measure other parameters; the variability of neonatal body weight was $\pm 12\%$, cerebral weight 11%, cerebral protein 14.5%, but cerebral DNA only 6% (Zamenhof, Guthrie, & van Marthens, 1976). Thus, the value of cerebral DNA at birth, which is the index of cell number, seems to be the most constant parameter. Is it because of the regulatory and corrective action of natural cell death? Is this cell number indeed a constant, characteristic of each species, as the outcome of the process of evolution?

Since evolution implies better adaptation to the environment, we would like to describe first a phenemonon which may be called "minievolution"; a periodic, seasonal adjustment of the brain cell number to environmental conditions. We have demonstrated this phenomenon in the neonatal chick (Zamenhof & van Marthens, 1971). As can be seen from Fig. IX.3, the amount of cerebral DNA, and therefore cerebral cell number per gram egg, is *not* constant, but varies with the season. The evolutionary driving force is the anticipated food availability, and the cue is the *speed of change* in the duration of daylight.[3] Thus, final cerebral

---

[3]Some seasonal variations can be also shown for neonatal rat brain (Zamenhof *et al.*, 1971), but our rat vivarium environment is too constant and does not resemble a natural environment.

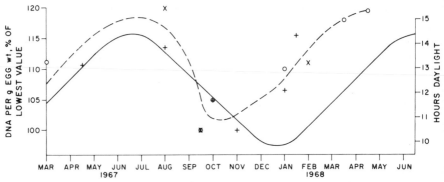

FIGURE IX.3. Seasonal variations in amount of newly hatched chick brain DNA (broken line, individual points) and in hours of Los Angeles daylight (full time) shown for the months in which eggs were laid. [From Zamenhof & van Marthens, 1971, reprinted by permission of University of California Press, Berkeley, California.]

cell number may not be constant and may respond to natural changes in the environment. Another example of such a natural response is the good negative correlation between brain weight (or brain DNA) and number in the litter. Venge (1950, pp. 61–67) was first to demonstrate a negative correlation between neonatal body weight in rabbits and the number per liter. Brain parameters were not studied, but as mentioned above, at birth they are correlated with body weights. Here, the cause of variability is presumably the variable amount of intrauterine nutrients and/or space. Obviously, the effect of such factors will be most pronounced right after the conclusion of the intrauterine life. Penrose (1961) estimates that for birth weight, the effect of all intrauterine environmental factors accounts for 62%, and all genetic factors only 38% (see also the review in Widdowson, 1968, p. 3). This situation may be reversed later in life. Neonatal brain weights have not been studied in this respect, but they are correlated with birth weights.

Another source of variability, caused by genetic or environmental factors or both, may be maternal performance. A strong positive correlation has been established between maternal blood flow to the placenta and placental and fetal weights (Duncan & Lewis, 1969; Wootton, McFadyen, & Cooper, 1977). Fetal brain weight has not been studied, but since it is correlated with both placental and fetal weight one can expect that brain weight will indeed vary with the maternal placental blood flow and with the efficiency and health of the mother in general. The effect of other environmental factors on neonatal brain weights will be further discussed in the last section of our chapter.

The variability of *adult* brain weights in different species due to genetic factors has, of course been, widely studied. However, neonatal cerebral weights, cerebral DNA, and cerebral protein of different strains of the same species have not been the subject of many reports. We have found that in rats as well as in rabbits, different strains have significantly *different* neonatal brain parameters—cerebral weight, cerebral DNA, and cerebral protein.

Rat strain S5B/PL was highly inbred, but was never selected for low brain or body weight (the selection was for resistance to chronic respiratory disease, CRD). Yet body weight and brain parameters at birth (Table IX.2) were significantly lower than for our albino Sprague-Dawley strain, which was bred as a closed colony in our laboratory for 30 generations. When adult, the females retained this significant difference, whereas males did not. In newborn rabbits (Table IX.3) all brain parameters in the small Dutch Belt strain were significantly lower than in the New Zealand white, but in the large body Flemish strain neonatal cerebral DNA was not different from New Zealand DNA, despite a 2

TABLE IX. 2
Body Weights and Brain Parameters of Two Strains of Rats

		Body weight[a] (gm)	Cerebrum		
			Weight (gm)	DNA (μg)	Protein (mg)
Sex	Strain				
Newborn					
Both	Sprague-Dawley	5.9 ± .65	.1597 ± .0123	610 ± 32	8.60 ± .86
together	S5 B/PL	5.2 ± .46	.139 ± .0109	582 ± 39	7.92 ± .80
	Δ[b]	− 12	− 13	− 5	− 8
	p	<.001	<.001	<.01	<.01
Adult					
Female	Sprague-Dawley	262 ± 43	1.206 ± .057	1103 ± 71	98.59 ± 6.44
	S5 B/PL	204 ± 12	1.173 ± .0279	1023 ± 45	93.84 ± 9.25
	Δ	− 22	− 3	− 7	− 5
	p	<.001	<.01	<.001	<.01
Male	Sprague-Dawley	415 ± 82	1.264 ± .0661	1071 ± 43	99.8 ± 6.44
	S5 B/PL	386 ± 30	1.2917 ± 0.0423	1038 ± 44	107.75 ± 15.52
	Δ	− 7	+ 2	− 3	+ 8
	p	NS	NS	NS	NS

[a]Mean ± S.D.
[b]Δ = difference to Sprague-Dawley in percent; p = probability; NS = not significant.

TABLE IX.3
Body Weights and Brain Parameters of the Newborns of Three Strains of Rabbits

				Cerebrum		
n^a	Strain	Gestation (days)	Body Weight[b] (gm)	Weight (gm)	DNA (μg)	Protein (mg)
34	New Zealand White	31	51.5 ± 10.6	1.0416 ± .1196	2002 ± 160	45.22 ± 6.51
9	Dutch Belt	31	32.3 ± 4.7	.8910 ± .0382	1644 ± 59	40.78 ± 2.89
	Δ^c		−37	−14	−18	−10
	p		<.001	<.001	<.001	.02>p>.01
21	Flemish	33	55.0 ± 14.1	1.2088 ± .1543	1950 ± 76	57.28 ± 7.47
	Δ^c		+7	+16	−3	+27
	p		NS	<.001	NS	<.001

a = number examined; both sexes together

[b] Mean ± S.D.

Δ = difference to New Zealand white, in percent; p = probability; NS = not significant.

day longer gestation. In adults, cerebral DNA and protein in Dutch belt and Flemish females were not different from New Zealand white females; however Flemish males were different from New Zealand white males.

All the strains were cross-fertile, that is, they were, by definition, of the same species. Neonatal DNA content in rats and rabbits is indicative of the final neuron number. Thus, one must conclude that not only brain weights, but also final neuron numbers in a species, are *not constant*. In the adult, the weight data may be obscured by sex differences. Fortunately, at birth, sex differences in the value of brain parameters are not significant (Zamenhof, van Marthens, & Grauel, 1972).

Why should neonatal brain parameters be higher in some strains of the same species? It could be because of the genetically determined better prenatal nutrition and greater intrauterine space. In fact, higher amounts of neonatal DNA are associated with greater neonatal body weight (Tables IX.3 and IX.4). It could be because of the genetically determined longer period of neuronal proliferation or shorter cell generation time (meaning more total cell divisions), and/or genetically determined larger "target tissue" resulting in lower natural neuronal death. As yet, no data are available in favor of any of these possibilities.

Genetic Manipulation of Brain Parameters

The first genetic manipulation that comes to mind is hybridization between strains of different size. This was the subject of many early publications (review in Venge, 1950), and the parameters studied were mostly body weight and size—seldom brain parameters (compare Wahlstein, 1975). Besides the expression of the hybrid genome as such, one could consider two other phenonmena: (*a*) maternal (environmental) influence that favors those fetuses whose *mother* belonged to the larger of the two strains (more intrauterine space, better prenatal nutrition); and (*b*) hybrid vigor (heterosis) that favors the fetuses of any genetically different parents. However, in our hands, crosses between *noninbred* rabbit strains of different size yielded offspring whose neonatal brain parameters were not significantly higher than the means for the two strains, even though neonatal body weights were higher. Thus, hybridization of the *noninbred* strains did not allow significant improvement of the values of parameters of an organ as conservative as the neonatal brain.

The other genetic manipulation would be selection for higher brain weights. Having heard about the beautiful results Wimer, Roderick, and

Fuller had with their strains of mice (Fuller & Geils, 1972, 1973; Fuller & Wimer, 1973; Roderick, Wimer, & Wimer, 1976; Roderick, Wimer, Wimer, & Schwartzkroin, 1973), we decided to study brain parameters of neonatal mice of these strains. We began this with the realization that neonatal brains are closer to the time of conclusion of neuronal proliferation and, therefore, are more indicative of neuronal population as such. Wimer kindly supplied the strains and his advice. The results of our work have been reported (Zamenhof & van Marthens, 1976).

The subjects were mice from the Roderick-Wimer SEL-16 lines, all descended from the same eight way cross of inbred strains. Lines C (control), H (high, called here high black [Hb]), and L (low) were used in our study. In addition, we used a new line, Hg (high grey), in which the grey coat color is associated with high adult brain weight. The Hg mice occurred spontaneously in our laboratory in strain Hb (one or two per 80 Hb newborns); when cross-mated, the Hg animals bred true (100% grey coat color). In all studies the males and females were represented in equal numbers.

In confirmation of the reports of Fuller and Geils (1972, 1973) the neonatal body weights in the L and C lines were practically identical, and the cerebral weights in the H lines were significantly higher than in the L line. On the other hand, in variance with Fuller and Geils, the body weights in the H lines were significantly higher than in the L line, and the cerebral weights in the C lines were significantly higher than in the L line. However, we must point out that perhaps 10–12 generations of selection intervened between their study and ours.

The DNA and protein contents of neonatal cerebra were significantly higher in H and C animals than in L animals. Since the cells at that time are mostly neurons, the H and C animals have significantly higher numbers of neurons than the L animals.

Neonatal cerebral weights of several animals at birth were more than two standard deviations above the mean for their line. The proportions of such animals were 3.1% in the L strain, 4.8% in the unselected control, and 4.2% in both H strains together. Because L and H strains were repeatedly selected for their brain weights until stabilization (Roderick, Wimer, & Wimer, 1976), genetic uniformity apparently removed very little neonatal variability. The remaining larger component of variability might have been *environmental* (intrauterine environment) superimposed on genetic differences in the bulk of the population.

The ratio of cerebral DNA/cerebral weight (an index of cell density) in all three lines was practically the same. Moreover, the ratios of cerebral protein/cerebral DNA (an index of cerebral protein content per cell or cell size), and cerebral protein/cerebral weight (an index of cerebral protein content per unit of cerebral volume) were also practically the same. These data indicate that the neonatal parameter that is highest in H cerebra and lowest in L cerebra is only cell (predominately neuron) number, and not cell size and density.

In the adult animals (equal proportions of each sex) the cortex and the cerebellum could be dissected separately. The determinations made on these brains indicated that all the differences (compared to L) that were significant for the whole cerebral hemispheres in the newborn were even more pronounced and remained highly significant in the cerebra and the cerebella of the adult animals. In addition, some of the differences in the ratios of DNA/weight, protein/weight, and protein/DNA also were significant.

The comparison of differences between the H strains and the L strain at birth and in adulthood suggests the following:

1. The differences in cell numbers (DNA) have increased considerably after birth. Because the postnatal DNA increase is essentially due to proliferation of glial cells (and of some nonneural cells), the numbers of these cells in the strains compared must differ even more than the numbers of neurons.

2. As compared with L, the Hb and Hg strains in adulthood not only have more cortical cells, but also higher cell density (DNA/weight) and higher protein density (protein/weight), though not larger cell size (protein/DNA).

3. The strain differences with respect to the cerebellum, an organ with mainly postnatal neuron proliferation, essentially follow the differences found in the cerebrum.

Thus, the animals of the H lines have values of brain parameters genetically higher than those of the L line; this conclusion applies not only to cerebral neuron number (neonatal DNA), but also to many other neonatal and adult brain parameters. These findings may be causally related to the reported differences in behavioral performance of these lines of animals.

Early Environmental Manipulation of Brain Parameters

The harmful effects of some prenatal environments, such as those resulting from maternal malnutrition or radiation, on brain weight and brain cell number of pups, have been the subject of many publications. The reader is referred to recent reviews on these subjects (Hicks & d'Amato, 1978, Zamenhof & van Marthens, 1974, 1978). Here we would like to discuss the concepts of *optimal* prenatal brain development and *enhancement* of this development, and hence, enhancement of brain cell number and brain weight.

When studying brain size, one must take into consideration the concept that the *actual* brain development is, in most cases, below the *optimal*, that is, below the genetic potential of the individual or the species. According to the recent study by Naeye, Blanc, and Paul (1973), "The larger brain size in newborns of mothers who were best nourished raises the possibility that fetal brain growth may reach its full genetic potential *only* under such circumstances of full nutrition [p. 502]." In addition to the more obvious question of what constitutes "full nutrition," at present it is difficult to ascertain whether a particular dietary regime, which does not give any symptoms of malnutrition, is also an optimal regime. Genetic differences in strains, in intestinal absorption, etc., may play a considerable role here. A diet optimal in one respect or at one time in development may not be so in other respects or at other times. In this section we concern ourselves with the conditions *optimal for prenatal brain development.*

The term "supernutrition" as distinct from "overnutrition" has been used by Williams (1971) to denote "quality above and beyond nutrition as it is ordinarily experienced" to provide "a completely suitable assortment ideally tailored to individual needs [p. 2,899a]." Although this concept has mainly qualitative connotations, the optimal *quantity* is also a part of supernutrition. For instance, Winick and Noble (1967) reported increases in the cell numbers of many organs, including the brain, by increasing the *quantity* of milk available to rat pups during nursing.

In this section, we will summarize the evidence that suggests that the quantity of nutrients normally allocated to a fetus may not be optimal and is subject, within genetic limits, to experimental improvement.

One work concerns the effects of pituitary growth hormone. In the case of maternal malnutrition during pregnancy, which results in malnourished fetuses, one may wonder whether the amounts of nutrients the mother is supplying to them is really all she can do for them; after all, she usually has ample nutrient reserves: fat, glycogen, muscle protein. If only she could mobilize them!

The levels of pituitary growth hormone are known to increase during pregnancy and during fasting. Perhaps this mobilizes maternal nutrient reserves; thus, mothers of similar genome but different pituitary development might produce offspring with different brain development.

In the case of maternal malnutrition, however, such natural mobilization is often not sufficient to produce normal offspring. Thus, an attempt was made to stimulate such nutrient mobilization by injecting pregnant females with additional growth hormone (Zamenhof, van Marthens, & Grauel, 1971). Such treatment of malnourished females produced nearly normal offspring. The improvements of the malnourished animals were highly significant. In addition, treatment of normally nourished females with growth hormone produced a significant increase in cerebral weight over and above the normal; this increase was not due to water, but to increased content of cerebral protein. As explained above, the primary action of this hormone might have been on the mother, by mobilization of maternal nutrient reserves, especially fat deposits. Thus, conceivably, each fetus received more nutrients that stimulated its prenatal brain development.

The improvement of early brain development upon administration of growth hormone to normal animals also has been demonstrated in the past (in tadpoles: Hunt & Jacobson, 1970; Zamenhof, 1941; in pregnant rats: (Clendinen & Eayrs, 1961; Zamenhof, 1942; Zamenhof, Mosley, & Schuller, 1966); and also more recently (Sara & Lazarus, 1974, 1975; Sara, Lazarus, Stuart, & King, 1974). Behavioral studies on rats indicate that the treatment of pregnant females with growth hormone results in a significant improvement of learning ability in the offspring (Block & Essman, 1965; Clendinnen & Eayrs, 1961; Croskerry & Smith, 1975; Ray & Hochhauser, 1969; Sara & Lazarus, 1974, 1975; Sara et al., 1974); however, various investigators give different interpretations of the cause of such improvement.

Another method to enhance prenatal brain development is to reduce the number of fetuses during pregnancy by surgical means: presumably such a procedure provides more nutrients and space for the remaining fetuses. One method for achieving this reduction consists in tying one of the two uterine horns (rat) prior to mating (van Marthens & Zamenhof, 1969). Another method, used in rabbits (van Marthens, Grauel, & Zamenhof, 1974), consists of destroying some implantation sites soon after implantation. The result is a significant increase in neonatal body weight, placental weight, cerebral weight, cerebral DNA (cell number), and cerebral protein. In the case of the rabbit, the increase in placental weight was up to 105%; in neonatal body weight up to 50%; in cerebral DNA (cell number) up to 21%; and in cerebral protein up to 46%. In the rat the increases in placental weights closely followed the degree of reduction of number of fetuses.

The constancy of neonatal cerebral DNA (cell number) in *normal* animals is probably the result of stringent regulatory mechanisms. Conceivably, neuronal proliferation includes a multitude of closely overlapping checks so that if one factor is enhanced the next one becomes the rate limiting step, and so on. Superimposed on that is the phenomenon of natural death of excess of neurons, which tends to regulate the final neuron number. Nevertheless, cases of enhanced brain development in selected *individuals* of genetically uniform strains can not only be produced experimentally, but can also occur naturally; possibly in natural cases many factors have changed in concert.

As can be seen from Figure IX.4, in a genetically uniform population animals from the same litter can sometimes be found that have brain DNA well above the range of others (more than two standard deviations) (Zamenhof & van Marthens, 1974). Such spontaneous occurrences are rare—approximately 2% of cases in the rat. The causes of such high DNA are completely unknown, but their occurrence indicates that the

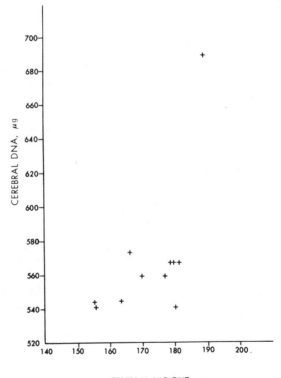

CEREBRAL WEIGHT, mg

FIGURE IX.4. Individual (+) neonatal rat cerebral weights and neonatal cerebral DNA (cell number), from one of the litters in which one fetus has cerebral DNA more than two standard deviations above the mean. [From Zamenhof & van Marthens 1974, reprinted by permission of W. Junk, b. v. Publishers, The Hague, The Netherlands.]

mechanism of regulation of DNA synthesis, cell number, and cell death in the prenatal brain are not completely precise and inviolable.

In a recent study (Zamenhof *et al.*, 1976), newborn rats with parameter values more than two standard deviations above the mean (outstandingly high [OH]) were identified in a normal population of 720 animals and were studied for correlations between the following parameters: body weight, brain weight, brain DNA (cell number), and brain protein (Table IX.4).

It was found that an animal OH on one parameter tends to have values for other parameters higher than the mean for the population. Some of these animals with OH values of cerebral weight, cerebral DNA, or cerebral protein came from litters whose mean values on these parameters was also OH ("OH litters"), and the percentages of such animals were significantly higher ($p < .001$) than would be expected if there were no correlations among the parameters. Thus, on a statistical basis, an individual with an OH cerebral cell number (DNA) at birth is likely also have a higher than average birth weight, and also to be from the litter OH with respect to cerebral cell number. Such findings may facilitate the search for these OH individuals. In the newborn rat cerebral cells are mostly neurons, and their number at birth is final or nearly final; thus, such an animal may well retain the superiority in neuron number when an adult. Other parameters, such as cerebral protein content, may not remain OH as adults, but nevertheless such superiority at birth may exert beneficial influences during postnatal neuron differentiation.

The normal occurrence of newborns with OH amounts of cerebral DNA (cell number) indicates that the remarkable constancy of this parameter at birth can be circumvented by natural causes. In the past, the occurrence of such OH animals has rarely been reported (Zamenhof & van Marthens, 1971, 1974), and the causes are essentially unknown.

It might be hypothesized that the occurrence of OH animals is due to their special genotype. Although at present this cannot be totally excluded, it must be pointed out that the rats used in the present study were bred as a closed colony for 33–37 generations; thus, *genetic* variability is not very likely to be the explanation of the occurrence of OH animals. This was also our conclusion regarding the neonatal variability in Roderick–Wimer mice. Variability in those lines remained, even after selection, until genetic stabilization. It has been mentioned in the section entitled "Variability of Brain Parameters" that for many species, including the human, heredity is not the main factor in determining the size of the newborn: the main factors seem to be environmental. How-

TABLE IX.4
Identification of OH Individual Newborns [a] and OH Litters [b] (rats)

	Entire population				OH with respect to			
	Body weight	Cerebral weight	Cerebral DNA	Cerebral protein	Body weight	Cerebral weight	Cerebral DNA	Cerebral protein
Individual animals								
Number	720	720	720	720	7	10	16	23
Percent of total	100	100	100	100	0.97	1.39	2.22	3.19
Mean value (mg) ± std. dev.	5978 ± 715	161.5 ± 17.5	.5597 ± .0344	8.758 ± 1.27	7900 ± 428	203.4 ± 5.78	.6464 ± .02	11.744 ± .40
Litters								
Number	81	81	81	81	0	2	1	3
Percent of total	100	100	100	100	0	2.5	1.2	3.7

[a] Parameter values more than 2 standard deviations above the mean for the entire population;
[b] more than 2 standard errors above the mean for the entire population, both sexes together and cerebrum without olfactory lobes.

ever, prenatal brain development has not been studied in this respect. The present finding that the newborns OH with respect to brain parameters also have body weights higher than the mean for the population suggests that for the neonatal brain, too, the causes may be environmental, such as the general optimal intrauterine conditions, including optimal prenatal nutrition. Such conditions might have prevailed for each OH litter, but might have been especially favorable for the OH fetuses within such litters. The improvement of newborn brain parameters by experimental improvements of intrauterine conditions has been discussed previously.

Summary and Conclusions

The list of factors necessary for proper brain functioning must be formidable. Several of them, especially the number of neurons, are involved in determination of brain volume and brain weight. Brain cell number, as determined by DNA content, is most indicative of neuron number if this cell number is determined at the end of neuron proliferation (birth in rats). When the sample size is sufficiently large, this cell number (DNA) is well correlated with neonatal brain weight, brain protein, head circumference, and even neonatal weight and placental weight. Later in life, some of these good correlations disappear.

The events that determine final neuron number include not only the extent of neuronal proliferation, but, after the latter is completed, the natural death of those neurons in excess of what is needed to synapse with "target tissue." We found that this natural neuronal death occurs also in cerebral hemispheres to the extent of approximately 20%, and is coordinated with the increase in the activity of DNA-degrating enzymes, and decrease in the activity of DNA-synthesizing enzymes.

Although neonatal brain parameters, especially human head circumference, are remarkably constant and characteristic of each species as determined by evolution, some variations occur naturally. One of them, which may be termed "minievolution," is a seasonal variation of neonatal brain cell number (DNA) in anticipation of food availability. Other factors may involve genetically and environmentally determined maternal performance (intrauterine space, maternal nutrition, maternal blood supply to placenta, etc.), as well as fetal performance (length of period of neuronal proliferation, cell death, etc.). It has been estimated (Penrose, 1961) that for birth weight the effect of all intrauterine environmental factors accounts for 62%, and all genetic factors accounts for only 38%; this situation may be reversed later in life. We have studied two rat strains and three rabbit strains, and we found within each of these species significant differences in their brain parameters, even though the strains were not selected for differences in brain weight; thus, constancy of brain parameters within species is not stringent. Hybridization of these strains did not give us a clear indication of hybrid vigor. It is of interest that *neonatal* brain parameters in rat are the same for both sexes.

We have also determined several neonatal and adult parameters in the Roderick-Wimer lines of mice selected for low (L) or high (Hb and Hg) adult brain weight, and in the unselected control line (C). Neonatal cerebral weight, DNA (cell number), and protein were significantly higher in the H and C lines than in the L line. The ratios of cerebral DNA/weight (index of cell density), cerebral protein/weight, and cerebral protein/DNA (index of protein content per cell or cell size) were at birth practically the same in all lines. In the adult animals all the differences were amplified, and some of the differences in the above ratios were significant for the cerebral cortex as well as for the cerebellum. These findings may be causally related to the reported superiority in behavioral performance of the H line.

We have further discussed the concept that actual brain development may be, in most cases, below the *optimal* (i.e., below the genetic potential). Manipulations to achieve optimal prenatal brain development may include optimal prenatal nutrition, mobilization of maternal nutrient reserves (e.g., by growth hormone), enhancement of fetal nutrition, and space available by operational reduction of the number of fetuses, etc.

We find that in a genetically uniform nonmanipulated population, animals from the same litter can sometimes be found that have brain DNA well above the range of others. In our further study, "outstanding" newborn rats with brain parameter values more than two standard deviations above the mean (outstandingly high [OH]) were identified in a *normal* population of 720 animals and were studied for correlations between these parameters. The animals OH on any one of these parameters were also higher than average on all the others, and some of these animals come from OH litters. Such findings may facilitate the search for OH individuals. The causes of the occurrence of OH animals are more likely to be environmental than genetic.

In conclusion, mechanisms exist to favor limitations in brain weight and brain cell number of a species; however, because of the multitude of genetic and environmental factors involved, these limits are not precise and inviolable, and can be manipulated.

References

Block, J. B., & Essman, W. B. Growth hormone administration during pregnancy: A behavioural difference in offspring rats. *Nature* (London), 1965, *205*, 1136–1137.

Clark, G. M., & Zamenhof, S. Correlations between cerebral and cortical parameters in the developing and mature rat brain. *International Journal of Neuroscience*, 1973, *5*, 223–229.

Clendinnen, G. B., & Eayrs, J. T. The anatomical and physiological effects of prenatally administered somatotropin on cerebral development in rats. *Journal of Endocrinology*, 1961, *22*, 183–193.

Cowan, W. M. Neuronal death as a regulative mechanism in the control of cell number in the nervous system. In M. Rockstein (Ed.), *Development and aging in the nervous system.* New York: Academic Press, 1973. Pp. 19–41.

Croskerry, P. G., & Smith, G. K. Prolongation of gestation by growth hormone: A confounding factor in the assessment of its prenatal action. *Science*, 1975, *189*, 648–650.

Dobbing, J., & Sands, J. Quantitative growth and development of human brain. *Archives of Disease in Childhood*, 1973, *48*, 757–767.

Duncan, S. L. B., & Lewis, B. V. Maternal placental and myometrial blood flow in the pregnant rabbit. *Journal of Physiology*, 1969, *202*, 471–481.

Fuller, J. L., & Geils, H. D. Brain growth in mice selected for high and low brain weight. *Developmental Psychobiology*, 1972, *5*, 307–318.

Fuller, J. L., & Geils, H. D. Behavioral development in mice selected for differences in brain weight. *Developmental Psychobiology*, 1973, *6*, 469–474.

Fuller, J. L., & Wimer, R. E. Behavior genetics. In D. A. Dewsbury & D. A. Rethlingshafer (Eds.), *Comparative Psychology: A Modern Survey.* New York: McGraw-Hill, 1973. PP. 197–237.

Hicks, S. P., & d'Amato, C. Effect of radiation on neural and behavioral development. In G. Gottlieb (Ed.), *Studies on the development of behavior and the nervous system, Early Influences* Vol. 4. New York: Academic Press, 1978. Pp. 149–186.

Hunt, R. K., & Jacobson, M. Brain enhancement in tadpoles: Increased DNA concentration after somatotropin or prolactin. *Science*, 1970, *170*, 342–344.

Hyndman, A. G., & Zamenhof, S. Thymidine phosphorylase, thymidine kinase and thymidylate synthetase activities in cerebral hemispheres of developing chick embryos. *Journal of Neurochemistry*, 1978, *31*, 577–580.

Hyndman, A. G., & Zamenhof, S. Cell proliferation and cell death in the cerebral hemispheres of developing chick embryos. *Developmental Neuroscience*, 1978, *1*, 216–225.

Margolis, F. L. DNA and DNA-polymerase activity in chicken brain regions during ontogeny. *Journal of Neurochemistry*, 1969, *16*, 447–456.

Naeye, R. L., Blanc, W., & Paul, C. Effects of maternal nutrition on the human fetus. *Pediatrics*, 1973, *52*, 494–503.

Penrose, L. S. Genetics of growth and development of the fetus. In L. S. Penrose, & H. Lang Brown (Eds.), *Recent advances in human genetics.* Boston: Little, Brown and Co., 1961. P. 64.

Ray, O. S., & Hochhauser, S. Growth hormone and environmental complexity effects on behavior in the rat. *Developmental Psychology*, 1969, *1*, 311–317.

Roderick, T. H., Wimer, R. E., & Wimer, C. C. Genetic manipulation of neuroanatomical traits. In L. Petrinovich & J. L. McGaugh (Eds.), *Knowing, thinking and believing.* New York: Plenum Publishing Co., 1976. Pp. 143–178.

Roderick, T. H., Wimer, R. E., Wimer, C. C., & Schwartzkroin, P. A. Genetic and phenotypic variation in weight and brain and spinal cord between inbred strains of mice. *Brain Research*, 1973, *64*, 345–353.

Sara, V. R., & Lazarus, L. Prenatal action of growth hormone on brain and behavior. *Nature* (London), 1974, *250*, 257–258.

Sara, V. R., & Lazarus, V. Maternal growth hormone and growth and function. *Developmental Psychobiology*, 1975, *8*, 489–502.

Sara, V. R., Lazarus, L., Stuart, M. C., & King, T. Fetal brain growth: Selective action by growth hormone. *Science*, 1974, *186*, 446–447.

van Marthens, E., Grauel, L., & Zamenhof, S. Enhancement of prenatal development by operative restriction of litter size in the rabbit. *Life Sciences*, 1972, *11*, 1,031–1,035.

van Marthens, E., Grauel, L., & Zamenhof, S. Enhancement of prenatal development in the rat by operative restriction of litter size. *Biology of the Neonate*, 1974, *25*, 53–56.

van Marthens, E., & Zamenhof, S. Deoxyribonucleic acid of neonatal rat cerebrum increased by operative restriction of litter size. *Experimental Neurology*, 1969, *23*, 214–219.

Venge, O. Maternal influence on birth weight in rabbits. *Acta Zoologica*, 1950, *31*, 3–148.

Wahlstein, D. Genetic variation in the development of mouse brain and behavior: Evidence from the middle postnatal period. *Developmental Psychobiology*, 1975, *8*, 371–380.

Widdowson, E. M. Growth and composition of the fetus and newborn. In N. S. Assali (Ed.), *Biology of gestation* (Vol. 2). New York: Academic Press, 1968.

Williams, R. J. "Supernutrition" as a strategy for control of disease. *Proceedings of the National Academy of Sciences, U.S.A.*, 1971, *68*, 2899a.

Winick, M., & Noble, A. Cellular response with increased feeding in neonatal rats. *Journal of Nutrition*, 1967, *91*, 179–182.

Winick, M., & Rosso, P. Head circumference and cellular growth of the brain in normal and marasmic children. *Journal of Pediatrics*, 1969, *74*, 774–778.

Wootton, R., McFadyen, I. R., & Cooper, J. E. Measurement of placental blood flow in the pig and its relation to placental and fetal weight. *Biology of the Neonate*, 1977, *31*, 333–339.

Zamenhof, S. Stimulation of the proliferation of neurons by the growth hormone: I. Experiments on tadpoles. *Growth*, 1941, *5*, 123–139.

Zamenhof, S. Stimulation of cortical cell proliferation by the growth hormone: III. Experiments on albino rats. *Physiological Zoology*, 1942, *15*, 281–292.

Zamenhof, S., Bursztyn, H., Rich, K., & Zamenhof, P. J. The determination of deoxyribonucleic acid and of cell number in brain. *Journal of Neurochemistry*, 1964, *11*, 505–509.

Zamenhof, S., Grauel, L., & van Marthens, E. Study of possible correlations between prenatal brain development and placental weight. *Biology of the Neonate*, 1971, *18*, 140–145.

Zamehof, S., Grauel, L., van Marthens, E., & Stillinger, R. A. Quantitative determination of DNA in preserved brains and brain sections. *Journal of Neurochemistry*, 1972, *19*, 61–68.

Zamenhof, S., Guthrie, D., & Clarkson, D. Study of possible correlations between body weights and brain parameters in neonatal and mature rats. *Biology of the Neonate*, 1974, *24*, 354–362.

Zamenhof, S., Guthrie, D., & van Marthens, E. Neonatal rats with outstanding values of brain and body parameters. *Life Sciences*, 1976, *18*, 1391–1396.

Zamenhof, S., & Holzman, G. B. Study of correlations between neonatal head circumferences, placental parameters and neonatal body weights. *Obstetrics and Gynecology*, 1973, *41*, 855–859.

Zamenhof, S., Mosely, J., & Schuller, E. Stimulation of the proliferation of cortical neurons by prenatal treatment with growth hormone. *Science*, 1966, *152*, 1396–1397.

Zamenhof, S., & van Marthens, E. Hormonal and nutritional aspects of prenatal brain development. In D. C. Pease (Ed.), *Cellular aspects of neural growth and differentiation*. Berkeley: University of California Press, 1971. Pp. 329–359.

Zamenhof, S., & van Marthens, E. Study of factors influencing prenatal brain development. *Molecular and Cellular Biochemistry*, 1974, *4*, 157–168.

Zamenhof, S., & van Marthens, E. Neonatal and adult brain parameters in mice selected for adult brain weight. *Developmental Psychobiology*, 1976, *9*, 587–593.

Zamenhof, S., & van Marthens, E. Nutritional influences on prenatal brain development. In G. Gottlieb (Ed.), *Studies on the development of behavior and the nervous system, Early Influences* Vol. 4. New York: Academic Press, 1978. Pp. 149–186.

Zamenhof, S., van Marthens, E., & Grauel, L. Prenatal cerebral development: Effect of restricted diet, reversal by growth hormone. *Science*, 1971, *174*, 954–955.

Zamenhof, S., van Marthens, E., & Grauel, L. Studies on some factors influencing prenatal brain development. In R. J. Goss (Ed.), *Regulation of organ and tissue growth*. New York: Academic Press, 1972. Pp. 41–60.

Chapter X

Fuller BWS Lines: History and Results

JOHN L. FULLER

Rensch (1956) and Jerison (1973), among others, have stressed the point that species with bigger brains, relative to their body size, are capable of more complex, or at least more modifiable, behavior. Brain size also varies among members of a species, although the behavioral implications of these differences have seldom been studied. Storer (1967) reported large variations in brain size among inbred mouse strains. These strains also differ in many aspects of behavior, but I cannot discern in these inbred animals any obvious relationship between variations in the physical dimensions of their brains and their adult behavior. It would be premature, however, to conclude that no correlations exist (Fuller & Wimer, 1966). In fact, the idea that genes must affect behavior through the mediation of the nervous system is almost self-evident. Thus, in the middle 1960s I discussed with my Jackson Laboratory colleagues, T. H. Roderick, C. C. Wimer, and R. E. Wimer, the possibility of selecting for a brain character and looking for behavioral correlates. We shortly went our separate ways but continued our common interest in the project. All of us were aware of the dangers of generalizing from a single set of selected lines and hoped that our parallel programs would support each other's. Roderick, Wimer, and Wimer (1976) have recently published an extensive review of their studies; some of their results and conclusions are presented in other chapters of this volume. This chapter is a status report of a similar selection and testing program carried out under my

187

DEVELOPMENT AND EVOLUTION
OF BRAIN SIZE

supervision at the State University of New York at Binghamton. I acknowledge with thanks Roderick's contribution of the original foundation stock, and his donation of additional animals from his selected lines for Jensen's (1977) comparative studies.

One may ask why brain size was chosen as the criterion for selection rather than a more dynamic trait, such as catecholamine content or the richness of dendritic branching. The answer is that our choice of brain weight was based primarily on ease of measurement and the resources available to us. We hoped that size variation would be associated with functional differences, and that if these appeared we could identify the specific factors affecting behavior.

The foundation stock for the Fuller Brain Weight Selection (BWS) was an eight-way cross of Jackson Laboratory inbred strains chosen by Roderick on the basis of diversity of origin and freedom from retinal degeneration. The mating plan was:

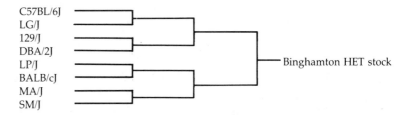

The procedure for the Binghamton breeding program was a variant of family selection. In an effort to reduce the possibility that selecting for big brains was really only selecting for big mice, we calculated for each of our lines, once they were separated, the regression of brain weight on body weight. Test litters were obtained from each mated pair—usually 10 per line—and the brain weight of each litter was evaluated with respect to the brain weight expected on the basis of body weight. Thus, for the high (H) line, animals chosen as breeders were siblings of those in prior litters whose brains were heavier than predicted by the regression equation for all litters in their generation. For the low line (L), breeders were chosen from families whose brains were light in relation to body weight. A medium line (M) was selected by breeding from families that deviated least from the predicted brain weight. In addition, an unselected control line, the Binghamton HET stock, was maintained by continuation of the original base stock from the eight-way cross.

The first three generations were reared at the Jackson Laboratory.

Later generations were born and maintained in the Psychology Department at SUNY—Binghamton. At generation 18, a complete set of matings was transferred to Martin E. Hahn at the William Paterson College of New Jersey. Selection ceased at generation 12, but there have been intermittent checks on the characteristics of the lines. Separation on the basis of brain weight has been well maintained.

The effects of selection on brain weight are shown in Figure X.1. The lines separated early and continued to diverge throughout the period of active selection. There is no real indication of reversion to the control level since selection ceased. In fact, the L line brains continued to decrease in size following relaxation of selection.

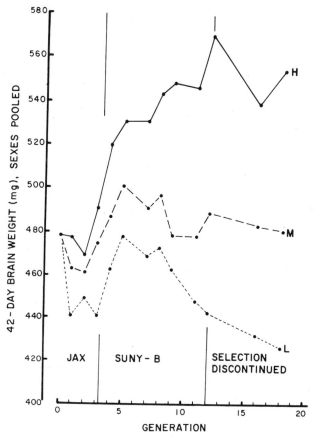

FIGURE X.1. Mean brain weights shown of 42-day old mice (sexes pooled) from start of selection through generation 18.

Quantitative Aspects of Selection

The selection procedure, though effective, was not well adapted for conventional methods of determining heritability. The parents for each generation were selected on the basis of measurements made on their younger siblings. Since there was considerable variation in brain weight within families, we cannot be sure that the individuals actually chosen for breeding were those best meeting the selection criterion. The brain weights of parents were determined when they were replaced by a new set of breeders at 100–200 days of age. The means are shown in Figure X.2. The curves are somewhat surprising. Average brain weights of the three selected lines rank as expected. However, there is no indication

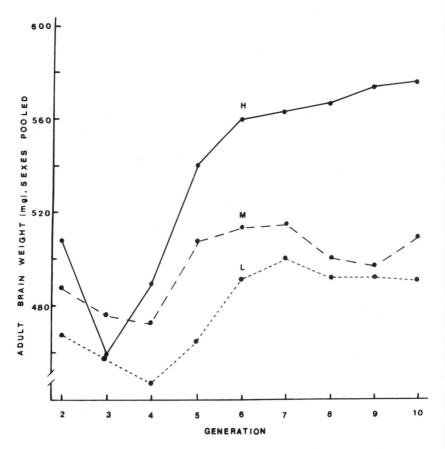

FIGURE X.2. Brain weights of adult breeders (100–200 days old), which are from generations 2–10.

that selection produced a reduction in the brain weight of adult L line mice; in fact, both L and M line mice of generation 10 have heavier brains than mice of generation 2. It is likely that the increment in the H line adult brain weight is similarly associated with factors unrelated to the selection criterion. The overall increments in all lines may be due to changes in housing and diet associated with the move from Maine to New York. The differences between the adult and the 42-day curves, however, suggest that different genes affect brain weight at the two ages.

It is of interest, therefore, to look at parent–offspring correlations within lines at various stages of the selection process (Table X.1). These correlations are of two kinds. For generations 5–6 and 17–18 they were computed from the midparent values and the means of all tested offspring. We have pooled sexes, since no reliable sex differences in brain weight have been found in most tests. For parental generations 5–7 and 8–10, midparent values were correlated with individual values of those offspring selected as parents for the next generation. Generations were pooled to obtain samples of suitable size. For these correlations, both parent and offspring brains were collected from adults. The data indicate that significant correlations within lines were found only through the first 7 generations of selection. This suggests that relatively few loci were involved; by generation 8, most genetic variation was between lines. This point is well demonstrated in Figure X.3, based on data from generations 17 and 18. The relationships of parent and offspring brain weights can be fitted to a straight line, along which there are three clusters of points, each corresponding to one of the BWS lines. Within the clusters there seems to be no evidence of a correlation.

TABLE X. 1
Parent–Offspring Correlations for Wet Brain Weight

	Generation(s)			
Line	5[a]	5–7[b]	8–10[b]	18[a]
H	.54*	.33*	.01	.19
M	.58*	−.17	−.11	−.01
L	.15	.27*	.21	.24

[a]Midparent adult, means of tested offspring.
[b]Midparent adult, breeding offspring.
*p<.05

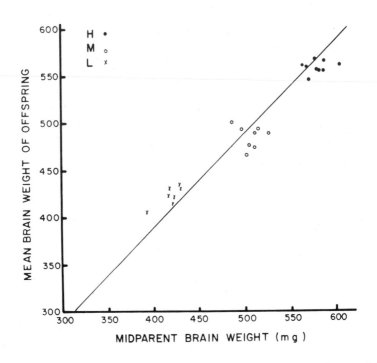

FIGURE X.3. Relationship between midparental brain weight and mean brain weight of 42-day-old offspring (generation 18).

Nevertheless, there seems to be some genetic heterogeneity remaining within the lines. After 3 generations of reverse selection beginning at generation 12, the brain weight of 42-day H line mice fell 19.5 mg (−3.9%) and that of the L line mice rose 22.3 mg (+5.0%).

Selection Differential

Our selection procedure was intended to detect those families from which individuals would be selected randomly to transmit the appropriate phenotype to their offspring. In practice, approximately one-half of the 8–12 pairs per generation in each line provided the offspring that became the breeders of the next generation. At the time families were chosen, the brain weights of the adult members were unknown. Later, when these animals were no longer required for breeding, their brains were removed and weighed, whether or not their offspring had been chosen to remain in the breeding program. We subtracted the mean brain weights of all parents in a generation from the mean brain weights of parents whose litters were selected for breeding. This provided a measure of the actual selection differential at the adult level (Table X.2).

Table X.2 has peculiarities that are difficult to explain. The cumulative selection differentials based on adult brain weights are in the expected order. However, the gains in the M and L lines run contrary to their negative selection differentials, and the gain in the H line far exceeds the cumulative differential. No plausible genetic hypothesis can explain these results. They must be attributable to environmental factors, but one can only speculate as to their nature. Obviously, it is imprudent to estimate heritabilities from the data. But despite this failure in the quantitative analysis of the selection procedure, it was successful in modifying brain weight within a few generations, although it was admittedly less efficient than conventional procedures.

TABLE X.2
Cumulative Selection Differential and Change in Brain Weight

Line	Selection differential[a] (mg) generations 2–10	Mean brain weight (mg)		
		Generation 2	Generation 10	Change
H	24.6	508	589	81
M	− 6.5	486	510	24
L	−20.0	467	492	25

[a]The selection differential at each generation was the mean brain weight of adults whose litters were chosen for continuation of the line minus the mean brain weight of all adults whose litters were evaluated.

Brain Growth Patterns in BWS Lines

We now turn to the matter of the patterns of brain growth over time in the BWS lines. Do L line brains lag behind H line brains from the start, or is there retardation of growth only during some specific age range? At birth, a mouse brain weighs approximately 100mg; 42 days later it has increased fivefold. The course of growth in the three lines at generation 7 is shown in Table X.3. It is apparent that at this stage of selection differences were small and inconsistent in direction at birth and at 4 days of age. Significant separation is apparent from the eighth day onward. In the current generations (20+) there appears to be a small but reliable reduction of brain weight and DNA content of neonate L mice, compared with H line neonates (Chapter XIII, this volume).

These data, combined with those from adults, suggest that selection has modified brain growth rate in more than one way. The rate of

TABLE X.3
Brain Weight from Birth to 42 Days—Generation 7, Sexes Pooled (in milligrams)

Age (days)	BWS-H			BWS-M			BWS-L			ANOVA		
	N	$\bar{X}$	SD	N	$\bar{X}$	SD	N	$\bar{X}$	SD	F	df	p
0	12	102.0	12.2	16	95.1	7.4	12	94.8	4.4	2.95	2,37	ns
4	20	196.8	12.4	18	187.4	25.3	12	206.1	17.6	1.01	2,47	ns
8	20	332.2	27.0	18	311.8	23.5	16	322.4	23.2	4.07	2,51	.05
14	20	465.6	17.7	20	423.0	18.6	16	416.9	19.0	39.45	2,53	.001
42	15	531.1	19.3	20	497.2	27.2	16	484.3	19.8	17.26	2,48	.001

growth in L line mice falls clearly behind that of H and M line mice at 8 days of age, and possibly even in neonates. However, growth may continue longer in the L line, so that the differences between the lines is slightly less in mature adults. Evidence for the latter statement comes from brain weight determinations made on breeding adults at ages 100–200 days. The mean increment in brain weight from 42 days to adulthood (calculated for generations 17–18) was greater in the L line (36.9 mg, 8.1%) than in the H line (25.1 mg, 4.3%), even though L brains are substantially lighter at both ages.

Body Weight and Fertility of BWS Mice

We have been concerned that the brain weight changes are simply a by-product of inadvertent selection for body size. There is no doubt that in the BWS lines, and in the Roderick, Wimer, and Wimer lines, body weight has moved in step with brain weight during selection. The data for the BWS lines are shown in Figure X.4. Brain weight in BWS mice, however, is not determined primarily by body weight. After adjusting brain weights for their covariance with body weight, 64% of variance at generation 5 was attributable to strain differences independent of body weight. At generation 18 the picture is similar. Correlations between mean brain weight and mean body weight of males for 10 generations, for which the data are most complete, ranged from −.528 to .652. None is significant when tested by a two-tailed t test.

Another important biological characteristic is fertility. This trait might have been expected to change under selection if: (1) brain weight were an important component of fitness; or (2) impaired by the inbreeding that is inevitable in a small scale selection program. Actually, as shown

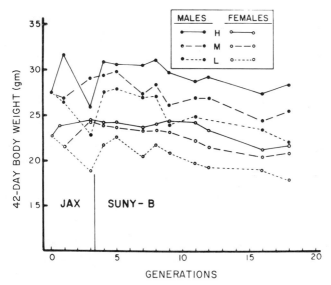

FIGURE X.4. Mean body weights of 42-day-old males and females of BWS lines plotted from start of selection through generation 18.

TABLE X.4
Mean Number of Living Young per Litter

	Generation			
Line	1–4	5–8	9–12	Mean
H	9.00	10.15	9.77	9.69
M	8.89	10.03	10.35	9.76
L	8.95	10.23	10.64	9.94
Mean	9.15	10.13	10.25	9.80

in Table X.4, fertility has increased slightly but significantly ($p<.01$) during selection. No reliable differences between lines were found at any age.

Behavioral Correlates

The selection program was undertaken primarily in the hope that changes in behavior would be correlated with changes in brain size. It is fair to say at this time that the results have been positive but not spectacular. I shall briefly review a number of the published studies dealing with the behavior of BWS mice, and then report two previously unpublished experiments.

Hahn, Haber, and Fuller (1973) found that L lines males isolated immediately after weaning were more aggressive than similarly treated M or H line males. Males of the three lines isolated 10 days after weaning (the intervening 10 days were spent with siblings) did not differ in amount or intensity of fighting. Fuller and Herman (1974) reported that H line mice were generally more advanced than M or L line mice in open-field activity, balancing on a rotorod, age of eye-opening, and edge avoidance. Practice speeded the development of these neuromotor capacities, but did not abolish strain differences. Later, Herman and Nagy (1977) showed that H line mice learned shock avoidance in a T-maze more quickly and retained the correct response more reliably than either of the other two BWS lines.

Ahroon and Fuller (1976) failed to find reliable differences in the rate of learning the correct path in a Lashley type III maze. They did, however, report subtle differences between the H and L lines in details of the learning process. H line animals persevered better than L line mice, once a correct response was made. The learning curves of young and adult H line mice were similar; L line youngsters were more erratic in acquiring a correct response pattern. Jensen (1977) carried out an extensive series of tests with the Roderick, Wimer, and Wimer, and the Fuller lines. He found statistically reliable differences between some of the lines on every task. Across the lines, however, there was no consistent relationship between brain weight and performance level. An analysis of data from the heterogeneous foundation stock animals, included in the experiment as controls, did detect a reliable positive correlation between high brain weight and good performance (Jensen & Fuller, 1978).

Jensen and Fuller conclude that heterogeneous stocks are more appropriate than either selected lines or sets of inbred strains for demonstrating correlations between diverse phenotypes such as brain size and learning ability. Selected lines are usually somewhat inbred, and inbreeding leads to nonfunctional associations of the alleles affecting structure with those affecting behavior. Such associations have led to erroneous claims for behavioral pleiotropy of genes regulating structure. They can also conceal pleiotropic effects of structure-regulating genes, since the genetic background on which a gene operates modifies its action. In a heterogeneous population, background differences are randomized and behavioral pleiotropy may be more readily detected. This problem could be overcome by using large numbers of independently derived BWS lines, or large arrays of inbred strains from a common source of high genetic heterogeneity. The financial, physical, and time requirements for such experiments exceed the resources of most experimenters.

Intertrial Interval and Water Maze Learning

Strains superior in learning one task are often only average, or even inferior, in others (Searle, 1949). Even changing the details of procedure on the same task, such as varying the temporal distribution of training trials, may have an important influence on strain differences. McGaugh, Jennings, and Thompson (1962) found that Tryon maze bright rats were superior to Tryon maze dull rats only when tested with short (30 sec) intertrial intervals (ITI). We considered it interesting to compare the effects of changing training schedules on maze-learning of three BWS lines. Two experiments were performed.

Experiment 1: Method

In the initial study, 24 male and 24 female mice, equally distributed among the three BWS lines, were assigned randomly to distributed practice (one trial per day) or massed practice (five trials per day with an ITI of 30 sec) in a recurved-T maze filled with water at 20°C (Waller, Waller, & Brewster, 1960). Subjects were dropped into the stem of the T and could escape by climbing a ladder placed at the end of one arm of the T. One arm of the T was painted black, the other white; one-half the subjects were trained with black positive, one-half with white positive. The position, right or left, of the correct side was varied according to the tables of Vandament, Burright, Fessenden, and Barker (1970). Training was discontinued when a subject made nine correct responses in 10 consecutive trials. Data were analyzed by a 3 (lines) × 2 (sex) × 2 (treatment) analysis of variance.

Experiment 1: Results

From their first trial, four subjects ran consistently to black, thus distorting the data. Since each of the four was from a different group, its score was replaced by the mean of the remaining three members of its group, with an appropriate reduction of the degrees of freedom. The number of trials to criterion was strongly affected by treatment (massed trials, 40.9); distributed trials, 35.4; $p < .001$). Differences between the mean scores of males (35.4) and females (30.6), and between the lines

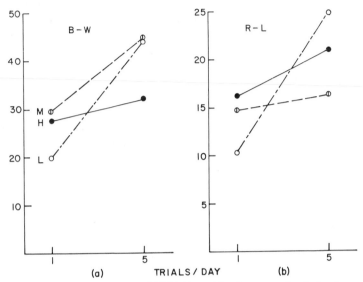

FIGURE X.5. Mean number of trials for BWS-H, M, and L mice to reach criterion for water-maze tests under two conditions: one trial per day and five trials per day. (a) Data are from a black–white discrimination task. (b) Data are from a right–left discrimination task.

(BWS-H, 29.5; BWS-M, 37.3; and BWS-L, 32.2) were not significant. Two of the interaction terms suggested a difference in the effect of changed schedule of training on learning. The mean difference score (massed minus distributed) was 22.3 for males and 9.2 for females. For the lines, the difference scores were as follows: BWS-H, 5.2; BWS-M, 16.9; and BWS-L, 25.0. The data for the lines are shown in Figure X.5a. The reliability of these interactions is marginal ($p < .10$), but it appears that BWS-H mice learn equally well under either training schedule, whereas BWS-M and BWS-L mice benefit from distributed practice.

Experiment 2

A second experiment was conducted with the same apparatus and procedures except that the subjects were required to learn a right–left discrimination in a maze painted uniformly gray. Correction was permitted when an error was made. Ten female mice from each of the three BWS lines were used as subjects. Each animal was given 10 trials with escape possible from both arms of the maze in order to become familiar with the task. Each was then trained to a criterion of 9 correct out of 10 consecutive trials, with escape possible only from the side least often chosen during the practice trials. As with the black–white discrimination task, one trial per day was more effective than five trials (mean trials to criterion; distributed, 13.9; massed, 21.2; $p<.01$). For the three strains, the increments in score associated with the massed trial procedure were the following: BWS-H, 5.3; BWS-M, 2.6; BWS-L, 14.1; ($p<.10$) (Figure X.5b).

The two experiments are consistent in showing that changes in training schedule influence BWS-L mice more than BWS-H mice. The BWS-M animals are intermediate. There is much variability in the data and neither study alone meets conventional criteria for reliability. More experiments are needed. But the high agreement between the experiments, each run by a different experimenter who was not informed of the strain identifications, encourages me to believe that the phenomenon is real. One could postulate that these presumed line differences in response to differing training schedules are associated with variable efficiency of short-term and long-term memory (Bovet, Bovet-Nitti, & Oliverio, 1969; McGaugh *et al.*, 1962). But factors associated with the physical and emotional stress of immersion could also be proposed legitimately as explanations. The area is certainly worth further study.

Audiogenic Seizure Susceptibility in BWS Mice

Observations on the course of behavioral development in the Roderick, Wimer, and Wimer lines (Fuller & Geils, 1973) and the Fuller lines (Ahroon & Fuller, 1976; Fuller & Herman, 1974; Herman & Nagy, 1977) suggest that the basic processes are similar in all lines, but that selection for brain weight has changed the timing of the appearance of new capacities. One problem with experiments on learning, and observations on neuromotor development, is the day-to-day variability often shown in the index behavior. Also, despite efforts to set objective criteria for rating activity and reflexes, a degree of subjectivity remains, particularly if one is trying to detect the first sign of a response. Audiogenic seizures have many advantages for developmental studies. The phenotype is unmistakable; it is manifested in clearly discrete levels of intensity; its frequency of occurence is known to be age related. For these reasons, a study was undertaken to determine if there were age-related differences in susceptibility to these seizures in the Fuller BWS lines.

Each subject was tested twice in order to determine both innate susceptibility to audiogenic seizures and sensitivity to priming (the induction of susceptibility by prior exposure to a sound stimulus that does not at the time produce a seizure) (Collins & Fuller, 1968; Fuller, 1975; Henry, 1967.).

Methods

In the first phase of the experiment, 55 litters from the three brain weight lines were taken from our colony. Large litters were reduced to eight young; when possible, with equal numbers of males and females. On Day 6 or 7, subjects were assigned at random to one of eight groups and toe-clipped for identification. Beginning on Day 12 and continuing through Day 19, the assigned member of each litter was weighed, placed in a test chamber and exposed to the sound of a doorbell (95–98 decibels) for 1 minute. Responses were recorded and later scored as: no seizure response (0); wild running only (1); clonic convulsion (2); tonic convulsion (3); fatal tonic convulsion (4). The scoring system was based on that of Henry and Bowman (1970). Two days after the first, or priming, trial, subjects were exposed to the bell for 1 min as on the initial trial. Bell ringing was terminated on all trials when an animal had a clonic seizure.

As this experiment progressed, it became evident that data were needed from older mice. Therefore, individuals from 32 additional litters were primed at Days 17 through 24 and tested for seizure susceptibility 2 days later. Except for the difference in the age of the subjects, all procedures were identical to those in the first phase.

Results

The most notable result of this experiment is shown in Figure X.6. Here the mean intensity scores of primed animals, aged 14–26 days, are shown separately by line. Their mean scores, when unprimed, at ages 14–24 days are represented by a single curve, since no significant differences between lines were found at any age. It is obvious that the majority of unprimed mice received scores of 0 or 1. However, when a convulsion occurred, it was as severe as those in primed animals.

From 14 to about 22 days, primed animals respond to the bell more intensely than do unprimed mice. This finding confirms previous experiments. More interesting for our purposes is the difference among the BWS lines from Day 19 through Day 22. On these days, the BWS-L line falls noticeably below the other lines. Analysis of variance confirmed the trend towards lower scores of L mice, with a borderline probability ($p < .10$) on each day. When the data were grouped by days

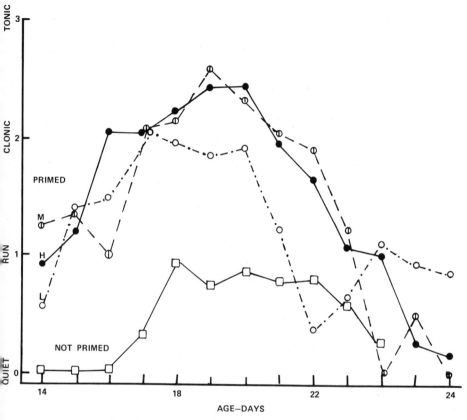

FIGURE X.6. Mean seizure intensity scores of primed and unprimed BWS mice 14–24 days of age.

(14–18, 19–22, and 23–26) and reanalyzed, the line difference for the middle period was highly significant ($p<.001$) (Table X.5). It may be objected that this analysis is based on a post hoc classification of the data, and it is true that the limits of the age ranges were determined after inspection of the data. However, the experiment was conducted to test the hypothesis that development of these lines is out of phase, and that differences in vulnerability to priming might define the period of the phase dislocation.

On only 4 consecutive days (19–22) do differences in seizure susceptibility of primed mice from the three lines approach significance. The orderliness of the data argue for their reliability and indicate developmental asynchrony in these lines.

TABLE X. 5
Mean Seizure Score[a] of BWS Mice at Three Age Ranges

		Age range (days)		
Line	Primed?	14–18	19–22	23–26
Combined	No	.28	.82	.56
Combined	Yes	1.57	1.93	.61
BWS-H	Yes	1.69	2.20	.68
BWS-M	Yes	1.56	2.26	.35
BWS-L	Yes	1.50	1.54	.73
		ANOVA of primed groups only		
	F	.49	8.68	1.31
	df	2,262	2,274	2,116
	p	.25	.001	.25

[a]No seizure, 0; running only, 1; clonic seizure, 2; tonic seizure, 3; fatal tonic seizure, 4.

Discussion

One interpretation of the data is that development of the nervous system is faster in BWS-L mice, so that the immunity to priming characteristic of most adults occur sooner. The idea that low brain weight mice mature earlier was proposed by Fuller and Geils (1972), on the basis of growth curves from the Roderick, Wimer, and Wimer lines. This concept is at odds with the idea that BWS-L mice are retarded. If so, they should retain their adolescent characteristics longer. It is also discordant with the finding that the brains of BWS-L mice seem to catch up with BWS-H brains between 42 days and late maturity. We seem to be dealing with a shift in the temporal programming of brain growth over a long period of life, rather than with a simple retardation or acceleration of the whole process.

Summary

Selection for high and low brain weight through sibling-breeding is successful, although there are difficulties in estimating heritability by standard methods. Changes in brain size are correlated with changes in body size of a somewhat lesser magnitude. Selection appears to operate through effects on the temporal patterning of brain growth. Behavioral changes also are correlated with changes in brain weight. For the most part these changes are rather subtle. A cause–effect relationship between the physical and behavioral characteristics of the BWS mice has not been demonstrated.

Acknowledgments

Many individuals not cited in the bibliography have helped in the care of the BWS lines and in the gathering of data concerning them. First among these is Patricia Wojdyla, who has had a major responsibility for the day-to-day management of the colony, coordination of experiments, and maintenance of records. She was a coinvestigator with me in the experiment on audiogenic seizure susceptibility in young mice. Lawrence Herman abstracted and organized the data on litter size. Debra Letai and Mary Healy conducted the water-maze experiments as independent study projects.

References

Ahroon, J. K., & Fuller, J. L. Performance characteristics of maze learning in mice selected for high and low brain weight. *Journal of Comparative and Physiological Psychology*, 1976, *90*, 1184–1190.

Bovet, D., Bovet-Nitti, F., & Oliverio, A. Genetic aspects of learning and memory in mice. *Science*, 1969, *163*, 139–149.

Collins, R. L., & Fuller, J. L. Audiogenic seizure prone (*asp*)—a gene affecting behavior in linkage group VIII of the mouse. *Science*, 1968, *162*, 1137–1139.

Fuller, J. L. Independence of inherited susceptibility to spontaneous and primed audiogenic seizures in mice. *Behavior Genetics*, 1975, *5*, 1–8.

Fuller, J. L., & Geils, H. D. Brain growth in mice selected for high and low brain weight. *Developmental Psychobiology*, 1972, *5*, 307–318.

Fuller, J. L., & Geils, H. D. Behavioral development in mice selected for differences in brain weight. *Developmental Psychobiology*, 1973, *6*, 469–474.

Fuller, J. L., & Herman, B. H. Effect of genotype and practice upon behavioral development in mice. *Developmental Psychobiology*, 1974, *7*, 21–30.

Fuller, J. L., & Wimer, R. E. Neural, sensory and motor functions. In Green, E. L. (Ed.), *Biology of the laboratory mouse* (2nd ed.). New York: McGraw-Hill, 1966. Pp. 609–628.

Hahn, M. E., Haber, S. B., & Fuller, J. L. Differential agonistic behavior in mice selected for brain weight. *Physiology and Behavior*, 1973, *10*, 759–762.

Henry, K. R. Audiogenic seizure susceptibility induced in C57BL/6J mice by prior auditory exposure. *Science*, 1967, *158*, 938–940.

Henry, K. R., & Bowman, R. E. Behavior-genetic analysis of the ontogeny of acoustically primed audiogenic seizures in mice. *Journal of Comparative and Physiological Psychology*, 1970, *70*, 235–241.

Herman, B. H., & Nagy, Z. M. Development of learning and memory in mice genetically selected for differences in brain weight. *Developmental Psychobiology*, 1977, *10*, 65–75.

Jensen, C. Generality of learning differences in brain-weight-selected mice. *Journal of Comparative and Physiological Psychology*, 1977, *91*, 629–641.

Jensen, C., & Fuller, J. L. Learning performance varies with brain weight in heterogeneous mouse lines. *Juornal of Comparative and Physiological Psychology*, 1978, *92*, 830–836.

Jerison, H. J. *Evolution of the brain and intelligence*. New York: Academic Press, 1973.

McGaugh, J. L., Jennings, R. D., & Thompson, C. W. Effect of distribution of practice on the maze learning of descendants of the Tryon maze bright and maze dull strains. *Psychological Reports*, 1962, *10*, 147–150.

Rensch, B. Increase of learning capability with increase of brain size. *American Naturalist*, 1956, *90*, 81–95.

Roderick, T. H., Wimer, R. E., & Wimer, C. C. Genetic manipulation of neuroanatomical traits. In L. Petrinovich & J. L. McGaugh (Eds.), *Knowing, thinking, and believing.* New York: Plenum, 1976. Pp. 143–178.

Searle, L. V. The organization of hereditary maze-brightness and maze-dullness. *Genetic Psychology Monographs,* 1949, *39,* 279–325.

Storer, J. B. Relation of lifespan to brain weight, body weight and metabolic rate among inbred mouse strains. *Experimental Gerontology,* 1967, *2,* 173–182.

Vandament, W. E., Burright, R. G., Fessenden, R. R., & Barker, W. H. Tables of event sequences for sequential analyses of data in psychological experiments containing two-class events. *Behavioral Research, Methods and Instrumentation,* 1970, *2,* 290–296.

Waller, M. B. Waller, P. F., & Brewster, L. A. A water maze for use in studies of drive and learning. *Psychological Reports,* 1960, *7,* 99–102.

Chapter XI

Learning Performance in Mice Genetically Selected for Brain Weight: Problems of Generality[1]

CRAIG JENSEN

The intent of this chapter is to examine the extent to which artificial selection based on brain weight in mice is associated with concommitant changes in learning performance. Attention will be directed primarily toward the brain weight selection programs carried out by John L. Fuller at the State University of New York at Binghamton, and by Thomas Roderick and Richard and Cynthia Wimer at The Jackson Laboratory, Bar Harbor, Maine. Summaries of the response to selection are available in this volume (see Chapters VII and X) and elsewhere (Fuller & Geils, 1972; Roderick, Wimer, & Wimer, 1976) and will not be reviewed here. The primary focus will instead be on the special problems posed by collateral pleiotropic effects of genes (Fuller & Thompson, 1960, pp. 77–79), and random fixation of alleles within the selected lines; the intent is to determine whether behavioral traits found in the selected lines may be attributed to variation in brain weight.

Assessment Problems Posed by Genetics

Pleiotropic Effects

A gene is said to have pleiotropic effects if it influences more than one character. The primary problem in trying to assess relations between a selected physiological character and behavior is to distinguish between

[1]This research was supported in part by Grant BMS 73-01499 from the National Science Foundation to John L. Fuller.

DEVELOPMENT AND EVOLUTION
OF BRAIN SIZE

lineal pleiotropic effects and effects due to collateral pleiotropism or to random fixation of alleles within lines (see Chapters VII, VIII, and X, this volume). While it may be easier to conceive of a lineal pleiotropic effect in which mice with bigger brains perform better on learning tasks, it is possible that the genes responsible for the differences in brain weight also determine differences in one or more of the following: brain neurotransmitters, blood supply to the brain, speed of neural transmission, body weight, or maternal behavior (see Chapter XIII, this volume). This list is not exhaustive, of course, but the main point is that differences in one or more correlated phenotypes may be responsible for a relation between brain weight and learning performance observed across the selected lines. Roderick *et al.* (1976) have used the term *indirectly conjoined trait* to refer to a character outside the pathway of primary interest, which has an influence on a particular phenotype. They point out that in order to control for indirectly conjoined traits, it is necessary to look for the most likely ones and show that they did not change during selection, or, if they did, they had no effect on behavior. Another approach is to incorporate the most likely indirectly conjoined traits in the selection criterion. For example, in trying to avoid body weight as an indirectly conjoined trait, Fuller (Fuller & Geils, 1972) based his brain weight selection (BWS) on deviations from a linear regression of brain weight on body weight.

Random Fixation

Random fixation of alleles within selected lines is likely under laboratory conditions in which inbreeding occurs, due to the small populations being used. Random fixation of alleles unrelated to brain weight within the selected lines could produce differences in task-specific abilities, thus obscuring the relation between brain size and learning performance. One way to circumvent this problem is to conduct several replicated selections. Finding the same correlated response in most of the selections would provide evidence for a pleiotropic effect and against random fixation. Using many replicated selections is impractical, however, because selection studies are time consuming and expensive. Another solution is to examine relations between brain size and behavior in genetically heterogeneous stocks. Because differences in variables affecting performance should be randomly distributed across subjects, relations between brain size and learning performance can be examined without the possible confounding effects of random fixation of alleles, and can thus provide further evidence regarding the existence of lineal or collateral pleiotropic effects.

Learning Performance in Lines Selected for Brain Weight

Subjects

All eight selected and unselected lines from the Fuller BWS selection (Fuller & Herman, 1973), and the two selections of Roderick (Roderick *et al.*, 1976), were available. A set of eight inbred strains were completely intercrossed, forming a heterogeneous foundation stock from which the Fuller BWS selection and one of the Roderick selections (SEL 17L–19B) were drawn. A different foundation stock, again resulting from the complete intercrossing of eight inbred strains, was used to form the second Roderick selection (SEL 16C–16H). From his foundation stock, Fuller used divergent selection to obtain a high (H) and low (L) line, and stabilizing selection to obtain a medium (M) line. The genetically heterogeneous foundation stock (HET) from which the H,M, and L lines were drived was also available for testing, which, with the M line, provided two control groups. The lines selected by Roderick included a low brain weight line (SEL 17L), its selected control (SEL 19B), a high brain weight line (SEL 16H), and its unselected control (SEL 16C). Thus, a total of two lines selected for low brain weight and two lines selected for high brain weight were available, as well as four control lines, one of which had been subjected to stabilizing selection. For further details regarding the origins of the two foundation stocks, see Jensen (1977) or Chapters VII and X, this volume.

Experimental Design

Although the number of replicated lines and the number of unselected mice are not large, they do permit conclusions about random fixation of alleles versus pleiotropic effects. For example, if high activity levels were found in both high brain weight lines, intermediate activity levels in the four control lines, and low activity levels in both low lines, strong evidence would exist for a pleiotropic effect (lineal or collateral) between brain weight and activity level. On the other hand, if no discernable relation between brain size and activity was found across selections, this would indicate that either no relation existed, or that random fixation of alleles within lines obscured it. Only easily measured phenotypes, which might prove to be indirectly conjoined traits, were assessed. Ambulation was measured in an open field, and activity level was measured in the shuttle box prior to both active avoidance and operant discrimination testing. Defecation was measured for all tasks except the water maze and passive avoidance, and body weight was measured approximately once a week throughout the experiment. Mean response rate over the 10 days of responding under the 1 min variable interval schedule of water reinforcement was used as a measure of motivation (see Clark, 1958).

The three unselected lines permitted relations between brain weight and learning performance to be examined without the possible confounding effects of random fixation of alleles; however, relatively few extreme values for brain weight were found, as compared to the extremes found between the high and low lines. Since brain weight differences were not extreme in the heterogeneous stocks, it was necessary to use tasks that were highly reliable. On each task, reliability was increased by testing the mice for relatively long periods of time, as compared to the usual time allotted for testing each mouse in most behavior–genetic studies. Table XI.1 shows the sequence of tasks and the number of sessions devoted to each. Reliability estimates for the various tasks were derived from the data of 93 mice that completed all

TABLE XI. 1

Task Order and Number of Sessions Each Procedure Was in Effect

Task	Sessions
1. Open field (2530 1x: 1 min each session)	4
2. Active avoidance[a]	
a. Assessment of activity level (light off; 20 min each session)	4
b. Assessment of reaction to CS (3 sec light on; 20 min)	1
c. Training (40 trials; 20 min each session)	12
d. Extinction (40 trials; 20 min each session)	6
3. and 4. Water maze (48 mice)	
a. Assessment of stimulus preference (black or white)	1
b. Training (problem is reversed whenever criterion of 9 correct in 10 trials is met)	29
OR	
3. and 4. Operant discrimination training (48 mice)[b]	
a. Assessment of operant level (light off; 20 min each session)	3
b. Response acquisition (light off; 40 reinforcements of .025 ml water)	1
c. Continuous reinforcement (40 reinforcements each session)	4
d. Continuous reinforcement—VI. 1 min (40 reinforcements per session)	2
e. VI 1 min (light on/light off; 40 min each session)	10
f. Discrimination training [S+ (light on)/S− (light off); 40 min each session]	30
5. Step-through passive avoidance training	5–16
	112–123

[a]Intertrial interval in b,c, and d controlled by a VI 31 sec tape.
[b]Stimulus duration in e and f controlled by VI 2 min tape.

phases of testing, and are presented in Table XI.2. Further details regarding these tasks are available in Jensen (1977).

When assessing learning performance in selected lines, it is important to remember that learning is inferred from performance. If all learning tasks are based on similar motivational, sensory, or activity substrates, indirectly conjoined traits or random fixation of alleles could influence performance across tasks, and thus bias the outcome of the behavioral assessments. In an attempt to avoid this problem, a different source of motivation was used for three of the four tasks, and different activity levels were required for optimal performance. In active avoidance, high activity level would tend to facilitate response acquisition (Fuller, 1970; Jensen, 1975). In the acquisition of discriminative responding in the operant chamber, high activity should exert minimal effects; yet in the acquisition of passive avoidance, high activity level should interfere with acquisition.

The final feature of this series of experiments was that "enriched environments" were provided for all mice from weaning (at 21 days of age) until the end of active avoidance testing (when the mice were about 80 days of age). Henderson (1970b) showed that genetic effects are expressed more fully when mice have been raised in enriched environments. For this reason, the enriched environments were provided to increase the probability of detecting a relation between brain size and behavior.

Since all the physiological and behavioral traits that could affect per-

Table XI. 2

Pearson Product–Movement Correlations (r) for Selected Dependent Variables

Task	Variable	r
Open field	Activity on Days 3 and 4	.59
Active avoidance	Activity on Days 3 and 4 prior to training	.85
	Number of avoidance responses on Days 1 and 2, 6 and 7, and 11 and 12	.33,.89,.79
	Number of avoidance responses on Days 3 and 4 of extinction	.77
Water maze	Number correct on Days 28 and 29	.57[a]
Operant discrimination	Mean relative S− response rate in five-session blocks 1 and 2, 3 and 4, and 5 and 6	.89,.90,.93
Passive avoidance	Latency on Days 2 and 3	.36

[a]Does not include mice that met criterion on Day 28 and therefore began a new problem on Day 29.

formance on these tasks are not known, the various features of the experimental design were probably not sufficient to overcome the problems of indirectly conjoined traits and random fixation. In addition, Jensen, Schmitt, Scheirer, & Cochran (1978) found that the active avoidance and operant discrimination tasks had little in common with the water maze and passive avoidance tasks; however, the extent to which these tasks sample learning ability in the mouse is also unknown. Nevertheless, it was felt that attempting to deal with these problems was better than ignoring them. Given these difficulties, the only way to evaluate the line differences in learning performance was to assume that if brain weight exerts large effects on learning, these effects will show up in spite of any differential task-specific abilities produced across the various lines by indirectly conjoined traits or random fixation of alleles. If a consistent relation between brain size and learning performance is not found across tasks and across selections, the relation between brain size and learning ability is not a strong one. The inclusion of the heterogeneous stocks permits the strength of the relation between brain size and learning to be assessed, even though it might not be apparent in the selected lines.

Line Differences

Possible Indirectly Conjoined Traits

The wet brain weight of each mouse was taken at the conclusion of passive avoidance training, when the mice were about 41 weeks of age. Following the procedure described by Wimer, Roderick, and Wimer (1969), dura mater, flocculonodular lobes, and hypophysis were removed, the optic nerve was cut at the chiasma, the trigeminal nerve was cut at the surface of the brain, and the spinal cord was cut at the base of the medulla, approximately 5 mm caudal to the cerebellum. Results for brain weight and characters possibly influenced by indirectly conjoined traits or random fixation of alleles within the selected lines are presented in Table XI.3.

The various brain weight lines within each selection differed, as expected, on average brain weight. The one exception to this statement was the BWS–L line, which did not differ significantly from either control line. A similar result for the BWS lines was also found for mice 8–21 days of age by Herman and Nagy (1977). For the results discussed here, this nonsignificant difference means that the H line must be superior in learning to the other lines, L, M, and HET, in order to support the hypothesis that brain weight is related to learning performance. With

TABLE XI.3

Line Means for Brain and Body Weight, Daily Means for Activity, Defecation, and Response Rate Measures during VI One Training[a]

	Brain weight (gm) (41 wks)	Body weight (gm) (41 wks)	Activity level			Defecation			Response rate
			Open field	Active avoidance (first 4 days)	Operant discrimination (first three days)	Open field	Active avoidance (first 4 days)	Operant discrimination (first 3 days)	
BWS Selection									
H	.573	40.1_a	59.4_a	$103.3_{a,b}$	$157.3_{a,b}$	$.7_a$	7.4_a	$3.1_{a,b}$	9.4_a
HET	$.528_a$	37.7_a	59.7_a	108.5_a	192.8_a	$.7_a$	7.6_a	3.9_a	9.1_a
M	$.529_a$	38.1_a	50.0_a	60.1_b	$111.7_{b,c}$	1.0_a	8.7_a	2.5_b	8.4_a
L	$.514_a$	34.6_a	49.5_a	60.5_b	108.4_c	$.7_a$	7.8_a	1.7_b	9.6_a
SEL 16C–16H selection									
16 H	.564	34.4_a	42.4_a	47.4	66.0	.8	7.5_a	2.0_a	11.1_a
16 C	.512	34.2_a	44.5_a	65.7	125.8	2.4	9.6_a	2.5_a	10.7_a
SEL 19B–17L selection									
19 B	.554	33.6_a	61.5	47.6	67.1	1.4_a	12.3	2.2	9.1_a
17 L	.481	31.7_a	68.0	65.6	107.4	1.2_a	9.5	3.7	10.9_a

[a]For each selection, means with common subscripts in each vertical column are not significantly different at the .05 level. Some of these data are from Jensen, C. Generality of learning differences in brain weight-selected mice, *Journal of Comparative and Physiological Psychology*, 1977, 91, 629–641. Copyright 1977 by the American Psychological Association. Reprinted by permission.

regard to indirectly conjoined traits, none of the measures reported in Table XI.3 show a statistically significant linear relationship, across selections, with brain weight. The assessements of activity level in both active avoidance and operant discrimination testing indicate that random fixation occurred for this character in all three selections. Since none of the measures in Table XI.3 shows a consistent relation, across selections, with brain weight, it is unlikely that a pleiotropic relation existed between brain weight and any of these measures.

Learning Performance

Results for all four learning tasks are presented in Table XI.4. To remove statistically the contribution of line differences in activity level from line differences in active avoidance training (Days 6–17), the number of avoidance responses was adjusted with an analysis of covariance (ANACOVA) procedure, with number of shuttle crossings on Days 1–4 as the covariate. Within the BWS selection, number of ANACOVA-adjusted avoidance responses increased with brain weight. In the SEL 17 L–19B and SEL 16 C–16 H selections, however, no relation between brain weight and active avoidance performance was apparent. Anderson's (1963) shape function was used to make the daily responses to extinction number relative to terminal acquisition and extinction performance, but none of the lines within the three selections showed reliable differences on this measure.

Mice from the SEL 16 C—16H selection were tested in the water maze, but their results are not presented because two SEL 16 C and three SEL 16H mice failed to meet criterion on the original problem. Median swimming speed on Day 1 was used as a covariate in analyzing both water maze measures, but the ANACOVA adjustment had virtually no effect on the line means. As with the shape function in active avoidance extinction, trials to first criterion in the water maze were unrelated to brain size. Number of reversals completed in 29 days did vary with brain size, but the relationship was not consistent across selections. Within the BWS selection, the L line successfully completed more reversals than the other three lines, thus producing a relationship between brain weight and learning performance that was quite different from the one found in active avoidance acquisition. Moreover, within the SEL 17 L–19B selection, the number of reversals completed increased with increased brain size.

For the operant discrimination, performance did not vary significantly within the BWS lines, but superior performance was again shown by the SEL 19 B line relative to the 17 L line. In the SEL 16 C–16 H selection,

TABLE XI.4
Learning Task Means for the Selected Lines[a]

	Active avoidance		Water maze		Operant discrimination: daily relative response rate in $S-$	Passive avoidance: trials to criterion
	Avoidance responses per day[b]	Shape function	Trials to first criterion	Number of reversals		
			BWS selection			
H	24.3_a	$.58_a$	51.2_a	2.8_a	$.60_a$	4.0_a
HET	$20.5_{a,b}$	$.14_a$	41.5_a	2.9_a	$.59_a$	6.2
M	20.6_a	$.42_a$	35.4_a	3.2_a	$.59_a$	3.8_a
L	15.2_b	$.35_a$	27.8_a	4.2	$.60_a$	3.9_a
			SEL 16 C–16 H selection			
16 H	15.4_a	$.09_a$	—	—	.48	5.1_a
16 C	13.2_a	$-.02_a$	—	—	.64	5.4_a
			SEL 19B–17 L selection			
19 B	15.2_a	$.28_a$	38.0_a	3.7	.58	5.8_a
17 L	17.6_a	$.46_a$	36.4_a	2.8	.55	5.2_a

[a]For each selection, means with common subscripts in each vertical column are not significantly different at the .05 level. Some of these data are from Jensen, Generality of learning differences in brain-weight-selected mice. *Journal of Comparative and Physiological Psychology*, 1977 *91*, 629–641.Copyright 1977 by the American Psychological Association. Reprinted by permission.

[b]Means after adjustment with analysis of covariance.

an inverse relation was found between brain size and discrimination performance.

For the passive avoidance task, the only significant difference in learning performance was found within the BWS selection, where the HET stock required more trials to meet criterion than the directionally selected lines. The use of escape latency on Day 1 as a covariate in assessing the line differences had virtually no effect on line means; thus, the differences on the trials to criterion measure were not seriously confounded with differences in escape latency.

Overall, the results for the three selections for brain weight offer little support for the hypothesis that learning ability increased with brain weight. Only within the SEL 17 L–19 B selection were the results consistent with the hypothesis. But even here there were too few significant differences to provide strong support since the superiority of the SEL 19 B line to the 17 L line easily could be the result of chance. The results for the other two selections provide even less support for the directional hypothesis. Of the three measures on which learning performance varied significantly within the BWS Selection, only one provided support for the hypothesis. The only significant performance difference found in the SEL 16 C-16 H selection was opposite to that specified by the directional hypothesis.

The only conclusions to be reached from the experiments with the selected lines were that brain weight was either unrelated to learning performance, or it was a relatively minor determinant of such performance. The task-specific abilities produced by collateral pleiotropic effects or random fixation of alleles might be more influential than brain weight. Fortunately, the use of unselected genetically heterogeneous mice allows a choice between these two conclusions, and rectifies what would otherwise be a serious deficiency of selection studies in general.

Brain–Behavior Correlations in Heterogeneous Stocks

The use of genetically heterogeneous stocks of mice permits the relation between brain size and learning performance to be assessed in spite of the possibility of confounded performance variables. Such variables are expected to be randomly distributed across subjects, and relations found in such stocks are therefore assumed to be functional ones. To determine whether any functional relations existed between brain weight and learning performance, data from the three heterogeneous stocks were pooled, and correlations between brain weight and learning performance were obtained.

As Table XI.5 shows, the signs of the three correlations between brain weight and learning performance for acquisition in active avoidance and in the water maze all indicate superior performance with increased brain weight. More specifically, negative correlations were found for both the active avoidance acquisition shape function and trials to first criterion in the water maze, while a positive correlation was found for number of reversals completed in the water maze.

In extinction, an interesting relation was found between the correlation for resistance to extinction and whether the response was paired with punishment. In the nonpunished active avoidance extinction and operant discrimination procedures, brain weight was positively correlated with resistance to extinction. In the water maze, however, the correlation between brain size and trials to criterion on the first reversal problem was negative ($r = -.23$; $r^2 = .05$, n.s.). In both the active avoidance and operant discrimination procedures, there was no direct punishment of the response undergoing extinction. In reversal learning in the water maze, an incorrect response was punished by a delay in escape from water. A tentative conclusion is that the correlation between

TABLE XI.5
Correlations between Brain Weight and Learning Performance[a]

Partialed variable	Active avoidance		Water maze		Operant discrimination: relative S− response rate	Passive avoidance: trials to criterion
	Training (shape function)	Extinction (shape function)	Trials to first criterion	Total criterions		
None	−.17	.37*	−.24	.40**	.42**	.07
	(.03)	(.14)	(.06)	(.16)	(.18)	(.00)
Open						.02
field	−.13	.26	−.20	.33	.32	
ambulation	(.02)	(.07)	(.04)	(.11)	(.10)	(.00)
Operant	−.17	.38*	−.22	.38*	.48***	.11
level	(.03)	(.14)	(.05)	(.14)	(.23)	(.01)
Body	−.21	.39*	−.29	.44***	.39*	.06
weight	(.04)	(.15)	(.08)	(.19)	(.15)	(.00)

[a]Numbers in parenthesis represent values for r^2. These data are from Jensen, C. & Fuller, J.L. Learning performance varies with brain weight in heterogeneous mouse lines. *Journal of Comparative and Physiological Psychology,* 1978, *92,* 830–836. Copyright 1978 by the American Psychological Association. Reprinted by permission.
 *$p<.05$
 **$p<.02$
 ***$p<.01$

brain size and resistance to extinction is positive when no punishment follows a response, and negative when responses were followed by punishment.

Examination of some of the possible indirectly conjoined traits in Table XI.6, showed that body weight, activity level, defecation, and motivation for water did not show significant correlations with brain weight. Thus, aside from the correlation with ambulation in the open field, these correlations were consistent with the life differences summarized in Table XI.3; they provided no evidence for any easily measured trait being indirectly conjoined with brain weight. In a recent review, Walsh and Cummins (1976) concluded that ambulation scores in an open field were not synonymous with activity level, and that such scores partially reflected learning and habituation. The moderate correlation of brain weight with ambulation in the open field, but not with measures of activity level, is consistent with their first conclusion. The decrements in the correlations between brain weight and learning performance, when ambulation in the open field was used as a covariate (Table XI.5), are consistent with Walsh and Cummins' second conclusion.

Although no significant correlation between brain weight and any measured, possible, indirectly conjoined traits was found, it was of interest to determine the degree to which some of the possible indirectly conjoined traits influenced the correlations between brain weight and

TABLE XI.6

Correlations of Brain Weight with Open Field Ambulation, Activity Level, Defecation, and Motivation Induced by Water Deprivation[a]

Measure	r
1. Body weight, 41 wks of age	.23 (.05)
2. Ambulation, photocell crossing in open field	.39* (.15)
3. Activity level	
a. Grid crossings during Days 1–4, active avoidance	−.02 (.00)
b. Swim speed on Day 1, water maze	.14 (.02)
c. Grid crossing during Days 1–3, operant discrimination	−.11 (.01)
d. Step-through latency on Day 1, passive avoidance	.11 (.01)
4. Defecation	
a. Open field	−.04 (.00)
b. Days 1–4, active avoidance	.20 (.04)
c. Days 1–3, operant discrimination	.10 (.01)
5. Response rate during VI 1 min, operant discrimination	.06 (.00)

[a]Numbers in parenthesis represent values for r^2. Some of these data are from Jensen C. & Fuller, J.L. Learning performance varies with brain weight in heterogeneous mouse lines. *Journal of Comparative and Physiological Psychology*, 1978, *92*, 830–836. Copyright 1978 by the American Psychological Association. Reprinted by permission.

*$p < .05$

learning performance. Therefore, partial correlations were used to hold operant level of responding and body weight statistically constant. The operant-level variables partialled out were, reading across Table XI.5, number of crossings in the 4 days prior to active avoidance training, number of avoidances on the final day of training, median speed of swimming during the 10 escape trials on Day 1 (used for both measures of performance in the water maze), mean response rate during nominal S- over the final 5 days of prediscrimination training, and step-through latency on Trial 1, respectively. In all cases, partialling out body weight or operant-level determinations from the correlation between brain weight and learning performance did not produce a large change (or a consistent increase or decrease) in the magnitude of the correlations. The correlations between brain weight and learning performance appear, therefore, not to be influenced by these variables to any important degree.

The present correlations replicate previous reports, summarized by Roderick *et al.* (1976), of superior performance in a water maze with spatial or brightness cues for mice with high brain weight, and of a positive correlation between brain weight and activity in an open field. In addition, the relation between brain weight and learning performance was extended to two new tasks. The generality of the relation between brain weight and learning performance was not an artifact of task similarity, since Jensen *et al.* (1978) found low commonality of the active avoidance task with both the water maze and the passive–avoidance task.

Conclusions

The correlations for the heterogeneous stocks indicate that brain weight in mice was associated with superior learning performance; the failure to find such a relationship across the lines selected for brain weight was due to the existence of task-specific abilities produced by collateral pleiotropic effects of the genes controlling brain weight or random fixation of alleles within the selected lines. This conclusion is consistent with selection studies based on a behavioral phenotype in which, in addition to the problems posed by collateral pleiotropic effects and random fixation, the selections were based on task-specific abilities. It is now obvious that such selection programs will almost certainly fail to find generality of behavior across tasks. The best known selection for intelligence in rats (Tryon, 1940) failed to produce rats that were superior on a variety of mazes to their so-called dull counterparts (see Searle, 1949). More recently, Satinder (1977) has subjected rat lines, selected for performance on an active avoidance task, to an extensive avoidance testing program; he concluded that the original selection was for task-specific abilities.

Selection programs based on a physiological phenotype such as brain weight would, at first glance, appear to avoid the problem of task-specificity found when a behavioral trait is subjected to selection pressure. Unfortunately, with the small populations typically found in selection programs, random fixation of alleles within the selected lines is very likely, and there is always the possibility that indirectly conjoined traits are present. Thus, it is unlikely that a general relationship between the physiological trait and behavior will be found, unless the animals are given an extensive battery of tasks. Testing for the hypothesized relation among genetically heterogeneous stocks is a more economical and less time-consuming method than selecting for either a physiological or a behavioral trait. Nevertheless, selection studies are useful because the response to selection provides evidence regarding the role of that trait in evolution. Naturally selected traits show high directional dominance, low heritability, and a slow response to selection; those traits that are unrelated to fitness, or that have an intermediate score associated with fitness, exhibit large additive genetic variance, high heritability, and a rapid response to selection (Broadhurst & Jinks, 1974). Unfortunately, with the practical limitations of time and laboratory space, selection studies are less useful in providing information regarding specific relations between psysiology and behavior, because many relations will be obscured by indirectly conjoined traits or random fixation of alleles. The dual problem of indirectly conjoined traits and random fixation require that the conclusions arrived at in any selection program be verified in heterogeneous stocks, or across many inbred strains.

With regard to one of the primary focuses of this volume, evolution of brain size, individual differences in brain size can have behavioral consequences. In mice at least, bigger brains are associated with superior learning performance. This is consistent with data obtained from a wide variety of species. Rensch (1956) found that for closely related species of different brain size, acquistion and retention of learned tasks increased with brain size. That brain size can be used to predict performance across species and across orders on an extradimensional shift problem has been shown by Riddell (Chapter V, this volume). When raised in standard cages or enriched environments, hybrid mice tend to have brains larger than the average of their parents (Hahn & Haber, 1978; Henderson, 1970a), which indicates that brain weight is a trait that has been subjected to selection pressure (Broadhurst & Jinks, 1974). Since learning performance increases with brain size, it seems reasonable to conclude that a larger brain confers a selective advantage upon an organism through its effect on learning ability. Thus, natural selection for animals with large brains may operate indirectly through the behavioral differences associated with different brain sizes.

Although the correlational data reported here are consistent with the hypothesis that learning performance increases with brain size, they do not conclusively show that number of "extra neurons" is responsible for the learning differences. Jerison (personal communication, 1978) has suggested that although some of the individual variation in performance must be associated with number of extra neurons, much of the variation within species may be associated with the arborization of neurons. The enrichment studies of Rosenzweig and his colleagues are consistent with this idea, since enrichment is known to increase aborization but not cell number (Diamond, 1976), and animals raised in enriched environments tend to perform better on at least some learning tasks (Davenport, 1976). Therefore, differences in learning performance, both within and across species, may be due to differences not only on number of extra neurons, but also perhaps to differences in arborization or other types of brain plasticity in response to environmental enrichment.

Future Behavior—Genetic Approaches to Brain—Behavior Relations

Any genetic approach to behavior that requires the testing of different genetic groups will be faced with the interpretive problems posed by task-specific abilities. Henderson's solution to this problem is to use a wide sampling of complex tasks, and a larger, more diverse sampling of genotypes than is found currently in most behavior–genetic investigations (see Chapter XVII, this volume). The latter recommendation is certainly appropriate, but with regard to the former, another approach may be more fruitful. As shown in Chapter V and here, the effects of brain size are apparent when the behavior under investigation is one of general biological significance, such as inhibition, acquistion, extinction, or discrimination learning. The findings reported here, that effects of brain size on behavior are apparent within genetically heterogeneous stocks but not across selected lines, further suggest that brain–behavior relations should be examined within heterogeneous stocks before more complicated group designs are attempted. The proposed strategy differs from Henderson's approach in that more different genotypes are represented per subject tested, and the tasks are designed to minimize the number of behavioral processes involved. Hopefully, both approaches will be used in obtaining further information regarding relations between variation in brain parameters and in behavior.

Acknowledgments

I gratefully acknowledge the valuable comments made by Richard G. Burright on an earlier version of this chapter. Thomas H. Roderick's contribution of parental stock from the SEL 17 L–19 B and SEL C–16 H selections is also gratefully acknowledged.

References

Anderson, N. H. Comparison of different populations: Resistance to extinction and transfer. *Psychological Review*, 1963, *70*, 162–179.

Broadhurst, P. L., & Jinks, J. L. What genetic architecture can tell us about the natural selection of behavioral traits. In J.H.F. van Abeelen (Ed.), *The genetics of behavior*. Amsterdam: North-Holland, 1974. Pp. 43–63.

Clark, F.C. The effect of deprivation and frequency of reinforcement on variable interval responding. *Journal of the Experimental Analysis of Behavior*, 1958,*1*, 221–228.

Davenport, J.W. Environmental therapy in hypothroid and other disadvantaged animal populations. In R.N. Walsh & W.T. Greenough (Eds.), *Environments as therapy for brain dysfunction*. New York: Plenum Press, 1976. Pp. 71–114.

Diamond, M.C. Anatomical brain changes indiced by environment. In L. Petrinovick & J.L. McGaugh (Eds.), *Knowing, thinking and believing*. New York: Plenum Press, 1976. Pp. 215–241.

Fuller, J.L. Strain differences in the effects of chlorpromazine and chlordiazepoxide upon active and passive avoidance in mice. *Psychopharmacologia* (Berlin), 1970, *16*, 261–271.

Fuller, J.L., & Geils, H.D. Brain growth in mice selected for high and low brain weight. *Developmental Psychobiology*, 1972,*5*, 307–318.

Fuller, J.L., & Herman, B. Effect of genotype and practice upon behavioral development in mice. *Developmental Psychobiology*, 1974, *7*, 21–30.

Fuller, J.L., & Thompson, W.R. *Behavior genetics*. New York: Wiley, 1960.

Hahn, M.E., & Haber, S.B. A diallel analysis of brain and body weight in male inbred laboratory mice (*Mus musculus*). *Behavior Genetics*, 1978, *8*, 251–260.

Henderson, N.D. Brain weight increases resulting from environmental enrichment: A directional dominance effect in mice. *Science*, 1970, *169*, 776–778. (a)

Henderson, N.D. Genetic influences on the behavior of mice can be obscured by laboratory rearing. *Journal of Comparative and Physiological Psychology*, 1970, *72*, 505–511. (b)

Herman, B.H., & Nagy, Z.M. Development of learning and memory in mice genetically selected for differences in brain weight. *Developmental Psychobiology*, 1977, *10*, 65–75.

Jensen, C. Active avoidance learning and activity level. *Behavior Genetics*, 1975, *5*, 98. [Also in Corrigendum, *Behavior Genetics*, 1976, *6*, 125]

Jensen, C. Generality of learning differences in brain-weight-selected mice. *Journal of Comparative and Physiological Psychology*, 1977, *91*, 629–641.

Jensen, C. and Fuller, J.L. Learning performance varies with brain weight in heterogeneous mouse lines. *Journal of Comparative and Physiological Psychology*, 1978, *92*, 830–836.

Jensen, C., Schmitt, J.C., Scheirer, C.J., & Cochran, T.L. Factor analysis of active avoidance and operant discrimination learning in mice. *Multivariate Behavioral Research*, 1978, *13*, 45–61.

Rensch, B. Increase in learning capacity with increase in brain size. *American Naturalist*, 1956, *90*, 81–95.

Roderick, T.H., Wimer, R.E., & Wimer, C.C. Genetic manipulation of neuroanatomical traits. In L. Petrinovich & J.L. McGaugh (Eds.), *Knowing, thinking and believing*. New York: Plenum Press, 1976. Pp. 143–178.

Satinder, K.P. Arousal explains difference in avoidance learning of genetically selected rat strains. *Journal of Comparative and Physiological Psychology*, 1977, *91*, 1326–1336.

Searle, L.V. The organization of hereditary maze-brightness and maze-dullness. *Genetic Psychology Monographs*, 1949, *39*, 279–325.

Tryon, R.C. Genetic differences in maze-learning ability in rats. *Yearbook of the National Society for the Study of Education*, 1940, *39*, 111–119.

Walsh, R.N., & Cummins, R.A. The open field test: A critical review. *Psychological Bulletin*, 1976, *83*, 482–504.

Wimer, C.C., Roderick, T.H., & Wimer, R.R. Supplementary report: Behavioral differences in mice genetically selected for brain weight. *Psychological Reports*, 1969, *25*, 363–368.

Chapter XII

Biochemical Correlates of Selective Breeding for Brain Size[1]

BRUCE C. DUDEK
PETER J. BERMAN

The Darwinian imperative to demonstrate evolutionary trends toward hominoid behavioral capacities was taken up with varying degrees of success (Bitterman, 1965) during the first century after Darwin's "The Expression of the Emotions in Man and Animals." As we continue toward the second century after Darwin, there appears to be a burgeoning interest in evolutionary aspects of brain–behavior relationships. In many cases, the focus of these investigations continued to be on intelligence and learning capacity. Improved behavioral methodology has helped recently in several instances to overcome some of the past confusion in this area (Masterton & Skeen, 1972; see also Chapter V, this volume). Exceptions to the emphasis on intelligence are inquiries into the evolution of sensory function (Masterton, Heffner, & Ravizza, 1969), and social behavior (Wilson, 1975). The work of Jerison (1973) has reemphasized the role of brain size as a useful evolutionary phenotype. While cross-species correlations of brain size and behavioral capacity have been impressive (Jerison, 1973; Chapter V, this volume), within-species studies have been less consistent. For example, considerable variability in brain size has been demonstrated in the mouse, and its genetic basis documented (Roderick, Wimer, Wimer, & Schwartzkroin, 1973). Variations in learning capacity have not shown a consistent cor-

[1]This work was supported by NSF Grant BMS 73-01499.

DEVELOPMENT AND EVOLUTION
OF BRAIN SIZE

relation with this morphological character (see Chapters I, V, and X, this volume).

This discrepancy between cross- and within-species studies is the focus of several other chapters in this volume, and has been a topic of interest in the literature (Van Valen, 1974). There is sufficient variation in both behavior and brain size for correlations to emerge. In fact, Warren (1973) has found that intraspecific variability in performance of learning tasks by Old World monkeys is frequently so great as to preclude cross-species comparisons. Intraspecific variability in behavior is a common occurrence and is based frequently on genetic factors (Fuller & Thompson, 1978).

The inconsistent relationship of these variables, brain size and behavior, is also a concern of this chapter. There are three general reasons why the size–behavior correlation might be so elusive. First, the behavioral phenotypes being studied may be inappropriate. This seems an unlikely explanation, however, since a wide variety of phenotypes have been evaluated in mice from two separate selective breeding programs and three heterogeneous stocks (Fuller, this volume; Jensen, 1977 and this volume; Jensen & Fuller, 1978, Roderick, Wimer, & Wimer, 1976; this volume). A second reason is that within a species, brain size is simply not related to behavior. This might be a plausible explanation, given the general assumption that neural organization, not mass, is the proximate cause of behavior. Size may only be an artifact. This alternative is difficult to accept, however, in the face of the large differences in brain size produced by selective breeding in the mouse (see Chapters V and X, this volume). The sheer magnitude of the difference between heavy- and light-brained animals strongly suggests organizational differences as well. A third alternative is that searches for positive brain weight-behavior correlations might have obscured more interesting questions. Studies by Jensen (1977), Ahroon and Fuller (1976), and Hahn, Haber, & Fuller (1973) have all shown differences among the three Fuller-BWS lines selectively bred for brain weight. These differences, however, did not follow a pattern related to brain size, and in fact, genotypic differences varied with task.

It is plausible that behavioral correlates of selection for brain size do exist, but that gross brain weight is not a sufficient predictor variable. An alternative approach is suggested by work of Fuller and Herman (1974), in which examination of developmental rates in the Fuller–BWS mice yielded consistent genotype–behavior correlations. Gradations in developmental rates were such that heavier-brained animals developed more rapidly. This suggests a genetic control of rates of neural development. At least one area of human behavior genetics has also examined this question. The Louisville Twin Project has studied the role of genetics in cognitive development. Wilson (1972) has reported that the patterns of infant mental development in monozygotic co-twins is more similar than in dizygotic co-twins. These findings were interpreted as evidence for genetic control over patterning of mental development.

Epstein (Chapter VI, this volume) has suggested that patterns of brain growth spurts and plateaus may predict behavioral development in many species. In view of these studies from divergent areas, it is our assumption that there may be genetic control of brain growth rates and correlated behavioral development. Furthermore, the timing and durations of critical or sensitive periods may differ among genotypes, such that the effects of early experience might differ in organisms differing in rates of neural development.

In order to begin to ask questions about correlated neural and behavioral growth, we have chosen to study the biochemical development of neural tissue from the Fuller–BWS lines. Our preliminary studies have examined DNA content as a measure of cell number, and protein content as a partial index of neural complexity. These simple characterizations should form a basic data base from which more detailed questions of genetic regulation of neural development can be asked. Additionally, we will present data of neurotransmitter content in these lines of mice. Investigations into development of neurotransmitter systems recently have become a frequent means of examination of functional development and its behavioral consequences (Lanier, Dunn, & Van Hartesveldt, 1976).

Brain Weight Development

Brain weights of mice from the Fuller–BWS lines are shown in Tables XII.1 and XII.2. The patterns of growth reveal several interesting characteristics. At birth, brains from mice of the High (H) and Medium (M) lines are nearly the same weight, whereas those from the Low (L) line are lighter. It is possible that the H brains do not weigh more because larger brains, and therefore skulls, would impair normal birth. This interpretation is consistent with the fact that skull size is the limiting factor in length of gestation. By postnatal day 21, wide separation of the brain weights among the lines is apparent. Thus, even though the phenotype for the original selection was 42-day brain weight, there is clear separation much earlier. This fact, along with other evidence mentioned (in Chapter X, this volume) suggested that rate of development varied among lines in an H>M>L fashion. This is certainly true in terms of amount of brain weight gained from birth to 21 days of age. Alternatively, consideration of percentage of adult values at each age provides a different picture. At birth mean values for M and L mice were 19.7% and 20% of mean adult values. However, mice from the H line had attained only 17% of the adult weight. At 21 days the values were 88.9%, 91.9%, and 93.8% for H, M, and L brains, respectively. In this sense, the degree of maturity may be inversely related to brain size. Perhaps at least some subsystems in the H line are slower to reach functional maturity. This may begin to explain Hahn's (this volume) failure to find consistent superiority of the H line and inferiority of the L line on measures of relative behavioral development prior to 21 days. Simply stated, functional maturity and greater weight might not be the same thing. After 21 days it is clear that H brains continue to gain more weight, both in gross and relative terms. From 21 days to 53–55 days the weight gains expressed as percentage of adult values are 11.1%, 8.1%, and 6.2% for H, M, and L mice, respectively. Thus Fuller and Herman's (1974) suggestion of an extended period of growth in the H mice seems to be accurate some 20 generations later.

Table XII.1 also presents data of dry brain weights of 21-day-old animals. The line differences in dry weights are marked ($p<.01$) and certainly elminate any possibility that the net weight differences are due

TABLE XII. 1
Whole Brain Wet Tissue Weights[a]

Age (days)	Line		
	H	M	L
0[b]	90.2 ± 1.2 (38)	89.3 ± 1.6 (35)	82.8 ± .9 (42)
21	470.7 ± 5.1 (15)	416.4 ± 3.1 (30)	388.2 ± 2.7 (27)
53–55	529.3 ± 6.1 (13)	453.0 ± 6.0 (18)	413.6 ± 4.2 (23)
	Dry weights[c]		
21	114.6 ± 11.9 (11)	91.9 ± 2.8 (10)	80.9 ± 1.0 (8)

[a]Data are expressed as mean mg tissue ± S.E.M. Numbers of samples are found in parentheses. Mice were from generations 20 and 21.

[b]Neonatal weights do not include cerebellum that weigh less than 5 mg at birth.

[c]We thank John Fuller for these data, which come from animals of the twelfth generation.

TABLE XII.2
Partitioned Brain Weights[a]

Age (days)	Line		
	H	M	L
21 cerebellum	57.6 ± 1.3	48.1 ± .9	47.5 ± .9
Remainder	414.0 ± 3.8	368.4 ± 2.5	340.7 ± 2.3
	(15)	(30)	(27)
53–55 cerebellum	66.2 ± 1.3	56.2 ± 1.1	51.2 ± 1.2
Remainder	463.2 ± 5.0	396.8 ± 5.2	362.3 ± 3.5
	(13)	(18)	(23)

[a]Data are expressed as mean mg wet tissue weight ± S.E.M. Numbers of samples are in parentheses.

solely to water content. If the mean dry weights for each line are expressed as a percentage of wet weight means, the values for H, M, and L brains are 24%, 22%, and 21% respectively. The higher percentage in the H line may in part result from a higher density of protein in the H brains (see following).

Table XII.2 presents data for brains partitioned into two parts: the cerebellum, and remainder. The pattern of greater growth in the H line after 21 days is apparent in both these parts. The cerebellum, which shows most of its growth postnatally, has reached 86%, 86%, and 92.7% for the H, M, and L lines respectively. Thus the L line appears to have achieved relatively more of its adult size at an earlier stage. The most striking aspect of the data from Table XII.2 is that by 21 days, both cerebellum and remainder of H mice weigh more than do those parts of M and L brains at 53–55 days. The large magnitude of line differences is thus reemphasized.

In general these data suggest that the relationship of the adult brain weight to developmental pattern is complex. While in some ways an H brain may gain weight more rapidly, it does so over a different time course than does the M brain, which also differs from the L brain. These subtleties in temporal growth patterns are likely to reflect differences in functional maturation as well.

Biochemical Characteristics

Procedures

Neonatal and adult (53–55 days) mice of the H, M, and L lines were obtained from generations 20 and 21. Subjects were sacrificed by decapitation and the brain was immediately removed and transferred to a watch glass over ice. Cerebella were rapidly dissected. The remainder of the brain from older animals was split longitudinally. The tissue was rapidly weighed, frozen on dry ice, and then stored at $-40°C$ until assay.

Cerebella from neonates were discarded, and from adults were used in the DNA-protein determinations, as was the remainder of the neonatal brain. Of the two adult hemispheres, one was used in DNA-protein determination, and the other in catecholamine determination. Two or three neonatal brains of same-sex animals from the same litter were pooled for assay purposes. Two or three samples were also pooled for cerebellar DNA-protein determinations.

Nucleic acid extraction and assay used a modification of the procedure of Howard (1974). Tissue samples were homogenized in cold acetone-ethanol (1/1, v/v) using a motor driven teflon pestle in a glass tube in ice (1 gm tissue/25 ml). The homogenate, less 10% for protein determination, was centrifuged at 12,000 × g for 15 min, and the supernatant was discarded. Extraction continued by resuspension of the pellet in chloroform-methanol (2/1, v/v) for 1 hour at room temperature. After centrifugation again for 15 min at 12,000 × g, the supernatant was discarded and the pellet was resuspended in chloroform-methanol (1/2, v/v) with 5% H_2O for 30 min at room temperature. After centrifugation at 12,000 × g for 15 min, the supernatant was discarded. The pellet was washed with 95% ethanol (ETOH), and placed on ice where it received two successive washes with cold 5% trichloroacetic acid. The pellet was resuspended in 4.5 ml of 5% trichloroacetic acid and placed in a shaking water bath at 90°C for 25 min. The sample was centrifuged for 25 min at 30,000 × g and the supernatant saved. The pellet was then resuspended in another 4.5 ml of trichloroacetic acid, the procedure repeated, and the supernatants combined for DNA determination.

DNA content in the pooled supernatants was assayed by Burton's method (1956). Standard curves were determined with salmon sperm DNA (Sigma Type III). Interference by RNA in the DNA absorption was nonexistent. Protein content was determined by the method of Lowry, Rosebrough, Farr and Randall, (1951). DNA estimates were derived as the mean of duplicate determinations. Protein estimates were derived as the mean of triplicate determinations.

Fluorometric determination of norepinephrine (NE) and dopamine (DA) were accomplished with modifications of standard procedures (Dudek, 1978). Nanogram estimates of the catecholamines were made from half brains of the male mice used for DNA and protein determinations. Estimations of whole brain content (minus cerebellum) were made by extrapolation on a wet tissue weight basis; ratios of transmitter to protein were also made for each sample.

Data Analysis

Whole brain (minus cerebellum) DNA and protein values were estimated by adjustment of single hemisphere values on a wet tissue weight basis, as was done for NE and DA. Ratios of the parameters and tissue weight were computed with these estimated values. Simple doubling of single hemisphere values resulted in nearly identical values for whole brain estimates, as did the weight adjustment procedure.

Analysis of variance was performed on each measure for each age group. Where appropriate, line and sex were included as factors. No analyses produced a significant effect of sex; the line by sex interaction also was not significant. Therefore, these effects will not be discussed further. Additionally, trend analysis of the line factor always was performed, and linear and quadratic components obtained. All significance levels reported represent tests of the linear component, except where the quadratic effect is discussed. In all cases where the linear component was significant, the overall effect of line was also significant.

DNA and Protein Content

Figure XII.1 presents DNA and protein data from young adult mice from the three selected lines. These data are from the whole brain minus cerebellum. Amounts of DNA per brain vary widely among the three lines ($p<.001$). Brains of H mice contained about 20% more DNA (and thus cells) than brains of L mice. The total difference in DNA between H and L brains represents about 18% of the average of the two lines. This figure is smaller than the 25% of average wet weight represented by the H–L difference. Thus, while cell numbers are highly different in the expected direction, not all the difference in weight is explained by this measure. Support for this statement may be found in the μg DNA/gm ratios (Figure XII.1). It is clear from the figure that cellular density is is inversely related to weight. Thus H brains have fewer cells per gram than M brains, which in turn have fewer than L brains ($p<.01$). Cell size therefore apparently changed, as well as cell number. A more direct estimate of cell size is the ratio of protein to DNA. This ratio (mg protein/μg DNA) also differed among the lines in an H>M>L fashion ($p<.01$). Total protein and protein density (per gm tissue) are also similarly different among the lines ($p<.05$ and $p<.01$ respectively). Predictably, the

H line increases in cell size and L line decreases are related to the amount of protein per cell.

Neonatal DNA measurements are probably a more precise index of neuron number than are adult DNA levels. In the mouse as in the rat, glial cell number at birth is minimal, and thus DNA content reflects only neurons and neuroblasts. At this age, the DNA content of H brains is larger, and in L brains it is smaller than in the M line ($p<.001$, see Figure XII.2). The difference between the lines is about 12% of their average

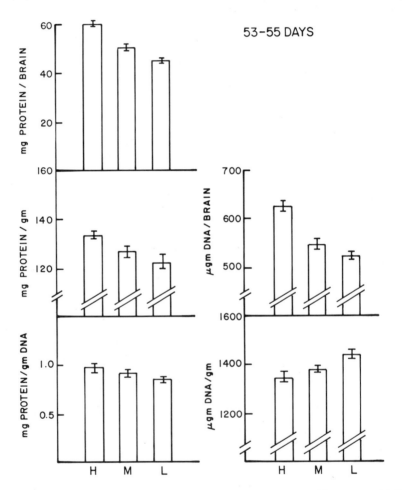

FIGURE XII.1 DNA and protein levels and concentrations are presented for young adult BWS mice. The histograms represent data from 13, 18, and 22 samples of H, M, and L mice respectively. Data are presented as means ± S.E.M., pooled across sex since no sex differences were observed.

values, substantially less than the 18% of young adults. This indicates that not all the differences in cell number of young adults are predictable from neonatal cell number. A substantial portion of the adult line differences in cell number must originate postnatally. Perhaps the postnatally developing cerebellum accounts for this added differential (see following). No significant line differences existed in the neonatal ratio of μg DNA/mg weight. Protein levels in the L line were lower than in H and M brains, which did not differ, as can be seen in Figure XII.2.

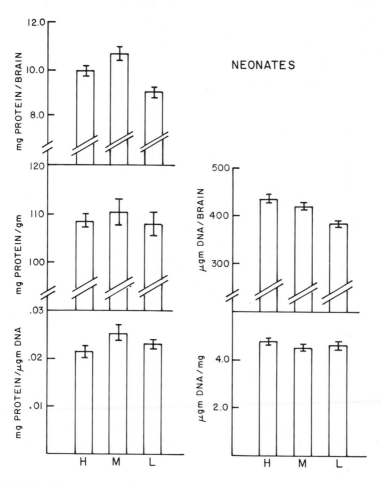

FIGURE XII.2. DNA and protein levels and concentrations are presented for neonatal BWS mice. The histograms represent data from 16, 8, and 17 samples of H, M, and L mice respectively. Data are presented as means ±, S. E. M., pooled across sex since no sex differences were observed.

Analysis of variance on this measure produced a significant quadratic trend ($p<.01$). This is the same pattern that neonatal brain weight followed in these lines. Thus, neonatal brain weight may be more related to protein concentrations than to cell number. Protein density (per gm tissue or per gm DNA) did not differ among the lines.

Cerebellar DNA and protein concentrations are shown in Table XII.3. DNA levels in cerebellum are not as precise an estimate of cell number, since purkinje cells are tetraploid. Thus line differences in total cerebellar DNA might reflect small differences in purkinje cell number, larger differences in diploid cell number, or a combination of the two. The observed line differences are nonetheless large and parallel to the weight differences. The difference between H and L cerebellar DNA represents about 25% of the average of the two lines, while the wet weight difference represents about 23% of the average weight. Thus the cerebellar weight differences are probably completely based on cell number. Accordingly, no line differences in cellular density would be expected, and in fact this is the case (μg DNA/100 mg; Table XII.3).

Protein content in cerebellum varied among lines in somewhat different fashion. High line cerebella contained greater than 50% more protein than either M or L cerebella, which did not differ (linear and quadratic components both significant, $p<.01$). This pattern of line differences was also seen in the density measures of mg protein/gm and mg protein/μg DNA; both showed higher concentrations of protein in H than in M or L samples (linear and quadratic components were significant, $p<.05$). This facet of protein distribution, in absence of cellular density or size differences in cerebellum, suggests the possibility of

TABLE XII.3
Cerebellar DNA and Protein[a]

	Line		
	H	M	L
μg DNA	477.52 ± 19.7 (6)	409.00 ± 12.3 (8)	394.25 ± 11.3 (8)
μg DNA/gm wet weight	7191.2 ± 304.3	7283.2 ± 213.3	7243.6 ± 193.1
mg protein	8.88 ± .05	5.64 ± .30	5.43 ± .39
mg protein/ gm wet weight	134.1 ± 8.0	101.4 ± 5.8	101.1 ± 6.3
mg protein/ μg DNA	.019 ± .001	.014 ± .0005	.014 ± .001

[a]Numbers present mean ± S.E.M. for each measure. Animals were 53–55 days of age. Numbers in parentheses are number of samples.

differences in the genetic regulation of cellular complexity. These lines may thus serve as a useful tool in the study of genetic control of postnatal cerebellar development, much as the neurological mutants have in the past (Caviness & Rakic, 1978).

In summary, these data provide several new insights into the characteristics of the Fuller–BWS lines. Although behavioral characterization has implied postnatal developmental differences among the lines, it is clear that adult differences in brain size are foreshadowed by neonatal DNA levels. Therefore, rates of neuroblast formation are surely different prenatally in the three lines. Adult size differences include not only changes in cell number, but also cell size. The postnatally developing cerebellum has much of the same pattern of line differences, with the exception of cellular density.

Neurotransmitter Characteristics

As the emphasis in this chapter has suggested, one of the major tasks of the neurosciences is understanding the mechanisms by which genetic and environmental factors act together to produce the complex pattern of neural communication. One such area of study has involved examining developmental trends in neurotransmitter systems. This reflects that the most basic problems in developmental neurobiology are questions regarding the establishment and maintenance of synapses. Such studies have examined the developmental patterns of neurotransmitter concentrations, neurotransmitter biosynthetic and degradatory enzymes, receptor binding capacities, as well as functional maturation (see Lanier et al., 1976 for review).

A large number of investigations have centered on the development of the catecholamine systems in brain tissue (Coyle, 1974). Norepinephrine and dopamine, although both present at birth in the mouse, show striking developmental increases that last well past weaning. Both are found at 20–40% of adult concentrations at birth, but their postnatal developmental patterns differ (Agrawal, Glisson, & Himwich, 1968; Alhava & Klinge, 1972). Norepinephrine attains adult levels by about 4 weeks after birth in the rat and mouse. Dopamine levels, however, continue a more gradual increase until postpuberty. These neurotransmitters may therefore prove to be fruitful in studies of correlated development of brain biochemistry and behavior.

Genetic involvement in regulation of catecholamine systems has also been demonstrated. Inbred strains of mouse have been shown to vary substantially in their content of biogenic amines (Sudak & Maas, 1964), as well as in the activities of the amine-related enzymes (Kessler, Ciaranello, Shire, & Barchas, 1972).

In the present set of studies, we have examined NE and DA content in the Fuller–BWS lines. We hoped to find genotypically based differences that might then serve as a starting point for investigations into genetic control of catecholamine development. Specifically, if transmitter levels are related consistently to brain size, then common mechanisms underlying brain weight development and catecholamine development might be postulated.

Table XII.4 depicts NE and DA results. It is apparent that whole brain levels of these two catecholamines are not regulated in the same way among the three lines. NE levels are constant in each line (ng/brain), and therefore concentration per gm tissue is ordered in a L>M>H fashion ($p<.05$). Concentrations of NE when expressed per mg protein are also ordered in the L>M>H fashion on ($p<.05$). This is to be expected, since protein levels among these lines were highly related to weight (see preceding). The regulation of dopamine levels was, however, in marked contrast to that of NE. DA levels per brain were highly different among the lines, with H animals containing the most, and L animals the least ($p<.01$) of this transmitter. Expression of DA levels on a wet weight or mg protein basis thus produced equivalencies among the three lines. This pattern of transmitter concentration is what one would normally expect from brain tissue. In fact, concentrations are usually expressed on a wet tissue weight basis. The implicit assumption is that regulation is based on the amount of tissue to be innervated. That is, we would generally expect a constant amount of transmitter per gm tissue. The failure of NE to follow this pattern is somewhat puzzling. This fact, as well as the differences in NE and DA patterns among the three lines, require further discussion.

TABLE XII.4
Catecholamine Levels[a]

		Line		
		H (6)[b]	M (7)	L (9)
ng/brain	DA**	325.6 ± 15.8	278.0 ± 18.3	244.7 ± 13.1
	NE	168.5 ± 10.7	164.3 ± 9.1	179.5 ± 14.4
ng/gm wet	DA	694.1 ± 28.7	701.5 ± 49.7	665.5 ± 38.8
weight	NE*	360.0 ± 24.0	415.9 ± 27.6	488.9 ± 39.5
ng/mg	DA	5.55 ± .35	5.58 ± .38	5.30 ± .34
protein	NE*	2.87 ± .21	3.33 ± .28	3.91 ± .35

[a]Data represent mean ± S.E.M. of male subjects of age 53–55 days.
[b]Numbers in parentheses are numbers of samples.
*$p<.05$ (linear component).
**$p<.01$ (linear component).

Differing levels of neurotransmitters may arise from a number of sources. If the numbers of neurons using a particular transmitter varied, we might predict that the content of that transmitter would also vary. Alternatively, number of terminals per neuron or amount of transmitter per terminal might differ among genotypes, thus producing different transmitter content. Support for the first possibility may be found in the work of Ross, Judd, Joh, Pickel, and Reis (1976). These investigators have demonstrated that differing amounts of tyrosine hydroxylase in dopamine neurons (of midbrain origin) from two inbred strains of mice has its basis in different numbers of these DA neurons. That is, CBA/J mice have fewer DA cells than BALB/cJ mice, and their tyrosine bydroxylase (TH) activities differ accordingly. Thus, these differing TH activities are not the result of differential arborization of DA containing axons, but simply the result of differing DA cell numbers. The activity of the rate limiting enzyme of DA synthesis, TH, appears to be under a control intrinsic to the DA cell, and not necessarily under the influence of target tissues. The Ross *et al.* (1976) study did not present data showing levels of dopamine in the brains of these mice, but parsimony would lead one to believe that the CBA-J strain, with fewer DA neurons, would also contain less DA.

The data under consideration from the BWS mice might very well be explained by a similar mechanism. We know from DNA estimates that overall cell number varies widely among the H, M, and L lines. The weight difference among the lines appears to be a general characteristic of all brain areas, and not only cortex or cerebellum for example (Dudek, unpublished data; this is also true of the Roderick–Wimer mice selected for brain size; see Wimer, this volume). It is plausible then that the number of neurons containing DA that arise in areas A9 and A10 (Ungerstedt, 1971) of the midbrain might also differ in an H>M>L fashion. These areas give rise to the nigrostriatal, mesolimbic, and mesocortical DA systems, which contain the bulk of brain dopamine (Moore & Bloom, 1978). We suggest that the BWS differences in DA content might result then from differing numbers of dopaminergic neurons. The primordial tissues that will give rise to the A9 and A10 areas begin to form about 1 week prior to birth in the rat (Lanier *et al.*, 1976). Further examination of the earliest development in BWS lines of these areas thus is suggested strongly.

The pattern of NE concentrations in the BWS mice clearly is reflective of a different developmental-regulatory mechanism than that just suggested for DA projections. At first glance this is most surprising, since both transmitters are catecholamines, synthesized by the same biochemical pathway that uses TH as the rate limiting enzyme (Axelrod,

1965). However, Joh and Reis (1975) have shown that the TH in DA neurons may not be the same form of TH present in adrenergic neurons. It is possible that different genes code for similar yet distinct forms of the same enzyme in the two types of catecholamine neurons. The probability of differential genetic regulation of this enzyme might be speculated on as a basis for the apparent differential regulation of the two catecholamines.

A more interesting possibility involves the manner in which the NE projections develop. The majority of brain NE (particularly cortical) arises from a comparatively small nucleus in the brain stem, the Locus Coeruleus (LC) (Lindvall & Bjorkland, 1974). Each nucleus (LC is bilaterally represented) contains only about 1500 cell bodies, but each cell may project in ascending and descending fashion, and innervate diverse areas in neocortex and subcortex. This extensive arborization of NE axons is the characteristic feature of LC cells. Thus NE levels might be related more closely to the extent of the plexiform innervation of target tissue than to LC cell number. Additionally it is suggested that the extent of this arborization is influenced by target tissues. Establishment of adrenergic innervation in the sympathetic nervous system is certainly influenced by extrinsic factors (Black, & Mytilineou, 1976) and the CNS may be no different (Bjorkland & Stenevi, 1972). Recently, Johnston Reinhard, and Coyle (1979) have concluded that the development of NE innervation of the neocortex is influenced by "local factors in the terminal field." This hypothesis of extrinsic control of NE development is consistent with the findings of the present studies. BWS-L mice showed the highest concentrations of NE (per gm weight and per mg protein). The L mice also have more cells per gram of tissue (μg DNA/gm). Therefore, in order to innervate the same number of cells in a gram of brain tissue in an L mouse and in an H mouse, more dense networks of NE terminals should develop in the brain of an L mouse. This hypothesis admittedly ignores the fact that cells in H brains may be larger than in L brains (see preceding), and larger innervation per cell might thus be required. Nonetheless this working hypothesis is exactly the type that we had hoped these preliminary data would suggest. Predictions of this hypothesis will be discussed below.

It seems then that DA and NE systems may be under differing kinds of control during development. The DA projections may develop under intrinsic control. Dopaminergic terminals, with functional DA synthetic enzymes, may even reach their terminal fields before postsynaptic functionality is achieved (Lanier *et al.*, 1976). NE projections alternatively may develop under considerable control of extrinsic factors in the terminal field. The establishment and perhaps maintenance of synapses using these two catecholamines may be a prime object for study of correlated development of brain and behavior. For example, chronic blockade of DA receptors during development might not have an effect on the maturation of the presynaptic terminal. This type of study, using chronic blockade of β-adrenergic receptors during development, would markedly alter adrenergic innervation, if the hypothesis were correct. This would be accomplished perhaps by a hindrance of "functional validation" (Jacobson, 1969) in the establishment of NE synapses. Correlated alterations in behavioral development following such treatment would then provide evidence for the types of behaviors influenced by that particular transmitter.

Conclusions

These data may be compared with similar parameters in the Roderick-Wimer selected lines (see chapters by Roderick, Wimer, and Zamenhof & van Marthens, this volume). In both selection studies, neonatal cell number was higher in heavy brained lines, but protein concentrations in neonates did not differ among lines. A substantial difference in adult parameters exists between the two selection programs. We have found differences in cellular density such that L brains have more cells per unit tissue (whole brain minus cerebellum). Zamenhoff and van Marthens (this volume) have found heavy brained adults to have greater cellular density. In addition, we find that not only do H brains have more cells, but the cells are larger. The Roderick–Wimer lines apparently do not differ in cell size. Protein density (mg protein/gm wet tissue weight) is greater in the H brains of each selection program. Comparisons of cerebellar parameters produce similar results, except that cellular density is equivalent across lines in both sets of selected lines.

Reasons for these biochemical differences between the two selection programs are not apparent. Biochemical procedures were very similar and therefore unlikely to be the source of the discrepancies. It should be noted that the major finding of both studies may be the large differences in cell number at birth. Thus, both selections have produced differences in prenatal rates of neuroblast formation, as well as postnatal growth differences, which seem to be reflected in behavioral development (see Fuller, this volume; Herman & Nagy, 1977). The major differences in cell density and cell size between the two selection programs could reflect differences in selection procedure (Fuller, this volume; Roderick, this volume).

In a large selective breeding program for body size in mice, Falconer,

Gauld, and Roberts (1978) have found that both cell number and cell size change as selection progresses. Heavy mice have larger and more numerous cells in a variety of tissues, although the brain was not measured. Perhaps of greater interest is the interpretation by Falconer and coworkers that selection for body weight operated by altering the timing of normal processes of cellular growth. This is precisely what has been suggested for the Fuller–BWS program. Thus both body weight selection and brain weight selection have altered cell number and cell size; the possibility that the same growth mechanisms might have been altered in each case is certainly of interest. Furthermore, the observed different patterns of neurotransmitter levels has again emphasized the developmental mechanisms by which these differences arise. It is our hope that these lines of mice will serve as useful tools in investigations of the development of neurotransmitter systems, as well as in correlated development of brain biochemistry and behavior.

Acknowledgments

We thank John L. Fuller, Peter J. Donovick, and Linda P. Spear for laboratory facilities and advice. We also thank John Guastella and John Brick for technical assistance.

References

Agrawal, H.C., Glisson, S.N., & Himwich, W.A. Developmental changes in monoamines of mouse brain. *International Journal of Neuropharmacology*, 1968, *7*, 97–101.

Ahroon, J.K., & Fuller, J.L. Performance characteristics of maze learning in mice selected for high and low brain weight. *Journal of Comparative and Physiological Psychology*, 1976, *90*, 1184.

Alhava, E., & Klinge, E. Age and brain catecholamine content as factors influencing amphetamine toxicity in mice. *Acta Pharmacologica et Toxicologica (Kbh)*, 1972, *31*, 401–411.

Axelrod, J. The metabolism, storage and release of catecholamines. *Recent Progress in Hormone Research*, 1965, *21*, 597–622.

Bitterman, M.E. Phyletic differences in learning. *American Psychologist*, 1965, *20*, 396–410.

Bjorkland, A., & Stenevi, U. Nerve growth factor: Stimulation of regenerative growth of central noradrenergic neurons. *Science*, 1972, *175*, 1251–1253.

Black, I.B., & Mytilineou, C. The interaction of nerve growth factor and trans-synaptic regulation in the development of target organ innervation by sympathetic neurons. *Brain Research*, 1976, *108*, 199–204.

Burton, K.A. A study of the conditions and mechanisms of the diphenylamine reaction for the colorimetric estimation of deoxyribonucleic acid. *The Biochemical Journal*, 1956, *62*, 315–341.

Caviness, V.S., & Rakic, P. Mechanisms of cortical development: A view from mutations in mice. *Annual Review of Neuroscience*, 1978, *1*, 297–326.

Coyle, J.T. Development of the central catecholaminergic neurons. In F.O. Schmitt & F.G. Worden (Eds.), *The neurosciences third study program*. Cambridge: MIT Press, 1974. Pp. 877–884.

Dudek, B.C. Dopaminergic involvement in the genetic modulation of neurosensitivity to alcohol. Doctoral dissertation, State University of New York at Binghamton, 1978. (Ann Arbor: University of Michigan microfilms.)

Falconer, D.S., Gauld, I.K., & Roberts, R.C. Cell number and cell sizes in organs of mice selected for small and large body size. *Genetical Research, Cambridge*, 1978, *31*, 287–301.

Fuller, J.L., & Thompson, W.R. *Foundations of behavior genetics*. St Louis: Mosby, 1978.

Fuller, J.L., & Herman, B.H. Effect of genotype and practice upon behavioral development in mice. *Developmental Psychobiology*, 1974, *7*, 21–30.

Hahn, M.E., Haber, S.B., & Fuller, J.L. Differential agonistic behavior in mice selected for brain weight. *Physiology and Behavior*, 1973, *10*, 759–762.

Herman, B.H., & Nagy, Z.M. Development of learning and memory in mice genetically selected for differences in brain weight. *Developmental Psychobiology*, 1977, *10*, 65–75.

Howard, E. Hormonal effects on the growth and DNA content of the developing brain. In W. Himwich (Ed.), *Biochemistry of the developing brain*, Vol. 2. New York: Marcel Dekker, 1974. Pp. 1–68.

Jacobson, M. Development of specific neuronal connections. *Science*, 1969, *163*, 543–547.

Jensen, C. Generality of learning differences in brain weight selected mice. *Journal of Comparative and Physiological Psychology*, 1977, *91*, 629–641.

Jensen, C., & Fuller, J.L. Learning performance varies with brain weight in heterogeneous mouse lines. *Journal of Comparative and Physiological Psychology*, 1978, *92*, 830–836.

Jerison, H.J. *Evolution of the brain and intelligence*. New York: Academic Press, 1973.

Joh, T.H., & Reis, D.J. Different forms of tyrosine hydroxylase in central dopaminergic and noradrenergic neurons in sympathetic ganglia. *Brain Research*, 1975, *85*, 146–151.

Johnston, M.V., Reinhard, G., & Coyle, J.T. Methylazoxymethanol treatment of fetal rats results in abnormally dense noradrenergic innervation of neocortex. *Science*, 1979, *203*, 369–371.

Kessler, S., Ciaranello, R.D., Shire, J.G.M., & Barchas, J.D. Genetic variation in synthesis of catecholamines. *Proceedings of the National Academy of Science, USA*, 1972, *69*, 2448–2450.

Lanier, L.P., Dunn, A.J., & Van Hartesveldt, C. Development of neurotransmitters and their function in the brain. In S. Ehrenpreis & I.J. Kopin (Eds.), *Reviews of neuroscience*, Vol. 2. New York: Raven Press, 1976. Pp. 195–256.

Lindvall, O., & Bjorkland, A. The organization of the ascending catecholamine neuron systems in the rat brain as revealed by glyoxylic acid fluorescence method. *Acta Physiologica Scandanavica, Supplement*, 1974 *412*, 1–18.

Lowry, O.H., Rosebrough, N.J., Farr, A.L., & Randall, R.J. Protein measurement with folin phenol reagent. *Journal of Biological Chemistry*, 1951, *193*, 365–285.

Masterton, B., Heffner, H., & Ravizza, R. The evolution of human hearing. *Journal of the Acoustical Society of America*. 1969, *45*, 966–985.

Masterton, B., & Skeen, L.C. Origins of anthropoid intelligence: Prefrontal system and delayed alternation in hedgehog, tree shrew, and bush baby. *Journal of Comparative and Physiological Psychology*, 1972, *81*, 423–433.

Moore, R.Y., & Bloom, F.E. Central catecholamine neuron systems: Anatomy and physiology of the dopamine systems. *Annual Review of Neuroscience*, 1978, *1*, 129–169.

Roderick, T.H., Wimer, R.E., Wimer, C.C., & Schwartzkroin, P.A. Genetic and phenotypic variation in weight of brain and spinal cord between inbred strains of mice. *Brain Research*, 1973, *64*, 345–353.

Roderick, T.H., Wimer, R.E., & Wimer, C.C. Genetic manipulation of neuroanatomical traits. In L. Petrinovich & J.L. McGaugh (Eds.), *Knowing, thinking, and believing*. New York: Plenum Press, 1976. Pp. 143–178.

Ross, R.A., Judd, A.B., Joh, T.H., Pickel, V.M., & Reis, D.J. Strain dependent differences in tyrosine hydroxylase in inbred mice are due to differences in number of dopaminergic neurons. *Neuroscience Abstracts*, 1976, Vol 2, part 1, 473.

Sudak, H.S., & Maas, J.M. Central nervous system serotonin and norepinephrine localization in emotional and nonemotional strains in mice. *Nature*, 1964, *203*, 1254–1256.

Ungerstedt, U. Stereotaxic mapping of the monoamine pathways in the rat brain. *Acta Physiologica Scandanavica*, 1971, *367* (supplement 10), 1–48.

Van Valen, L. Brain size and intelligence in man. *American Journal of Physical Anthropology*, 1974, *40*, 417–424.

Warren, J.M. Learning in vertebrates. In D.A. Dewsbury & D.A. Rethlingshafer (Eds.), *Comparative psychology, a modern survey*. New York: McGraw Hill, 1973. Pp. 471–509.

Wilson, E.O. *Sociobiology, the new synthesis*. Cambridge: Belknap Press, 1975.

Wilson, R.S. Twins and early mental development. *Science*, 1972, *175*, 914–917.

Chapter XIII

Fuller BWS Lines: Parental Influences on Brain Size and Behavioral Development[1]

MARTIN E. HAHN

As described by Rosenzweig in this volume, the relationship between brain and behavior has been a classic problem for behavioral research. In general, early work in this area was designed to establish the relationship between brain and behavior by discovering what mental states accompanied or predisposed particular behaviors. As the area of research expanded, with the inclusion of new ideas and methods, the central question became a more general one of what brain characteristics accompanied or predisposed behavior. Any number of brain parameters might be associated with behavior, including: brain size, brain weight, number of cells, types and numbers of interconnections, types and properties of neurotransmitters, etc.

With the rediscovery of Mendel's work, the influence of synthetic evolutionary theory, and an application of developmental principles, the concept of brain–behavior relationships again expanded. Instead of viewing the relationship in terms of static parameters, it is now seen that brain and behavior are subject to the interaction of genetic and environmental variables, and that the relationship of brain and behavior changes over time. For the current study of brain and behavior, an investigator must deal with a complex of factors including genes, environmental stimuli, brain parameters, development, and behavior.

[1]The work reported in this chapter has been partially supported by NSF Grant Ser 76-13098.

DEVELOPMENT AND EVOLUTION
OF BRAIN SIZE

One approach to the brain–behavior complex was taken by Tryon (1940), who bred rats selectively for "bright" or "dull" performance in a specialized maze. This behavioral selection was successful, since bright and dull lines were separated with no overlap by generation eight (Tryon, 1942). Subsequent research on Tryon's lines has indicated that the behavioral and physiological parameters of his lines were not attributable to a simple bright-dull distinction. Searle (1949) studied Tryon's bright and dull lines and found that they performed in a fashion opposite to expectation on several mazes other than Tryon's. The lines also differed considerably in emotional and motivational characteristics. Another interesting feature observed with the descendants of Tryon's lines was that bright rats were far more susceptible to environmental enrichment than were the dull line animals (Rosenzweig, Krech, Bennett, & Diamond, 1962).

Detailed behavioral, anatomical, and chemical studies of the descendants of Tryon's lines were reported by Rosenzweig *et al.* (1962). They found that behavioral and brain chemistry differences existed in the S_1, S_3, and other lines, and that the relationships between behavior and chemistry were understandable but complex. The findings of Tryon, Searle, and Rosenzweig's group indicate that genetic selection has strong potential for altering brain and behavioral characteristics, but precisely determining the relationships between brain and behavior is extremely difficult.

From collaboration within Rosenzweig's group came another approch to studying brain and behavior; selection for a brain character and examination of the behavioral consequences. Roderick, Wimer, and Wimer (1976) began with inbred foundation stocks of mice and through crossing procedures obtained a heterogeneous population. They then bred together animals whose siblings had high or low brain weights and rapidly (three generations) had lines differing considerably on brain weight. Behavioral studies using the Roderick lines have demonstrated several interesting phenomena. High line animals showed greater locomotor activity and performed better in discrimination learning, active avoidance learning, and reversal learning (Elias, 1969, 1970; Wimer & Prater, 1966; Wimer, Roderick, & Wimer, 1969). Perhaps the most interesting finding, however, was that the high and low lines differed in developmental rates for both brain weight and behavior (Fuller & Geils, 1972, 1973). Prenatal and postnatal brain weight was affected, but most of the growth differential occurred during the postnatal period. A simple hypothesis of facilitated and suppressed maturation in the high and low brain weight lines, respectively, was probably not warranted in this case, since Fuller and Geils (1972) found that the brains of both lines contained less water than an unselected control population. These data suggest that both high and low lines were maturing more rapidly than the control line (Fuller & Geils, 1972).

In another selection on a different base population reported in Fuller and Herman (1974), Fuller selected mice for sibling breeding on the basis of brain weight without the correlated effects of body weight. He was able to separate high, medium, and low lines in less than five generations of selection, and when he began behavioral testing, discovered that his lines varied in rates of sensory and motor development (Fuller & Herman, 1974). In particular, Fuller and Herman observed that the high line matured more rapidly than either the medium or low line on several behavioral measures, including tactile and visual forelimb placing, edge avoidance, disappearance of fixed pivoting, rotorod balancing, and eye opening.

In addition to the observed early sensory and motor differences, other differences have been seen during the periods on which social stimulation and isolation affects later social behavior. Hahn, Haber, and Fuller (1973), using Fuller's BWS (brain weight selection) lines, discovered that one type of social rearing produced adults from each strain that varied little in several measures of aggression and aggressiveness. Given a different type of social rearing condition, the same lines differed dramatically on aggression measures. Although adult members of the Fuller BWS lines differ on some characteristics, Jensen (1977; this volume) reports that no consistent relationships between brain weight and learning performance exist.

The findings of Roderick, Fuller, and colleagues that genetic selection for brain weight produced a number of behavioral differences are quite important as a preliminary thrust into the brain–behavior complex. However, the work to date has not successfully specified the nature of the relationship between brain weight selection and behavioral differences in the selected lines.

Models of Pathways from Selection to Behavior

A number of models might be constructed to aid understanding of the relationship between selection and behavior. Figure XIII.1 illustrates several possible routes between selection and behavior. Two notes on this figure are necessary. First, the diagram is not exhaustive, but attempts to present exemplary relationships based on currently available data. Second, the various routes from selection to behavioral differences are not necessarily muturally exclusive. For example, it is possible that brain weight selection altered brain weight, which in turn resulted in altered rates of sensory-motor development in the young animals of the three Fuller lines. Differential social experiences in those young animals resulted in differential adult social behavior, as found in Hahn, Haber, and Fuller (1973). It is also possible that variance in adult behavior is

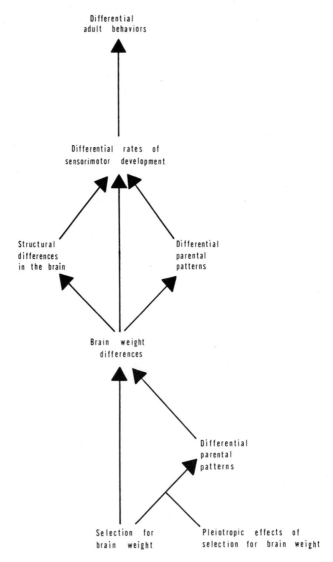

FIGURE XIII.1. Models presented of the relationship between brain weight selection and behavior.

the result of several components; for example, selection may have operated on brain weight *per se*, and the genes for brain weight acted pleiotropically on parental behavior. Acting together, these two effects of selection may have altered rates of sensory-motor development, and so on.

Alternative Hypotheses

The general objective of the reported research was to collect data that will aid in determining which model, (or models, or aspects of several models), leads to the best understanding of the relationship between brain weight selection and behavior. In order to pursue this objective, two alternative hypotheses for the relationship between brain weight selection and behavior were proposed.

1. Selection for heavy and light brains acts in a straight forward fashion by increasing and decreasing brain size. Changes in gross brain size are underlain by increases and decreases in subbrain components (functional units, numbers or complexity of cells, numbers of interconnections, etc.). Changes in subunit numbers result in increased or decreased behavioral capability, for example, learning and developmental rates.
2. Brain weight selection carried linked, pleiotropic, or epistetic acting genes that acted indirectly on parental or nutritional variables, which altered brain weight, development, and behavior in the brain weight selected lines.

These alternative hypotheses suggested an often used experimental strategy—fostering procedures. The literature on the influence of maternal care on the offspring of mice has demonstrated a number of interesting phenomena. For example, among the subspecies of the genus *Peromyscus, Peromyscus maniculatus bairdii* differed from *P.m. gracilis* in the time spent with pups in the nest and in the number of nest visits (King, 1958). It is known that the traits of pups can be altered by the stimulation of maternal care. King and Eleftheriou (1959) have shown that manipulation of pups during the neonatal period affected their adult performance in a learning situation. Lagerspetz and Wuoinin (1965) have shown (using *Mus musculus*) that fostering of pups of a line selected for high aggressiveness to a line selected for low aggressiveness, reduced aggressive tendencies in the fostered pups. Fostering in the opposite direction produced more aggressive animals. The effect of the male parent may also be an important influence on the developing offspring, but little research has been done on this topic. One study by Smith and Simmel (1977) indicated that fostering to a nonfather male altered the exploratory and agonistic behaviors of developing mice. Further, in this study, the genetic strain of the fostered father was also a determinant of the pups' later behavior. Though the exact mechanisms by which the parents influence their offspring are not known, Noirot (1964) has demonstrated that some maternal behaviors (pup retrieval and nest building) were induced by ultrasonic distress calling. The purpose of the present study was to assess the effects of cross-fostering on brain weight at 42 days and rates of sensory-motor development from 3–18 days.

Effects of Fostering Procedures on Brain Weight and Behavioral Development

Subjects

In early February, 1976, I received the entire third litter of each BWS line (generation 18) from Dr. John Fuller's colony at SUNY Binghamton. From these animals, I established 10 breeding pairs for each BWS line by random mating of males and females within each line. In order to accommodate the large subject needs at various times in the project and to protect the foundation stocks from experimental procedures, I established extra breeding pairs as needed (again using random mating within lines). After an experiment requiring additional parents was completed, those additional parents were killed. The subjects of the current experiments were the first litters of the 10 foundation breeders of the H and L lines, and the first litters of the 20 additional breeding pairs from the H and L line of the twentieth, twenty-first, and twenty-second generations of the BWS lines. The entire twentieth generation was used for brain weight data, the twenty-first generation was split between brain weights and development, and the twenty-second generation was used entirely for developmental data. Progeny of the breeders of all generations were assigned to one of three rearing conditions:

1. Cross-fostered—H pups to L parents and L pups to H parents
2. In-fostered—H pups to H parents and L pups to L parents
3. Control—Animals received the handling necessary for fostering but were returned to their nest without fostering.

All primary breeding pair progeny were reared in the control fashion. Progeny from the additional breeders of each line were assigned at random to fostered or cross-fostered at 1–2 days of age only, and fostering occurred between litters that were born the same day or 1 day apart only. All liters were culled to eight animals, with runts selectively culled. High line litters averaged 6.5 animals, and low line litters averaged 7.3. Animals assigned to the brain weight condition remained with their parents until 21 days of age, at which time they were placed with like sex siblings and remained with siblings until 42 days of age. At 42 days of age, their body and brain weights were measured, using the procedure described by Fuller and Herman (1974).

Measurement of Developing Behaviors

The animals assigned to behavioral testing began at the age of 3 days; the battery of tests employed by the Fuller and Herman (1974) "practiced" group to assess sensory-motor development. Those test procedures were as follows:

1. Open field activity—begun at 3 days of age
2. Type of locomotion—begun at 3 days of age
3. Righting time—begun at 3 days of age
4. Edge avoidance—begun at 3 days of age
5. Eye-opening—begun at 8 days of age
6. Auditory startle—begun at 8 days of age
7. Rotorod balancing—begun at 8 days of age

Tactile and forelimb placing used by Fuller and Herman were not tested, because they could not be measured objectively.

Before looking at the results, it is appropriate to discuss briefly the proper control group for comparison with a cross-fostered group. Fostering involves a social situation, that is, the results of fostering arise from an interaction between pups and parents. For example, increased materal care giving may result from better mothers, or from pups who ultrasound more, or a combination of the two. Thus, depending on the dynamics of pup–parent interaction an infostered group may or may not adequately "control" for the cross-fostering procedure. It is safe to say that fostering itself has effects, as demonstrated by Ackerman, Hofer, and Weiner, (1977) whose fostered pups had lower body weights and reduced survival to food deprivation compared to pups who stayed with their biological parents. The best solution may be fostering all pups to standard parents, an extrapolation from Fuller and Hahn (1976), but the solution adopted here is to compare cross-fostered groups to both nonfostered control and infostered groups.

Effects of Line and Rearing Procedures on Brain and Body Weights

As previously noted, brain and body weight measurements were made on mice from the twentieth and twenty-first BWS generations. In all, there were 495 mice with about 40 animals for each line, sex, and condition. Figure XIII.2 illustrates the effects of line and rearing on brain weight. As suggested by the means and standard deviations, there was no overlap between high and low lines. High control brains of both sexes were about 140 mg heavier than low controls of the comparable sex. Cross-fostering reduced the difference between male control high and low mice by 17% and between female highs and lows by 14%. Analysis of variance and Duncan multiple range tests supported these observations by showing that in H line males, there was a significant

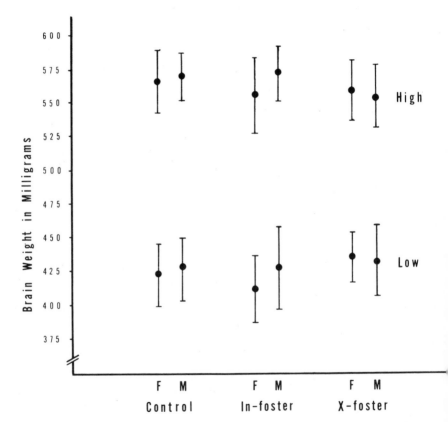

FIGURE XIII.2. Mean brain weights of Fuller BWS lines shown after fostering manipulations; standard deviations are indicated by vertical lines.

effect of rearing. In the H line males, the brains of cross-fostered mice were significantly lighter than infostered ones, while in-fostered brains were not different from controls. In H line females, there was a significant overall effect due to rearing.

In the L line, for males there was a significant overall effect of rearing. The brains of cross-fostered males were heavier than controls, and brains from in-fostered animals were not different from controls. In L line females, there was a significant overall effect of rearing; cross-fostered and in-fostered animals did not differ from controls, but brains of cross-fostered animals were significantly heavier than in-fostered ones.

Figure XIII.3 illustrates the effects of fostering procedures on body

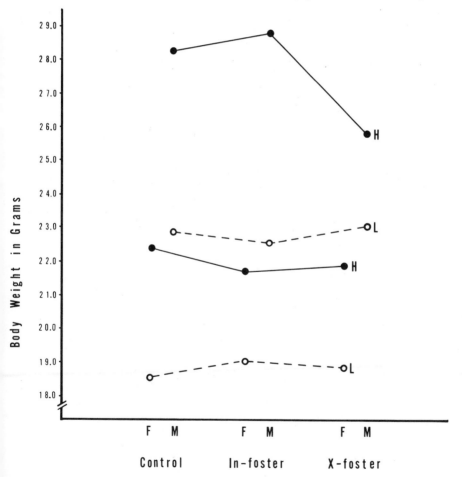

FIGURE XIII.3. Mean body weights presented of Fuller BWS lines after fostering manipulations.

weight. There was some overlap in body weights between the H and L lines, but the differences between them were highly reliable. H line control males were about 5 grams heavier than the L line control males. Cross-fostering reduced this difference by 51%. In females, there was a 4 gm difference between the H line and L line controls. Cross-fostering reduced the difference in female body weight by 21%. Analysis of variance and Duncan multiple range tests supported these observations. In H line males, there was a significant overall effect due to rearing. Cross-fostered males were different from controls and in-fostered males. There was no difference between controls and in-fostered animals. In H line females, there were no significant changes due to rearing procedures.

In the L line, there was no overall change in males due to rearing, but the cross-fostered males were heavier than the in-fostered ones. In L line females, there was a significant overall rearing effect. Cross-fostered females were heavier than controls, and controls did not differ from the in-fostered females.

Brain weights were not different between males and females within lines and conditions except in the L line control and H line in-fostered groups, where male brains were heavier than females. In all groups, male body weights were heavier than females.

The results of rearing were similar in direction for brain and body weights, but body weights changed more as a result of rearing procedures. The overall correlation between brain and body weights was + .588. Correlations between brain and body weights within rearing and sex groups varied, but not systematically as a function of either rearing or line.

Effects of Rearing Procedures on Behavioral Development

As was already noted, developmental measurements were made on mice from the twenty-first and twenty-second BWS generation. There were 540 animals tested in all, with approximately 90 animals for each line and condition. Because of similarity in development to 18 days, males and females were not differentiated, so means represent both sexes. In our rearing procedures, litters were not split; entire litters were assigned to the three rearing conditions. There were 13 litters in each of the six groups. Since most of the developmental tests produced nominal data, for example, met or did not meet criterion on that day's testing, analysis was done by obtaining within-cell error between litters within a group. In other words, for analysis each litter was treated as an *n* of 1.

The development of locomotion was observed for amount (number of squares entered in the open field) and type (fixed pivoting, crawling, and walking). In general, as the animals aged, their locomotion increased, and the mode of movement changed from fixed pivoting to crawling to walking.

LOCOMOTOR ACTIVITY

Figure XIII.4 illustrates the development of locomotor activity from Days 3–18 in all groups of the study. Inspection of the figure indicates apparent line effects: H line was more active during the early Days (3–9) and later Days (15–18), with an intermediate period (10–14) in which a line effect did not appear. There was a suggestion of a rearing effect, since cross-fostered H and L mice resembled each other more than they resembled their respective control groups for most of the 15 days during which activity was measured.

In order to test the effects of line and rearing 2 × 3 ANOVAS and Duncan multiple range tests were employed with the minimum *p* value for significance set at .05. Those analyses revealed line differences on Days 3–6 and 16–18. There was a rearing effect on Day 5 and 16. There were no significant interactions between line and rearing.

Duncan multiple range tests add support for a slight fostering effect, since on Days 3, 4, 5, 7, and 17, control H line animals exhibited more activity than the L line controls. On no days did the in-fostered H line and L line animals differ. On Day 15, cross-fostered L line animals differed from H line cross-fostered animals on activity, but on no other day did their activity levels differ.

FIXED PIVOTING

Figure XIII.5 illustrates the results of fixed pivoting, the first type of locomotion to appear in infant mice. Apparent in this figure is a line effect on Day 3 and Days 6–11. There appear to be no fostering effects in the L line, but the H line cross-fostered group behaved like the L control group on Days 4–8.

Analysis by a 2 × 3 ANOVA revealed a significant line effect on Days 3,6,7, and 8. There was neither an overall fostering effect nor interaction of fostering and line on any day. Some support was found for a fostering effect in the H line; there was a significant difference between cross-fostered H and both in-fostered and control H line mice on Day 7. On

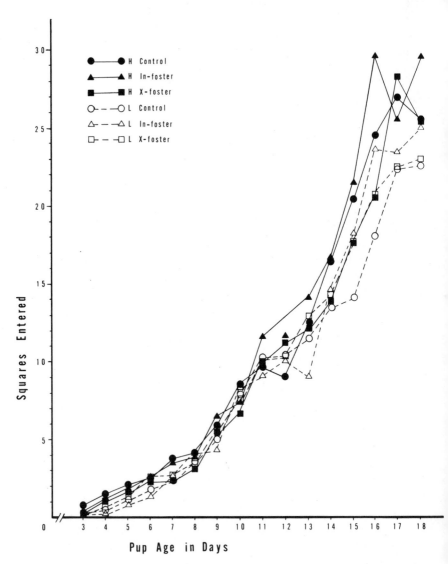

FIGURE XIII.4. Locomotor activity bound in Fuller BWS lines after fostering manipulations.

Days 4 and 6, H line cross-fostered mice differed from in-fostered animals but not from controls.

CRAWLING

Figure XIII.6 illustrates the effects of line and rearing on crawling, the second type of locomotion to appear in infant mice. The figure shows

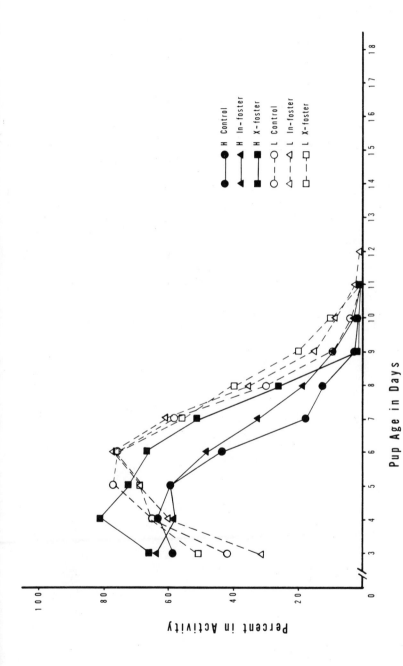

FIGURE XIII.5. Fixed pivoting of Fuller BWS lines after fostering manipulations.

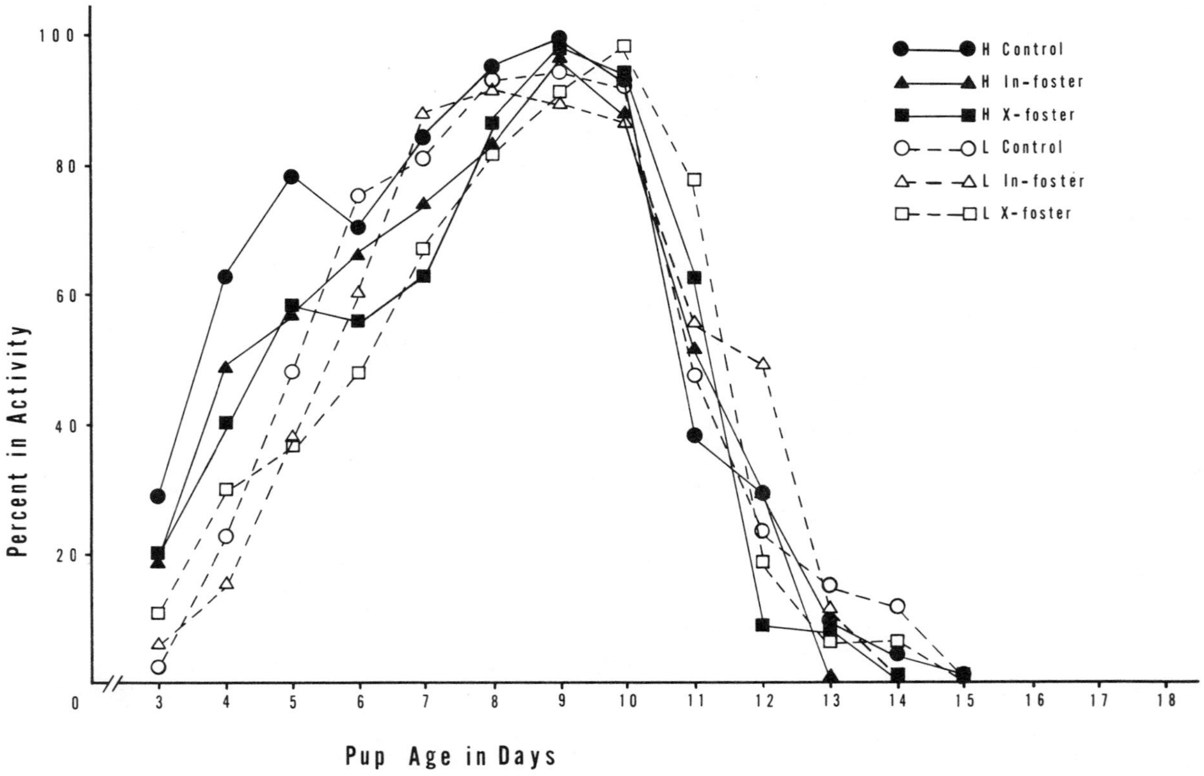

FIGURE XIII.6. Crawling shown of Fuller BWS lines after fostering manipulations.

that H line mice exhibited more crawling than L line early in the period, but the effect disappeared by Day 6. There appear to be fostering effects on Days 3–7, since the H line cross-fostered group exhibited a pattern more like the L cross-fostered group than the H line control. Following Day 7, neither line nor rearing seemed to make any consistent contribution.

Analysis of variance revealed significant line effects on Days 3–5. On those days, there were neither main effects of rearing nor interactions between line and rearing. Duncan multiple range tests showed H line controls to differ from L line controls on Days 3–5; cross-fostered H and L mice were different from their respective controls on those days, and the cross-fostered H and L mice were not different from each other.

WALKING

Only a brief summary of the results of walking, the third type of infant locomotion, is presented here. The results duplicated those of fixed pivoting and crawling, that is, the H line walked more rapidly than the L line, and cross-fostering eliminated much of the difference between the lines.

EDGE AVOIDANCE

For edge avoidance, a mouse was placed with its forelimbs one-half way across the edge of a horizontal platform. In order to meet criterion, the mouse was required to move backward from the edge within a given time period. Accomplishment of this task required perception of the edge, aversion to it, and backward crawling to escape the edge. Figure XIII.7 illustrates the results in this task. Data points in this graph represent the cumulative percentage of mice to reach criterion (retreat from the edge in 10 sec or less on 2 successive days). There was a clear difference between H line and L line control and in-foster groups on Days 4–8, with the H line meeting criterion sooner than the L line. In addition, the cross-fostered low group closely resembled the H line control group, which suggested a one-way fostering effect.

Analysis of variance revealed a line effect on Days 4–8 and a fostering effect on Days 5–7. There were no significant interactions. Duncan multiple range tests added the information that there was no difference between the rearing groups of H line on any day. In the L line, the control and in-foster groups differed only on Day 7. Control and cross-fostered L groups did not differ, and the L cross-fostered group did not differ from the H control group on any day. L line in-fostered and cross-fostered groups differed on Days 5–7.

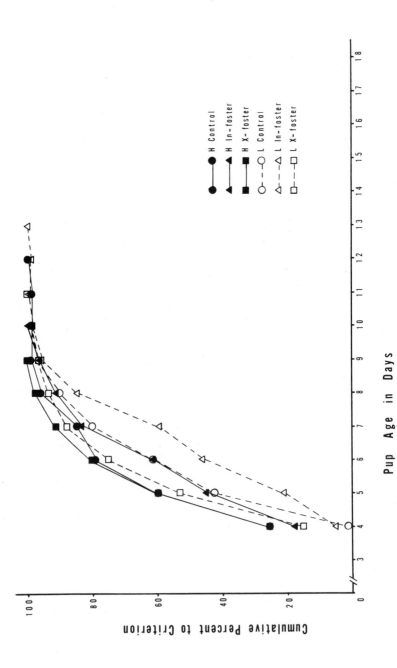

FIGURE XIII.7. Edge avoidance of Fuller BWS lines that occurs after fostering manipulations.

RIGHTING TIME

For the measurement of righting time, a mouse was placed on his back on a smooth sheet of Plexiglas. The length of time required for all four feet to return to the plastic surface was recorded. Animals were run to a criterion of righting in less than .5 sec. Figure XIII.8 illustrates the effects of line and rearing condition on righting time. Data points on the graph represent the cumulative percentage of mice to reach criterion. There appears to be a powerful line effect, as L line mice reached criterion more rapidly on each day the behavior was measured. There seems to be no rearing effect in either line.

Analysis of variance supports these observations, since there was a highly reliable line effect on Days 5–10 with no significant rearing effect or interaction. Duncan multiple range tests did not reveal any fostering effects in either line.

ROTOROD

The final measure to be discussed is rotorod performance. Beginning at 8 days of age, pups were placed on a moving 25mm diameter, knurled, aluminum rod. Initially, the rod moved at 1 revolution per minute (rpm) and in order to remain on the rod, the mouse had to perceive motion and respond by moving forward. After the pup remained on the rod for 30 seconds at 1 rpm, the speed was increased to 5 rpm. The mouse met criterion by remaining on the rod for 30 sec at 5 rpm. As can be seen in Figure XIII.9, the results of rotorod performance are similar to those for righting time. There appears to be a strong line effect, since the L line animals reached criterion sooner than the H line animals. Further, as for righting time, there does not appear to be a rearing effect.

Analysis of variance revealed a highly reliable line effect; L line animals were faster to criterion than H line animals on Days 11–16. There was no rearing effect and no interaction, and Duncan multiple range tests did not reveal any fostering effects within either line.

Summary and Conclusions

A survey of the results of the present study indicates three primary results. First, not surprisingly, the large brain and body weight differences observed in the Fuller BWS lines by Fuller and Herman (1974) are still present, some 16 generations later. Second, differential rates of behavioral development, also observed by Fuller and Herman, are still present in the H and L lines, with the H line developing more rapidly

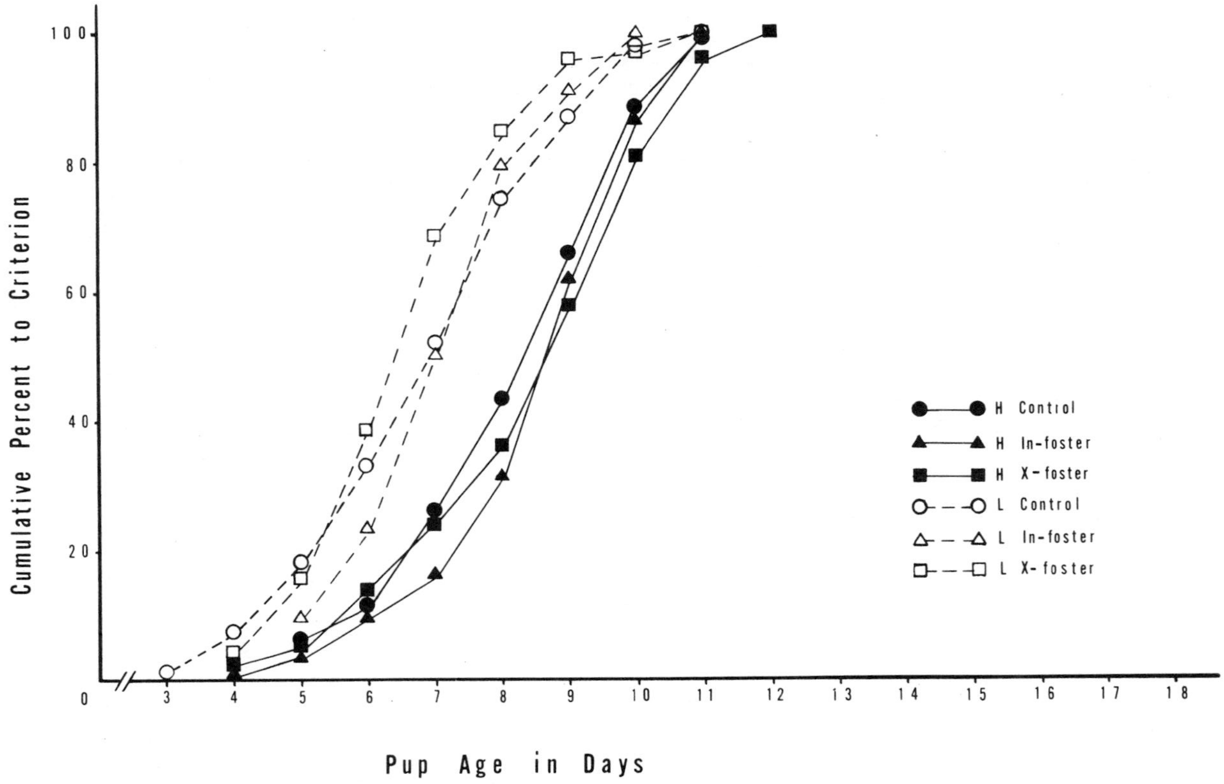

FIGURE XIII.8. Righting time of Fuller BWS lines seen after fostering manipulations.

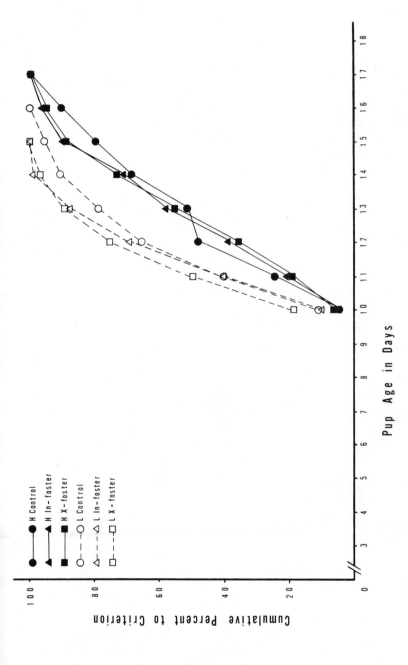

FIGURE XIII.9. Rotorod performance of Fuller BWS lines seen after fostering manipulations.

on most tasks. Third, cross-fostering procedures were successful in altering brain weights, body weights, and developing behaviors in the H and L lines. Taken together, these findings indicate that a simple understanding of the relationship between behavior and brain weight selection, based solely on either the direct effects of selection or the correlated responses to selection, cannot be supported. An explanation combining aspects of both simple hypotheses will be suggested, but first, a more detailed summary of my findings and a comparison of the present results to those of Fuller and Herman are necessary.

The present results indicate that large brain and body weight differences remain between the H and L lines from the selection project. Furthermore, cross-fostering procedures were successful in altering brain and body weights. L line animals reared by H line parents had increased brain and body weights compared to controls. Likewise, H line animals reared by L line parents had lower brain and body weights than controls. These effects were not due simply to the fostering procedures, because cross-fostered animals were generally different from the in-fostered and the nonfostered control groups.

For behavioral measures, the situation was somewhat more complex. The line of the animal had an effect on each measure studied, with the H line developing more rapidly than the L on all measures except righting time and rotorod ability. Fostering had varied effects on behavioral development. On locomotor activity and crawling, fostering had symmetrical effects. H line control pups were more active and showed crawling more rapidly than did the L line. Cross-fostering attenuated that effect—L line pups reared by H line parents showed increased activity and more rapid crawling than the L line controls. The converse held for the H line animals, as cross-fostering reduced their activity and crawling development. On two other behavioral measures, fixed pivoting and edge avoidance, there was a one-way effect. On fixed pivoting, H line controls developed the behavior more quickly than the L controls, but cross-fostering the H line animals eliminated the effect. The L line was not affected by fostering. On edge avoidance, the H line developed more rapidly than the L line, but L line cross-fostered animals developed in a manner similar to H line controls. On the final two behavioral measures, righting time and rotorod, L developed more rapidly than did the H line, and there were no effects on development due to fostering.

A comparison of the present results to those of Fuller and Herman (1974) reveals similarities and differences. Both studies found the H line to develop more rapidly than the L line on locomotor activity (open field activity), fixed pivoting, and edge avoidance. Such similar results might best be explained as genetic characters of the lines that were fixed early in selection and have remained through six generations of selection and nine generations of random mating within line.

There were also differences between the studies, as the present study found the L line to develop more rapidly than the H line on righting time and the rotorod. Fuller and Herman found no line differences on righting time, and the H line met criterion more rapidly than the L on rotorod. The difference between the current results and those of Fuller and Herman is more difficult to explain than the similarity.

The preceding results leave two phenomena to be explained. First, why have there been changes in the relationship between brain size and rate of behavioral development in the Fuller BWS lines since the 1974 study of Fuller and Herman? Second, why was cross-fostering successful in modifying brain and body weights and some aspects of behavioral development?

I think there is a common answer to these questions—correlated characters—that has been discussed by others in this volume (see chapters by Jensen and by Roderick). As discussed by both Jensen and Roderick, correlated characters (sometimes called conjoined characters) are those that are carried along during selection, because they are linked or in some other way related to those genes being selected directly. Thus, in the present case, genes that were selected because of their influence on brain weight had a correlated effect on body weight, (even though the selection criterion used by Fuller was biased against that event), and had an effect on parental behaviors. Clearly, H line parents are different from L line parents, since they strongly influenced brain and body weight and behavioral development in pups they reared.

Furthermore, since correlated characters are not likely to be tied one-to-one to the selection characters, their influence should be seen to build more gradually over generations during selection. In the present case, changes in behavioral development occurred between the fifth and twenty-first generation of selection, and this change could well be explained by the increased influence of correlated characters over the course of selection.

This result is not unique. Jensen (Jensen & Fuller, 1978; this volume) has shown that variation in brain size is related positively to variation in learning ability in heterogeneous mice, as would be expected on the basis of cross-species studies. This orderly relationship apparently breaks down, however, when heterogeneous stocks are subjected to selection for extremes of brain weight. Jensen (this volume) argues that the reason for the breakdown is the influence of correlated and/or randomly fixed characters.

In order for a model of the relationship between brain weight selection and behavior to be accurate for the Fuller BWS lines, it must show that brain weight selection was not the sole determinant of brain weight or behavior. The effects of parental behavior (whether due to pleiotropic gene action, linked genes, or genes randomly fixed within the lines) on the lines were considerable, and provide an interesting environmental effect on brain size and behavior that should be investigated further.

One might argue, on the basis of the preceding, that lines of animals selected for some characteristic are not really useful in the study of that characteristic, because the unknown influence of correlated characters and/or random fixation of genes within the selection lines rules out any straight forward conclusions. While that may hold for some selections, I argue that it does not hold for the Fuller BWS lines. In the Fuller BWS lines, brain size reliably predicted performance on most behavioral measures tested in this study. Furthermore, early environmental events influenced brain size and developing behaviors. Thus, the lines could be used to investigate the effects of genetic, environmental, and G × E variables on brain size and behavior. In addition, both genetic and environmental variables influenced brain size. The specific changes that resulted from the two influences should be described and compared in the manner described by Wimer, and by Greenough and Juraska in this volume. Studies along these lines are currently underway in my laboratory.

Acknowledgments

I would especially like to thank my student Paul Shrenker, who assisted on all the studies being reported. The following students have all been of assistance in data collection and reduction: Karen Glovinsky, Kathy Harland, Stan Kelman, Sam Kopec, Jacqueline Lavooy, Maria Lavooy, Kevin Macaluso, Mary Ann Murray, Kenny Poole, Fran Rogalski, and Irene Wallace.

References

Ackerman, S.H., Hofer, M.A., & Weiner, H. Some effects of a split litter across foster design applied to 15 day old rat pups. *Physiology and Behavior*, 1977, *19*, 433–436.

Elias, M.F. Differences in spatial discrimination reversal learning for mice genetically selected for high brain weight and unselected controls. *Perceptual and Motor Skills*, 1969, *28*, 707–712.

Elias, M.F. Spatial discrimination reversal learning for mice genetically selected for differing brain size: A supplemental report. *Perceptual and Motor Skills*, 1970, *30*, 239–245.

Fuller, J.L., & Geils, H. Brain growth in mice selected for high and low brain weight. *Developmental Psychobiology*, 1972, *5*, 307–318.

Fuller, J.L., & Geils, H. Behavioral development in mice selected for differences in brain weight. *Developmental Psychobiology*, 1973, 6, 469–474.

Fuller, J.L., & Hahn, M.E. Issues in the genetics of social behavior. *Behavior Genetics*, 1976, 6, 391–406.

Fuller, J.L., & Herman, B. Effect of genotype and practice upon behavioral development in mice. *Developmental Psychobiology*, 1974, 7, 21–30.

Hahn, M.E., Haber, S.B., & Fuller, J.L. Differential agonistic behavior in mice selected for brain weight. *Physiology and Behavior*, 1973, 10, 759–762.

Jensen, C. Generality of learning differences in brain-weight-selected mice. *Journal of Comparative and Physiological Psychology*, 1977, 91, 629–641.

Jensen, C., & Fuller, J.L. Learning performance varies with brain weight in heterogeneous mouse lines. *Journal of Comparative and Physiological Psychology*, 1978, 92, 830–836.

King, J.A. Maternal behavior and behavioral development in two subspecies of *Peromyscus maniculatus*. *Journal of Mammalogy*, 1958, 39, 177–190.

King, J.A. & Eleftheriou, B.E. Effects of early handling upon adult behavior in two subspecies of deermice, *Peromyscus maniculatus*. *Journal of Comparative and Physiological Psychology*, 1959, 52, 82–88.

Lagerspetz, K., & Wuorinen, K. A cross fostering experiment with mice selectively bred for aggressiveness and non-aggressiveness. *Reports Psychological Institute*, University of Turku, 1965, No. 17.

Noirot, E. Changes in responsiveness to youth in the adult mouse: The effects of external stimuli. *Journal of Comparative and Physiological Psychology*, 1964, 57, 97–98.

Roderick, T.H., Wimer, R.E., & Wimer, C.C. Genetic manipulations of neuroanatomical traits. In L. Petrinovich & J.L. McGaugh (Eds.), *Knowing, thinking and believing*, New York: Plenum Press, 1976.

Rosenzweig, M.R., Krech, D., Bennett, E.L., & Diamond, M.C. Effects of environmental complexity and training on brain chemistry and anatomy: A replication and extention. *Journal of Comparative and Physiological Psychology*, 1962, 55, 429–437.

Searle, L.V. The organization of hereditary maze-brightness and maze-dullness. *Genetic Psychology Monographs*, 1949, 39, 279–325.

Smith, M.L., & Simmel, E.C. Paternal effects on the development of social behavior in *Mus musculus*. *Developmental Psychobiology*, 1977, 10, 151–159.

Tryon, R.C. Genetic differences in maze-learning ability in rats. *39th Yearbook National Social Studies Education* (Part 1). Bloomington, Illinois: Public School Publishing, 1940.

Tryon, R.C. Individual differences. In Moss, F.A. (Ed.), *Comparative psychology*. New York: Prentice-Hall, 1942.

Wimer, C. & Prater, L. Behavioral differences in mice genetically selected for high and low brain weight. *Psychological Reports*, 1966, 19, 675–681.

Wimer, C. Roderick, T.H., & Wimer, R.E. Supplementary report: Behavioral differences in mice genetically selected for brain weight. *Psychological Reports*, 1969, 25, 363–368.

Chapter XIV

Responsiveness of Brain Size to Individual Experience: Behavioral and Evolutionary Implications[1]

MARK R. ROSENZWEIG

Does training influence the size of an individual's brain? Are differences in brain size among individuals of the same species correlated with intelligence? Are interspecies differences in brain size and in relations between brain size and body size correlated with differences in intelligence among species? These questions which occupy us in this volume are not new; in fact, all of them had been raised by the eighteenth century. I plan, therefore, to devote part of my paper to recalling some of the history of thought and research on these topics. We will see that some valuable early insights were forgotten and had to be rediscovered, and some early findings have not yet been completely assimilated. Noting some of the speculations and investigations of our early predecessors may provide us with a base for measuring progress, and may indicate some of the difficulties that have confronted researchers in this field.

After the historical introduction, I will review briefly some of the recent research that demonstrates that experience or training can alter brain size and other cerebral measures. Next, I will take up some of the hypotheses proposed to account for effects of differential experience of brain measures, and I will present some previously unpublished results that can be used to test between the arousal hypothesis and the learning

[1] The research has been supported in part by the Division of Biomedical and Environmental Research of the U. S. Department of Energy through the Lawrence Berkeley Laboratory and by National Institute of Mental Health Grant R01 MH 26704.

263

DEVELOPMENT AND EVOLUTION
OF BRAIN SIZE

hypothesis. Finally, I will consider briefly some hypotheses concerning benefits that may accrue to organisms whose brains are structurally plastic—benefits that may have led to evolution in this direction.

Historical Background

Certain questions about relations between brain anatomy and intelligence go back to classical antiquity—as when Erisistratus (around 300 BC) suggested that the more convolutions the cerebrum shows, the more intelligent is the species. But major concern with relations among brain anatomy, body size, and intelligence came only with the wave of European exploration beginning in the fifteenth century, and the ensuing attempt to assimilate and to systematize knowledge about the many new animal species discovered. A long-standing belief held that man, the most intelligent of animals, had the largest brain; this was upset in the latter half of the seventeenth century, when it was found that the elephant has a larger brain than the human being. When Karl Linneaeus (1707–1778) introduced his system for classification of plants and animals in 1735, he not only provided a basis for relating and comparing species, but his system also gave fresh impetus to the collection of new species.

Thus when Albrecht von Haller (1708–1777) wrote his classic text, *Elements of Physiology of the Human Body* in 1760, he included considerable data from comparative anatomy. Haller adopted the practice of stating brain weight as a fraction of body weight. This ratio placed man above the other large mammals, but rodents turned out to have brain–body weight ratios as great or greater than that of man. Haller noted that reports of different investigators often gave rather different ratios for the same species; further, the ratio decreases when an individual puts on weight, because brain weight remains constant while body weight varies. So shortcomings of the brain/body weight ratio were revealed over 200 years ago, and more were to appear, yet this ratio is still occasionally employed.

Can Mental Exercise Influence Growth of the Brain?

Whether exercise can induce growth of the brain appears first to have been discussed in correspondence between the prominent Swiss naturalist, Charles Bonnet (1720–1791), and an obscure Piedmontese anatomist, Michele Vincenzo Malacarne (1744–1816). Malacarne had asserted that individual differences in ability among men are correlated with individual differences in brain structure: In the brains of men of greater memory, sagacity, and vivacity, he claimed to have found greater numbers of folds in the cerebellum than in brains of the less endowed (Bonnet, 1783, Vol. 7, p. 140). Intelligence was said to be correlated with the number of folds in the brain, but in the cerebellum rather than, as

Erasistratus had long ago suggested, in the cerebrum. Note that the claimed relation was with a specific part of the brain rather than with the whole brain. Malacarne then agreed to undertake an experimental test of Bonnet's hypothesis that mental exercise might induce brain growth. His experimental design anticipated in important respects one that we began to use in the 1950s (without knowing of the earlier work). Malacarne chose as subjects two littermate dogs, and also pairs of birds, including parrots, chaffinches, and blackbirds, each pair coming from the same clutch of eggs. In each pair, one individual received intensive training and the other received none. After a few years of this treatment, Malacarne sacrificed the animals and compared the brains of the trained and untrained members of each pair.

The results of this experiment were published in a book, *Neuroence-falotomia*, 1791. I have not been able to obtain a copy of this work, but a one-paragraph review of it appeared in the *Journal de Physique*, Paris (1793, *43*, p. 73). The review indicates that the experiment furnished positive results—the trained animals were said to show more folds in the cerebellum than the untrained, in keeping with the earlier observations on individual differences among human brains.

It was doubtless with Malacarne's experiment in mind that the prominent German physician, Samuel Thomas von Soemmering (1755–1830) wrote the following passage in his major book on human anatomy published in 1791:

> *Does use change the structure of the brain?*
> Does use and exertion of mental power gradually change the material structure of the brain, just as we see, for example, that much used muscles become stronger and that hard labor thickens the epidermis considerably? It is not improbable, although the scalpel cannot easily demonstrate this. [1971, Vol. 5, p. 91. In the edition of 1800, the last phrase was changed to "although anatomy has not yet demonstrated this" (p. 394)].

Thus Soemmering was not convinced that Malacarne had found changes in the brain with exercise, although he still considered Bonnet's question worth mentioning. I have not found subsequent references to Malacarne's research, and it seems not to have been continued, (nor has much of the later research concerned possible relations between the cerebellum and intelligence, although Greenough and Juraska reported some new data on effects of experience on the cerebellum in this volume).

Almost exactly a century after Malacarne's work, a more specific hypothesis was formulated about effects of experience and training on the brain. Just about the time that the neuron doctrine was formally enunciated by Waldeyer (1891), several investigators proposed that learning occurs through modifications in the functional contacts between neurons. These junctions did not yet have a specific name; it was only in 1897 that Sherrington proposed the term "synapse." Perhaps the first person to propose that learning is due to a change in neural junctions was the Italian psychiatrist Eugenio Tanzi (1893). He surveyed recent advances in neurohistology and hypothesized that learning produces anatomical changes in interneural contacts and that these changes serve as a mechanism for memory.[2] Ramon y Cajal, apparently independently of Tanzi, went somewhat further in his Croonian lecture to the Royal Society of London (Cajal, 1894). He stated that the higher one looked in the vertebrate scale, the more the neural terminals and collaterals ramified. Also, during development of the individual neuronal branching increased, probably up to adulthood. And he held it very probable that mental exercise also leads to greater growth of neural collaterals. Near the end of his paper he delivered a picturesque set of analogies:

> The theory of free arborization of cellular branches capable of growing seems not only to be very probable but also most encouraging. A continuous pre-established network—a sort of system of telegraphic wires with no possibility for new stations or new lines—is something rigid and unmodifiable that clashes with our impression that the organ of thought is, within certain limits, malleable and perfectible by well-directed. mental exercise, especially during the developmental period. If we are not worried about putting forth analogies, we could say that the cerebral cortex is like a garden planted with innumerable trees—the pyramidal cells—which, thanks to intelligent cultivation, can multiply their branches and sink their roots deeper, producing fruits and flowers of ever greater variety and quality [pp. 467–468].

Although Cajal thus hypothesized changes in neuronal branching with experience, he did not hypothesize correlated changes in brain volume. We will return to this point later in the section entitled "Limits to Cajal's Foresight [p. 276]."

Sherrington, in the same chapter in which he named the synapse, also related synaptic contacts to learning in a striking way:

> Shut off from all opportunity of reproducing itself and adding to its numbers by mitosis or otherwise, the nerve cell directs its pent-up energy towards amplifying its connections with its fellows, in response to the events which stir it up. Hence, it is capable of an education unknown to other tissues [Foster & Sherrington, 1897, p. 1117].

[2]Kandel (1976, p. 476) has proposed a different candidate for priority: "The first suggestion that learning is due to a change in synaptic function was made by Lugaro (1899) . . ." But in his next sentence, Kandel writes, "Several years later Tanzi (1893) formulated a more specific hypothesis for learning based on a synaptic change due to usage." Actually Lugaro had published on this topic as early as 1895, but his suggestions appear to be extensions of the work of Tanzi, and Lugaro was a junior colleague of Tanzi, so priority seems to remain with Tanzi.

Tanzi (1893) was confident that investigators would soon be able to test by direct inspection the junctional changes that he hypothesized to occur with development and with training. About 80 years were to intervene, however, before the first results of this sort were announced (Cragg, 1967; Diamond *et al.*, 1975; Møllgaard, Diamond, Bennett, Rosenzweig & Lindner, 1971; West & Greenough, 1972).

Soemmering Relates Brain Size to Body Size and to Intelligence

The importance of Soemmering to research on this topic does not rest chiefly on his comments on Malacarne's research. Soemmering grappled with the problem of relating brain size both to body size and to intelligence, and his cogent remarks were to influence many later thinkers and investigators. In 1778 he proposed that man has a larger brain than any other animal, if the brain is measured in relation to the size of the cranial nerves. Soemmering came back to the question of how large a brain the body needs in another book published in 1785 and translated (in part) into English. Since this work appears to have influenced, directly or indirectly, many later investigators, a few of the main passages will be quoted here from C. White's translation:

> It was formerly taken for granted that man possessed a larger brain than any other animal. To prove this, it was usual to compare the weight of the brain and of the body in man, and in the most common domestic animals. Thus far theory bore the test of experiment. But physiologists, desirous of establishing the fact on a wider induction, were involved in no small perplexity. They found, on this principle, that birds stood higher in the scale than man; and that seals (*cetacea*) and more especially the smaller quadrupeds, as the mouse, squirrel, etc., possessed an infinitely larger brain, in comparison with their body, though certainly not with respect to the organs of sense, or that part of the head which forms the face [White, 1799, clx–clxiii].

Soemmering noted that body weight is not a good basis on which to compare brain weight, since the body can be affected much more by disease, fatigue, or accumulation of fat than can the brain: "A comparison of the size of the brain with that of the nerves, is not only attended with less difficulty, but promises important conclusions [White, 1799, p. clxiv]." Such a comparison is carried out in a paper by Krompecher and Lipak (1966), in which the ratio of brain weight to spinal cord weight is given for 24 mammalian and 6 avian species.

Soemmering further suggested that part of the brain is required for basic sensory and motor functions and that the remainder is related to intelligence:

XLIII . . . it appears to me that a very small proportion of the brain is requisite to enable [the nerves] to perform the functions of vegetation, or mere animal life.

XLIV . . . A being, therefore, that, in an eminent degree possesses more than is necessary for this purpose, may be presumed to inherit a superior capacity of intellect.

XLV . . . Considered in this point of view, man, who in any other light holds but a middle station, stands confessedly at the head of the animal world. Apes of every description . . . are, in this respect greatly inferior to him . . . Setting apart, therefore, a portion of their encephalon sufficient for these uses, the brain of these animals dwindles, in comparison with the human brain, almost to a cypher.

Animals of various kinds seem to posses this superabundant portion of brain in a greater or lesser degree, in proportion to their sagacity or docility [White, 1799, pp. clxiv–clxv].

This insight—that only part of the brain is required for sensory and motor functions and that the remainder is related to intelligence—was to reappear in the writings of many prominent investigators to the present, but usually without acknowledgment of their predecessors.

Extension of the Brain—Intelligence Relation to Fossil Animals

Georges Cuvier (1769–1832) not only accepted Soemmering's proposed relations between brain size and intelligence, but he also extended them. In 1800 Cuvier published what has been called "the first truly complete work in the history of comparative anatomy. Whereas his predecessors . . . had at best applied comparison to select groups of animals, he consistently attempted to employ it in his study of every known animal or species [Coleman, 1964, p. 62]." In later editions, Cuvier emphasized neuroanatomy by adopting the nervous system as the primary character for classification. He declared in 1807 that "the nervous system is the essence of the animal. It is by its means that [the animal] exists, that it has an individuality . . . The other organs are destined to maintain it or to satisfy its needs: digestion, circulation, respiration, locomotory system. Nevertheless, in its turn it maintains and animates them [Coleman, 1964, p. 91]."

Cuvier pioneered in the study of fossil animals. He was the first to reconstruct fragmentary fossil remains, employing his extensive knowledge of comparative anatomy and his principle of correlation of parts. Moreover, Cuvier initiated paleoneurology in 1804 when he recognized a fossilized brain case in the brittle skull of an *Anoplotherium,* an extinct pachyderm whose bones were found in Montmarte. From his description of the brain, Cuvier did not hesitate to estimate the animal's intelligence: "[The brain] was proportionately rather small and flattened horizontally; its hemispheres did not show convolutions but one saw only a shallow longitudinal depression in each. *All the laws of analogy permit us to conclude that the animal was greatly lacking in intelligence.* In order to make the conclusion anatomically rigorous, one ought to know the forms of the base of the brain and especially the proportion of its width to that of the spinal cord, but this base is not conserved in our mold [1822, p. 44; italics added]."

The last sentence quoted from Cuvier undoubtedly refers to Soemmering's claim that intelligence of species is related to the ratio of bulk of the cerebrum to the bulk of the cranial nerves or of the spinal cord. Cuvier cited this rule in a detailed consideration of relations of brain anatomy to intelligence in his comparative anatomy of 1800. In the same work he noted that "man is the animal whose brain case is the largest and whose face is the smallest; . . . the more animals depart from these proportions, the more stupid or the more ferocious they are [p. 4]." Although as a comparative anatomist Cuvier was chiefly interested in brain–behavior relations among species, he also indicated that some of the same relations held true among men: "We see examples among us every day, even though the differences among men in this respect are much smaller than the differences that one can see among different species of animals [1800, Vol. 2, p. 4]." Furthermore Cuvier noted that people have always used these anatomical relations as indications of intelligence. Thus the ancients made their statues of heroes and gods with exaggerated foreheads. Furthermore, Cuvier stated, people even extended these indications to animals and often do so incorrectly. Thus the elephant and the owl both have thick frontal bones that give them the appearance of larger brain cases than they actually have. It is for this reason, Cuvier held, that both of these animals are popularly considered to be more intelligent than they really are.

Continuing Belief in Relation of Head Size to Intelligence

Physiologists and anatomists attacked the claims of the phrenologists that mental faculties could be related to conformation of the skull. Nevertheless even the harshest critics of phrenology did not contest the existence of a clear relationship between brain size and intelligence. Thus François Magendie (1783–1855) wrote as follows:

> The volume of the brain is generally in direct proportion to the capacity of the mind. We ought not to suppose, however, that every man having a large head is necessarily a person of superior intelligence, for there are

many causes of an augmentation of the volume of the head beside the size of the brain; but it is rarely found that a man distinguished by his mental faculties has not a large head [1831, pp. 103–104].

Paul Broca (1825–1880) made several studies on the hypothesized relations of brain size to intelligence and to education. Thus, he attempted to improve Parchappe's investigation of 1836 concerning effects of education on brain size. Parchappe had found larger head measurements among 10 professors and magistrates that among 10 laboring men of the same age. Broca pointed out that in Parchappe's results one could not separate innate factors from education. Parchappe had taken as his educated group men who were not only trained, but who were also above average in achievement. Perhaps, Broca reasoned, outstanding laborers would also have had larger heads than the average of their group. Broca chose in 1861 to compare male nurses and interns. Internships, he stated, did not require special ability but were open to most hard-working students, so interns should be representative of the class of men who continue their education. Broca seems not to have considered that there must still have been real differences in the initial selection of his two groups. (The difficulty of establishing adequate control groups has continued to plague research in this area and has invalidated most of the work that has been done with human subjects. With animals, such research becomes feasible, but special precautions must nevertheless be taken, as we will point out later.) Broca's results, like those of Parchappe, showed greater skull diameters in the educated group, and again the differences appeared especially in the frontal region of the skull.

When measurements of intelligence began to be made in the twentieth century, they revealed only low relations between cranial size and intelligence, yet the older beliefs died hard. Thus, Karl Pearson reported that at the turn of the century Galton "was very unhappy about the low correlations I found between intelligence and size of head . . . it was one of the few instances I noticed when impressions seemed to have more weight with him than measurements [Pearson, 1924, p. 94, Note 2]." G. A. Miller claims that "to the day he died [Galton] was unwilling to admit that the size of a man's skull had no value as a measure of his intelligence [1962, p. 137]." But we should note that Pearson's evidence on intelligence came from teachers' ratings, not from formal testing, and Galton's "impressions" may have been of equal value.

A recent review by Van Valen (1974) shows only a few studies that have correlated head size with intelligence test scores. The observed correlations ranged from .08 to .22, but Van Valen argued that when allowance is made for errors inherent in the methods used in these studies, the results indicate that the true correlation between intelligence and brain size may be as high as .3. Jerison (personal communication) criticized Van Valen's argument, but he also mentioned unpublished analyses indicating the reality of a small positive correlation (.1) between head circumference and intelligence, after the influence of height is partialled out. One of these analyses was performed on data for American school children by Jerison, and the other was performed on English data by Passingham.

The Allometric Relation of Brain Weight to Body Weight

It had become clear by the end of the eighteenth century that brain weight should not be related directly to body weight; nevertheless it was apparent that there was a regular progression of brain weight with body weight, especially when one compared animals of similar form such as small and large carnivores. The nonlinear form of the relation between brain weight and body weight was stated in the nineteenth century, but current writers often refer to some later or secondary source. Thus a research article of 1977 cited a paper of 1972 that referred to Kroeber's (1948) anthropology textbook as the source for the statement that the relationship of brain size to body size in mammals is analogous to the relationship of the surface area to the volume of the body; body weight increases as a cubic function, whereas the brain weight increases as a squared function, as one goes from small to large animals. Kroeber did not cite sources for this in his textbook, but we can trace the concept back to an unlikely source—the study of an extinct sea mammal by a young Russian naturalist.

In 1867 Alexander F. Brandt (1844–19—[3] was studying the Stellar's sea cow or *Rhytine*, an aquatic mammal of Siberia that had become extinct in the preceding decade, and he was comparing it with related forms, the dugong and the manatee. The sea cow at twenty feet was the largest of the three animals and had the greatest absolute brain weight but the smallest relative brain weight. (The sea cow actually had a greater brain weight than man.) Brandt was unwilling to concede that these cerebral differences proved that there were differences in intelligence among the three species. "Anthropology has shown how difficult it is to draw conclusions about the relation that exists between the cerebral mass and psychic faculties [p. 530]." Perhaps it was having to

[3] I have been unable to find the date of death of A. F. Brandt, but he lived a long and productive life, publishing two books in the 1920s, one on sex behavior in 1924, and one on feminism in 1929.

reconstruct the animals from their skeletal measures (as he describes) that made Brandt keenly aware of their linear and volumetric relations. He then put Haller's rule—smaller animals have proportionately larger brains—into juxtaposition with the recently acquired knowledge that smaller animals have higher respiratory rates. Since the nervous system was being implicated more and more in the control of bodily functions, Brandt concluded that smaller animals with higher metabolic rates would need relatively larger nervous systems, as in fact they do possess. Going beyond metabolic considerations, Brandt also noted that the sensory surface of small animals is greater compared to their volume than in large animals. Presumably, then, the number of sensory nerves and the mass of the sensory centers of the brain should be related to the body surface rather than to body weight. Again, Brandt suggested that the number of muscle nerve fibers probably varies with the cross-section rather than with weight of the muscle—another relation of the nervous system to a surface rather than to a volume. Brandt seems to have stopped just short of stating that brain weight is related to the two-thirds power of body weight.

Although Brandt's hypothesis was cited by several investigators—for example, Bischoff (1880)—it was not tested or extended until 1892. In that year not only was the relation of brain weight to body weight finally stated explicitly and tested, but a suggestion was also made for incorporating intelligence into the relationship. These steps were taken by Otto Snell, a German physician. Snell (1892) did not credit Brandt or any other predecessor with originating this line of thought, but he did cite Bischoff as his source for human brain weights, so he probably knew of Brandt's hypothesis. At the outset of his article, Snell stated that the weight of brain depends on two factors, body size and intellectual activity. Considering only somatic function, brain weight should be related to the body surface, or to body weight to the two-thirds power. To take psychological activity into account, a further factor is required. Thus

$$h = k^s \cdot p$$

where h = brain weight, k = body weight, s = somatic exponent, and p = the psychological factor. Snell argued that s must be about the same in all healthy adult warm-blooded animals. To estimate s empirically, rather than to assume that it is .67, one can take pairs of species that are rather similar in body form and in mental ability but that differ in body size. Assuming p to be equal for both members of the pair,

$$s = \frac{\log h_1 - \log h_2}{\log k_1 - \log k_2}$$

Putting the known body weights and brain weights into this equation, s can be found.

Snell noted that since one cannot measure mental ability exactly, and since there is variability in the data, it is necessary to take an average of many different pairs of species. Snell did not report the species or numbers that he used, but the average value of s turned out to be about .68, close to the value predicted a priori. Once s is found, then p, the psychological factor, can be calculated for any species. Snell gave values of p and relative brain weights for 19 species of mammals and 24 species of birds. The values of p seemed to Snell to accord rather well with his impressions of the mental endowments of the various species: "If you order animals according to the size of the psychic factor, you obtain a series that starts with the most highly endowed animals and gradually descends to the least gifted [p. 446]."

Snell noted three qualifications to this work: (a) Mental ability of animals cannot be measured accurately enough to equate animals exactly; (b) Individuals of a species may differ considerably in weights, so that the average of many individuals should be taken; (c) Finally, more meaningful relations might be obtained by studying weights of parts of the brain rather than the whole brain. All three points were well taken, and research is only beginning to catch up with them.

Effects of Differential Experience on Brain Measures

The hypothesis formulated by Bonnet late in the eighteenth century, and posed again in more specific form by Tanzi, Cajal, and Sherrington late in the nineteenth century, has been confirmed over the last two decades: Differential experience does lead to measurable changes in the brain, including growth of cerebral tissue. Only a brief survey of these findings will be presented here, since several rather extensive recent reviews are available (Greenough, 1976; Rosenzweig & Bennett, 1977, 1978).

Most of the experiments on this subject have involved placing laboratory rodents for periods lasting from a few weeks up to a few months in differential environments—environments either enriched or impoverished in comparison to the usual animal colony cage. The enriched environments have usually included both more social stimulation and a greater variety of inanimate objects than the colony cage; that is, 10–12 animals are placed in a large cage with a variety of stimulus objects, "toys." In some experiments, the social stimulation and the inanimate stimulation have been varied separately (Rosenzweig & Bennett, 1976); social stimulation cannot account for the full enrichment effect (Rosenzweig, Bennett, Herbert, & Morimoto, 1978). For impoverished experience, the subject is placed alone in a colony cage, instead of having one or two cagemates as in the standard colony situation.

Effects on Brain Weights

Typical results in terms of brain weights are the following, when littermate rats are compared after exposure to the enriched condition (EC) versus the impoverished condition (IC): Rats with EC experience show greater weight of total brain by about 2%; this is statistically significant in most experiments, since the effect is highly reproducible and variability of brain weights is low. The overall brain difference is due chiefly to effects in the cerebral cortex; the cortex shows a difference of about 5%, while the rest of the brain differs by only about 1%. A very stable measure that yields highly significant differences between groups is the cortical/subcortical weight ratio. Because both cortical weight and subcortical weight are correlated with body weight, the ratio tends to eliminate the influence of body weight and to provide, in effect, a covariance on body weight. Within the cerebral cortex, the occipital area shows the largest difference between EC and IC, the occipital effect often amounting to 8% or more.

The results just described have been found in experiments in which starting ages ranged from 25 to 290 days and in which duration of differential experience ranged from 30 days to over 100 days. (See Table 17.1 of Bennett, 1976, for specific results with a variety of starting ages and experimental durations.)

The fact that the differences in weights are not found uniformly through the brain but occur mainly in certain regions of the cerebral cortex is reminiscent of Snell's (1892) suggestion that more meaningful brain–intelligence relations might be found by studying parts of the brain rather than the whole brain. Nevertheless, some recent investigators continue to use the weight of the whole brain or of the entire forebrain as their measure.

We should note that evidence of structural plasticity with differential experience is not limited to rats. It has also been found in laboratory mice, in gerbils (Rosenzweig & Bennett, 1969), and in feral deermice.

I was glad to hear about Dudek's unpublished research (personal communication) in which he found that mice bred for high brain weight are still capable of further increasing their brain weight in response to enriched experience. Experiments on the effects of differential experience or training on brain measures have used mainly rodents, but Greenough is now pursuing such studies with monkeys, in collaboration with G. Sackett and several students.

Interpretation of Brain Weight Effects in Terms of Cellular Changes

The occurrence of changes in weights of brain, and especially of cerebral cortex, as a function of exposure to different environments is interesting, but more refined anatomical analyses are required if we are to progress toward the level of understanding cellular functions. Fortunately a number of further anatomical observations have been made. We will mention a few of them briefly, and Greenough describes others in the following chapter. Clearly, more work of this sort is needed.

Greenough and collaborators found greater branching of dendrites in EC rats than in their IC littermates (Greenough, 1976). This also is a regional effect, occurring with greater magnitude in the occipital cortex than in the other cortical regions measured. Globus, Rosenzweig, Bennett, and Diamond (1973) found that the number of dendritic spines per unit of length of dendrite was significantly greater in EC than in IC rats. This effect was localized even within neurons, the difference in spine density on basal dendrites amounting to 9.7% ($p < .01$), on oblique dendrites, 3.6% ($p < .05$), and no effect occurring on apical dendrites. Along with this increase in the dendritic tree, it was found that the cross section of the neuronal cell bodies was significantly larger in EC than in littermate IC rats (Diamond, 1967). Presumably the cell body must be more active metabolically to support a larger dendritic arborization, and such an increase in biosynthetic function was supported by the finding of greater amounts of RNA in cortex of EC rats, as compared with IC littermates (Bennett, 1976). A greater diversity of species of RNA molecules has also been found in EC than in IC rats (Grouse, Schrier, Bennett, Rosenzweig, & Nelson, 1978). Enriched experience may also cause an increase in the number of glial cells to minister to the more active neurons; evidence for increase glial–neural counts has been reported in EC versus IC rats (Diamond et al., 1966; Szeligo & Leblond, 1977) but on the other hand greater total DNA (and thus a greater number of cells) is not found regularly in EC versus IC rats (Rosenzweig *et al.*, 1978).

Putting this evidence together, we attribute the increase in cortical bulk with enriched experience largely to the growth of neural ramifications. Presumably the interconnectedness of cortical neurons increase; this may reflect both greater redundancy (and thus greater effectiveness of some circuits), and the establishment of novel circuits.

Limits to Cajal's Foresight

When Cajal (1894) postulated that mental exercise would lead to greater branching of neurons and establishment of new functional contacts, he also considered an obvious objection: "You may well ask how the volume of the brain can remain constant if there is a greater branching and even formation of new terminals of the neurons. To meet this objection we may hypothesize either a reciprocal diminution of the cell bodies or a shrinking of other areas of the brain whose function is not related directly to intelligence [p. 467]."

This example shows that even the great Cajal could score as low as one out of four with his hypotheses. As we have just seen, he was correct in supposing that the dendritic trees of neurons can increase their branching and connections as a result of training or enriched experience (Globus *et al.*, 1973; Greenough, 1976). But Cajal was wrong in believing that the brain kept its volume constant while neural branching increased. Our data have demonstrated small but reliable increases in brain weight with training or enriched experience (e.g. Bennett, 1976, Table 17.1). And Cajal was wrong again in hypothesizing that neuronal cell bodies might shrink to compensate for increases in the branches. Actually a larger cell body is required to perform the metabolic function of a larger dendritic tree, and the cell bodies of cortical neurons develop greater cross-section areas in rats from an enriched environment, as compared with measures on littermates in an impoverished environment (Diamond, 1967). Cajal's final hypothesis in this set was probably incorrect too, since all the regions into which we have dissected rat brains have shown increased weights in those from enriched environments. Some regions increase more than do others, and some have appeared to decline in experiments where the EC rats weighed less than IC rats; when the influence of body weight was partialed out, all brain regions increased with enriched experience. Thus the cerebral changes as a consequence of experience are even stronger than Cajal foresaw 80 years ago.

Hypotheses to Account for Effects of Differential Experience on Brain

From our first work on effects of differential experience on brain measures (Rosenzweig, Krech, & Bennett, 1961), we have attempted to test alternative hypotheses to account for these findings, and other laboratories as well as our own are continuing in this effort. We originally turned to the differential environments as a way of providing animals with differential opportunities to learn. We had found that giving rats formal training appeared to alter cortical acetylcholinesterase (AChE) activity. We hoped to test this apparent effect of training more clearly and to enhance the magnitude of the results by providing round-the-clock opportunities for self-paced learning over a period of several weeks. When we obtained differences in cortical AChE following exposure to enriched or impoverished laboratory environments, we were inclined to attribute them to differential learning. Nevertheless, in our first publications we tested alternative hypotheses and showed that neither the greater handling of the EC rats nor their greater amount of locomotor activity could account for the observed effects (Krech, Rosenzweig, & Bennett, 1960; Rosenzweig et al., 1961).

During the last 16 years, many alternative hypotheses have been proposed, and quite a few have been tested. There is no need to discuss most of them at length here, because they have already been reviewed elsewhere (Greenough, 1976; Rosenzweig & Bennett, 1977, 1978). Let us simply note some of the frequently mentioned alternatives that research has allowed us to reject. Thereafter we will consider two further alternatives about which we will also present some unpublished findings.

Tests of Several Hypotheses

1. Stress is frequently offered as an explanation for the cerebral effects—either "isolation stress" in IC or the stress of information overload in EC. Neither IC rats nor EC rats show enlargement of the adrenal glands in comparison with littermate SC rats; it is unlikely that these rather mild treatments involve appreciable amounts of stress. Furthermore, imposition of overt stress daily for 30 days on IC or EC rats did affect adrenal weights, but did not alter EC versus IC cerebral effects in measures of brain weights or AChE activity (Riege & Morimoto, 1970). Therefore the cerebral effects of differential experience cannot be attributed to stress.

2. Hormonal mediation is probably not required for production of the cerebral effects. Not only do EC and IC rats not differ in adrenal weight/ body weight or in thyroid weight/body weight, but hypophysectomy does not prevent the development of typical cerebral differences between rats in EC or IC (Rosenzweig, Bennett, & Diamond, 1972).

3. Speeded maturation in an enriched environment has been suggested as a possible cause of cerebral differences observed between rats in EC and IC environments. This might seem able to account for some of the characteristics of EC rats, such as greater weight of cerebral cortex and greater branching of dendrites. But on other measures, EC rats resemble young animals more than do IC rats; for example, the cortical/ subcortical weight ratio declines with age, but it is higher in EC than in IC rats. Furthermore, most of the EC–IC differences can be induced even when the differential treatment is initiated in adult animals, so speeded maturation is clearly not the cause of these effects.

4. Deprivation or distortion of sensory input have been demonstrated to alter aspects of perceptual functions, receptive fields of cortical neurons, and even cortical anatomy. We believe, however, that this does not provide a general model for neural events in learning or for effects of differential experience. Three criteria enable us to distinguish the effects of sensory deprivation or distortion from those of differential experience of the EC–IC sort: The effects of differential experience occur even in adults; they require direct interaction with stimuli; and they do not require severe deprivation or distortion of stimulation. In contrast, the sensory effects occur only during a limited period of development; they have been reported to be produced by simple passive exposure to stimuli, and severe departures from normal stimulation are required to alter sensory development.

The "Developmental Theory of Environmental Enrichment"

Among the most active investigators in this field are Roger Walsh, Robert Cummins, and their collaborators. Not only have they conducted many empirical studies and published a variety of novel findings, but they have also been ingenious in suggesting alternative hypotheses. In the spirit of "strong inference" (Platt, 1964), we have attempted to test some of their hypotheses; the fact that the results do not seem to us to support these hypotheses does not lessen our esteem for the scientists who conceived them. Let us turn first to the "developmental theory" published in 1977 by Cummins, Livesey, Evans, and Walsh. In the following section we will consider the "arousal hypothesis" of Walsh and Cummins (1975).

Cummins *et al.* (1977) stated that they were led to their developmental theory by the following observations: They rank-ordered EC rats in terms of forebrain weights and also rank-ordered IC rats in the same way, then they examined brain weight differences between EC and IC rats of the same ranks. "The enrichment-isolation difference [was] apparent only between animals ranked low in brain weight. This relationship was found in seven of the nine studies. . . ." The two exceptions showed a significant correlation between brain weight and body weight, whereas the other seven studies did not. "Having thus found a significant confounding variable for forebrain weight in groups 30a and 30c, its influence was removed by forming a ratio of forebrain weight to body weight. When this ratio was used in the ranking procedure, groups 30a and 30c now showed the largest enrichment-isolation effect between the animals ranked low in brain weight [p. 693]."

The model elaborated by Cummins *et al.* (1977) holds that some cerebral neurons depend upon environmental stimulation for full development. Figure XIV.1 will help to explain this model. With low levels of environmental stimulation such as are found in the impoverished condition (IC), most animals will show brain weight values near the baseline, but for a few of these animals even the "low level of stimulation may be adequate to produce development comparable to that achieved by others in the enriched environment." Such impoverished-experience rats "could thus approach the developmental ceiling." Overall, the values of the impoverished group would tend to cluster in the lower part of their distribution. On the contrary, among enriched-experience animals, the brain weight values would tend to approach the "genetically

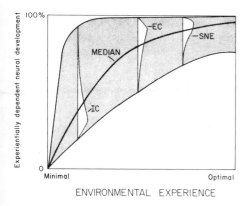

FIGURE XIV.1. Model for experientially dependent neural development is modified from Cummins *et al.* (1977, Figure 2). Results of our experiments do not support this model, as is described in the text.

determined ceiling" and therefore are grouped more closely above their median than below it. Also, the variance of brain values of the impoverished-experience rats should exceed that of the enriched-experience rats.

It occurred to us that data from some of our experiments should provide a more searching test of the model than was afforded in the original presentation, for three main reasons:

1. Whereas Cummins *et al.* (1977) used weight of forebrain as their only brain measure, we could also use other brain weight measures that are more sensitive to differential experience than is forebrain weight. We have shown previously that the effects of differential experience are largely restricted to the cerebral cortex, so inclusion of subcortical forebrain tissue only dulls the measure and adds error variance.

2. In seven experiments, we had assigned rats not only to enriched (EC) and impoverished (IC) laboratory environments like those of Cummins *et al.*, (1977), but also to a seminatural outdoor environment (SNE) that leads to significantly greater brain development than does EC. Comparisons of cerebral effects of SNE versus IC should provide stronger tests of the model than comparisons of effects of EC versus IC, since SNE is closer than EC to the optimal condition, as can be seen in Figure XIV.1.

3. The history of research in this area indicates the impropriety of using the ratio of brain weight to body weight that Cummins *et al.* (1977) employed in the two groups that did not show the low rank effect. We decided to test with our data whether forming this ratio does, in fact, remove the relationship of brain weight to body weight or whether, as we suspected, it would actually increase the correlation between the brain measure and body weight.

From the model, the following specific tests can be applied to the results of each experiment:

1. The variance of scores of the IC group should exceed the variance of scores of the EC group: $\sigma^2_{IC} > \sigma^2_{EC}$. Since our experiments include the SNE Condition as well as the IC and EC conditions, we can add the following two tests.

2. $\sigma^2_{EC} > \sigma^2_{SNE}$.

3. $\sigma^2_{IC} > \sigma^2_{SNE}$. This should be the strongest of the three tests involving variances, since the environmental conditions are furthest apart.

To perform the next five tests, brain weights are first rank-ordered for each condition within an experiment.

4. Among the IC animals, the variance among brain weights above the median (upper half—UH) should exceed the variance among weights below the median (lower half—LH). IC: This is shown in the hypothetical frequency distribution for the IC group in Figure XIV.1. (One of the standard ways of measuring skewness would probably be preferable to this idiosyncratic method employed by Cummins *et al.*)

5. Among the EC animals the variance should be smaller in the upper half than in the lower half. EC: $\sigma^2_{UH} < \sigma^2_{LH}$ This and the next point are also illustrated in Figure XIV.1.

6. The prediction made for EC animals should hold even more strongly for SNE animals. SNE: $\sigma^2_{UH} < \sigma^2_{LH}$

The enrichment-impoverishment differences in brain weights should be larger among the lower ranked than among the higher ranked animals.

7. The difference is larger between EC and IC rank-ordered pairs that fall below the median (LH) than between pairs that rank above the median (UH): EC–IC differences, LH > UH.

8. Similarly for differences between rank-ordered SNE and IC pairs: SNE-IC differences, LH > UH.

Before attempting to test the model, it must be decided whether to employ brain weights or brain weights divided by body weights. Unlike Cummins *et al.* (1977), we found a significant correlation between fore-brain weight and body weight in most groups. Among our 21 subgroups of rats (3 conditions × 7 experiments), 16 yielded correlations significant at beyond the .05 level of confidence, and 12 of these were significant at beyond the .01 level. The mean correlation of forebrain weight and body weight (using the *r* to *z* transformation) was .72, and the lowest coefficient found for any group was .44. One reason why Cummins *et al.* reported low correlations (below .22 in most cases) is that they cal-culated their correlations on combined groups of EC and IC rats. Such pooling obscures the within-group correlations, because differential ex-perience produces opposite effects on brain weights and body weights: Rats placed in EC develop greater brain weights but lesser body weights than littermates placed in IC. We have obtained from Cummins the correlations calculated separately for each of their EC and IC subgroups; these calculations show a mean correlation of .50, with 8 of the 18 coefficients significant at or beyond the .05 level. Thus the correlation of forebrain weight with body weight is more general and substantial than was indicated in the 1977 publication of Cummins *et al.* For their 6 subgroups in experiments of 30-day duration—the same duration we employed—the mean correlation found by Cummins *et al.* was .69, and five of the six correlations were statistically significant.

Since brain weights correlate reliably with body weights, can the "confounding influence" of body weight be removed by dividing forebrain weight by body weight, as Cummins *et al.* (1977) proposed? To test this, we calculated correlations for forebrain weight/body weight versus body weight for each of the 21 subgroups. These correlations were all strongly negative, the mean being −.93. In 19 of the 21 cases, the magnitude of the correlation was greater between forebrain/body weight and body weight than between forebrain and body weight; thus, using the brain/body weight ratio strongly increased the influence of body weight. We therefore employed brain weights as such in our main tests of the model.

Whether or not the statistical formulations of Cummins *et al.* (1977) are correct, it is still a matter of interest to see if their observations could be replicated. Is the enrichment–isolation difference found only between animals ranked low in brain weight? We did not find this to be true in our data for EC–IC comparisons for either forebrain weight or total cortex weight; only two out of seven experiments showed greater EC–IC differences for low-ranked than for high-ranked pairs. The results were only slightly more favorable to the hypothesis when we compared SNE with IC rats; here the differences favored the low-ranked pairs in four out of the seven experiments. In fact, none of the hypotheses detailed above found clear support in our data. Whereas there was a tendency (five out of seven cases) for forebrain weight values to cluster more closely above than below the median for the EC and SNE rats, as predicted, this was equally true for the IC rats, which runs counter to the prediction. We even tested forebrain weight divided by body weight to see if this would yield positive results, as reported by Cummins *et al.* Results of tests with these transformed data agreed with predictions in only 24 out of 56 possible cases, whereas those for raw forebrain weights yielded 30 out of 56 agreements.

It thus appears that whichever of the brain weight measures was employed, and whether the comparisons involved EC and IC or the stronger SNE condition, agreements with the model remained at the level of chance and did not support the theory. We cannot explain why our data do not conform to the model of Cummins *et al.*, but the least that can be said is that their theory lacks generality and has not stood up to the test of reproducibility in similar experiments performed under slightly different conditions and with a different strain of rats. This lack of agreement does not invalidate the general proposition that some cerebral neurons are dependent for their development upon environmental stimulation, and we would agree with this statement.

The Arousal Hypothesis

Walsh and Cummins (1975) proposed that the arousal response is "a fundamental mechanism" in production of anatomical and biochemical changes in brain as a consequence of "exposing animals to environments rich in sensory stimuli." Let us consider whether the "arousal theory" or "arousal hypothesis" (it is called both by Walsh & Cummins, 1975, p. 988) is stated in testable form, whether information is available concerning some of the proposed experimental tests, and whether alternative hypotheses have been eliminated by tests.

The statement of the arousal hypothesis appears to lack clarity in two main respects: (*a*) "Arousal" is not defined precisely; (*b*) Arousal is proposed as being only one of several mechanisms involved in the production of the cerebral changes, but it is not made clear whether the various mechanisms contribute independently or by interaction.

Walsh and Cummins state, "A single definition of arousal is extraordinarily difficult to pose because, as has already been indicated, the state of arousal can be estimated in so many different ways . . . It is not our intention to limit the definition of arousal but rather to suggest that no matter how it is defined, it will involve a transitory state of generalized neurological excitation [p. 989]."

It is not clear that such a transitory state, even if it is elicited repeatedly, will call for long-lasting structural changes in the brain—unless habituation to the arousing stimulation occurs. Walsh and Cummins state that habituation is a consequence of the stimuli that cause the arousal reaction. If the cerebral changes are to be attributed to habituation and to the fact that with repeated presentation of stimuli the rate of habituation increases, then the argument would seem to switch away from arousal and to learning, since habituation is considered by many to be a form of learning.

The possibility of independent contributions to the cerebral changes by various mechanisms appears when Walsh and Cummins "conclude that learning is almost certainly involved in the production of brain changes resulting from environmental stimulation in general and from environmental complexity in particular but that the extent of this contribution is almost entirely unknown [p. 988]." On the other hand, these

authors state in their conclusion, "The final picture, therefore, will probably be one of multiple interactive mediating mechanisms, perhaps with
arousal as a central process [p. 995]."

TESTS OF AROUSAL HYPOTHESIS

Perhaps the most testable form of Walsh and Cummins' hypothesis
is the following: "A combination of activation of sensory systems and
nonspecific activation, or arousal, underlies some proportion of the differential brain effects [p. 988]." A test of this form of the hypothesis
would appear to be available in the results of the experiment of Ferchmin, Bennett, and Rosenzweig (1975). In this experiment, littermate rats
were placed in one of three conditions—the Enriched Condition (EC)
with 12 animals placed in a large cage with a variety of stimulus objects
that were changed daily, the Impoverished Condition (IC) with single
animals in small bare cages in an isolation room, and the Observer
Condition (OC) in which each animal was placed in an individual hard-
ware cloth cage inside a regular EC cage. The OC rats shared the varied
sights, sounds, and smells that were available to their EC littermates.
Four times each day for 30 days, each OC cage was removed from one
EC cage to another. This treatment aroused the OC rats, and they remained aroused for some time as the EC rats in the new EC cage sniffed
and examined them. Thus the OC rats, in comparison with their IC
littermates, were aroused several times each day in a context of varied
sensory stimulation. Yet the combination of sensory stimulation and
repeated arousal over the 30-day period failed to produce measurable
brain differences between OC rats and their IC littermates; both OC and
IC rats did differ significantly from their EC littermates. These results
indicate the necessity for direct interaction of rats with a varied environment if brain effects are to be produced; merely "exposing animals
to environments rich in sensory stimuli" does not appear to be sufficient
cause for brain changes, even when coupled with arousal. The results
run counter to the statement of the arousal hypothesis.

When direct interaction with varied stimulus objects is possible, then
a sufficient degree of arousal may be necessary to produce the cerebral
effects of enriched experience. Results supporting this interpretation
were found when we sought to determine whether exposure of individual rats to an enriched environment for 2 hours per day would result
in similar cerebral effects to those found with groups in EC. The initial
observations were disappointing. Single rats showed much less activity
and interaction with the environment than did grouped rats; the single
animals tended to stay in a corner of the cage and eat, groom, or rest.
We therefore tried to prime the activity of the individual rats, either by

giving them small doses of methamphetamine before putting them in EC, or by putting them in EC during the dark hours of their daily cycle (when rats are more active), or by combining the drug with the dark hours (Rosenzweig & Bennett, 1972). These treatments were effective in promoting exploratory behavior and interaction with the environment. Arousal alone had little effect, since giving the drug to rats that were kept in their home cages caused only small cerebral differences from rats given control injections of physiological saline solution. But arousal in combination with the opportunity—not just for sensory stimulation—but for direct interaction with varied stimuli produced brain values very similar to those of rats placed in groups in the complex environment.

Since these results demonstrate that isolated rats can develop cerebral effects of enriched experience, it is obvious that isolation as such does not prevent the maturation of "environmentally dependent" neurons. Such findings indicate why we use the term "impoverished condition" rather than speaking of "isolation" as Cummins et al. (1977) do. (Note the difference between the labelling of the low stimulation condition in Figure XIV.1 of this chapter and in the comparable Figure 2 of Cummins et al., 1977.)

A further test proposed by Walsh and Cummins (1975) is this: "*The selection of subjects based on their endogenous arousability prior to the differential rearing conditions. One would predict a positive correlation between arousability and the magnitude of the environmentally induced change. Selection for arousability could be based on either behavioral or physiological parameters [p. 994].*" We had conducted a pilot experiment of this sort in 1971 but did not carry the work further when the initial experiment showed no indications of effects. Animals were selected for arousability by rating their rearing and locomotor behavior after placement in a novel compartment. The animals were separated into three groups—highly responsive to the novel environment, moderately responsive, and weakly responsive. Twelve highly responsive rats were placed in one EC cage for a 30-day period, 12 moderately responsive rats in another EC cage, and 12 rats of low responsiveness in a third EC cage. The experiment was run in our usual manner, with varied stimulus objects being placed in each EC cage each day. At the end of the 30-day period the rats were sacrificed and brain measures were taken. Not only were there no significant differences between groups, but there were not even suggestions of differences that would have encouraged us to continue this sort of experiment. Perhaps a different method of selecting animals for arousability will be found to yield more positive results.

A further attempt to test the arousal hypothesis and to separate effects of arousal from effects of learning will be reported after we have considered recent experiments testing the learning hypothesis.

The Learning–Memory Hypothesis

As was mentioned at the start of the section entitled "Hypotheses to Account for Effects of Differential Experience on Brain," we originally began using the differential environments in order to provide animals with differential opportunities to learn, and we hypothesized that the cerebral effects reflected differential learning and memory storage. Although many alternative hypotheses have since been tested to account for these effects, no alternative explanation has been strongly supported, and several could be rejected on the basis of experimental results. The learning-memory hypothesis remains viable and is supported by a variety of observations, as has been discussed by Greenough (1976) and by Rosenzweig and Bennett (1978).

One set of observations supporting the learning-memory hypothesis has been that a few experiments reported that formal training brings about cerebral changes similar to those caused by experience in enriched environments. In experiments of this sort, a crucial factor is the design of control conditions against which the presumed effects of learning can be measured (Greenough, 1976). Some recent experiments of our group seem to have met this criterion well, so I will describe them briefly here. (A full account of these experiments has now appeared: Bennett, Rosenzweig, Morimoto, & Herbert, 1979.) Also, a modification of these experiments is being employed in a test of the arousal hypothesis versus the learning hypothesis, as will be mentioned shortly.

These experiments included a novel condition—individual in complex maze, I-CM—in which individual rats ran self-paced trials in mazes, shuttling between a food station and a water station. The maze was contained in a plastic box inserted as a story in the same sort of cage that is used for EC (Figure XIV.2). The floor of the box was 15 cm above the floor of the cage. Food was placed as usual on the floor of the cage, but the water spout was available only above the plastic box. The rat therefore had to climb up into the plastic box through an open corner hole and out through a hole in another corner of the top to get from food to water. Each rat was moved from one cage to another each day, and it found a new pattern of barriers in the plastic box every day over a 30-day period. Each I-CM rat had littermates in the standard EC and IC environments.

Results showed that the I-CM rats differed significantly from their IC littermates in brain weights and in brain RNA ($N = 70$ per condition). These effects were about half as large as the EC-IC differences obtained in the same experiments. The last several experiments ($N = 26$ per condition) included a more stringent control to test whether the cerebral effects observed with I-CM might be due to the exercise of climbing into and out of the plastic box, the exposure to a series of large cages, etc. The control condition was exactly like I-CM except that the plastic box contained no barriers; this condition was therefore called individual in empty box—I-EB. In contrast to the effectiveness of the I-CM treatment, I-EB was almost completely ineffective in altering brain values. Thus these experiments demonstrate more clearly than heretofore that training causes significant modifications in brain measures.

A version of the plastic maze experiment is now being used to test the arousal hypothesis versus the learning-memory hypothesis. In these experiments, littermate rats are being placed in I-CM or I-EB for only 90 minutes per day over the 30-day period. The rats receive a small amount of food in their individual home cages, but they are hungry when they are placed in the large cage, and they spend most of the 90 minutes eating, drinking, and locomoting. Thus, these subjects are active and aroused during their daily 90 minutes in the apparatus, and they spend the rest of the day quietly in standard home cages. If arousal

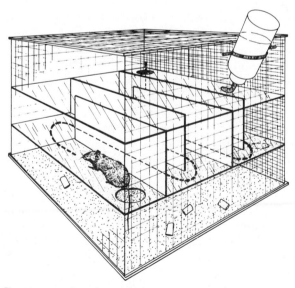

FIGURE XIV.2. Plastic maze placed as a story in a large cage; the rat runs self-paced trials to shuttle between the water bottle above the maze and food pellets below the maze. See the text for further description and for effects of this experience.

is the central mechanism in inducing brain effects, then rats from I-CM and I-EB should develop equivalent brain values, and both should differ from IC littermates by the same amount. If learning is the crucial factor, then the I-CM rats should differ more from IC littermates than should I-EB rats. Preliminary results appear to support the second alternative; further work is now in progress.

Possible Benefits of Structural Plasticity

In research on relations between neural processes and behavior, much attention is being given currently to relatively simple organisms such as *Aplysia*. In such an organism many of the individual neurons are identifiable, the neural circuits underlying some behaviors have been traced completely, and plastic functional changes have been demonstrated to occur at identified synapses without any structural concommitants. If an organism with fixed wiring of the nervous system can show adaptive behavior, as is true of *Aplysia*, what factors may have led to the evolution of organisms in which the connections among neurons can be modified by experience so that even the weight of the brain can vary?

Jerison (1973) has stated that it would be difficult to imagine a prewired central nervous system that was prepared, ready-made, for all the eventualities that an organism faces: Yet it appears that not only many molluscs but also many arthropods (Krasne, 1976) have prewired systems in which plasticity nevertheless occurs through changes of "gain" at certain neural junctions. Are there reasons why this solution may not have been sufficient for vertebrates, or at least for mammals, in which structural as well as functional plasticity seems to occur?

Before continuing we should note that this apparent contrast between invertebrates and vertebrates may not hold when more extensive observations have been made. Perhaps even relatively simple molluscs like *Aplysia* will be found to show structural plasticity in the nervous system when this possibility is investigated; after all, it is not very many years ago that structural plasticity was first found in mammalian brains. And even if simple molluscs do not show anatomical changes in the nervous system as a function of experience, such changes may be found in molluscs like the octopus that have relatively large brains and that are capable of rapid and complex learning.

These characteristics—a large brain and capacities for complex learning—suggest three ways in which structural plasticity of brain in response to environmental challenges may be advantageous and may therefore have been selected in evolution. Let us examine these hypotheses briefly.

First is the hypothesis that structural plasticity in response to environmental demand is advantageous because it spares the organism some of the evolutionary cost of carrying a large amount of genetic information. To specify all of the detailed connections in the brain of a mammal would require an enormous amount of genetic information, and the mathematician Bremermann (1967) has argued that this would entail an evolutionary disadvantage. He points out that in order to be able to evolve speedily, a species should have as few genes as possible, and in this regard $E.coli$ is superior to a mammal. On the other hand, in order to be able to organize complex structures and intricate patterns of behavior, a species needs many genes. These two requirements are thus antagonistic, and different living systems represent various compromises. Bremermann has attempted to estimate the amount of information that would be necessary to specify the details of neural circuits in the mammalian brain, and he has concluded that it would be greater than the genetic information available for the entire body. The need for genetic information is reduced to the extent that information acquired from the environment, during typical experiences, can help in the processes of organizing the nervous system.

The hypothesis may seem plausible, but a major difficulty should be noted. The presumed advantage is for preservation of a population rather than for the reproduction of individuals having a certain genetic characteristic; thus it would be an example of what has been termed *group selection* leading to *biotic evolution*, rather than *genic selection* leading to *organic evolution* (Williams, 1966). Williams has argued forcefully that various supposed biotic adaptations are spurious or inconclusive, that there is no strong evidence of mechanisms for maintaining evolutionary plasticity, and that natural selection, which functions to maximize the genetic selection of individuals, remains the only acceptable explanation for the maintenance of adaptation.

The second hypothesis to be examined is based on the idea that, for an organism that must deal with a complex environment determined partly by chance, a completely predetermined nervous system will not be adequate, and therefore neural plasticity is required. Whereas the hypothesis of Bremermann emphasized the typical features of the environment that are usually present and that can thus contribute to the common development of members of a species, the second hypothesis emphasizes ways in which the environment can differ significantly even for members of the same species. Three examples will be given. First is the fact that higher social animals must interact with fellows who differ noticeably from each other, but whose characteristics depend upon the lottery of meiosis. Thus there is no way for an individual to be equipped with just the behaviors suited for interaction for the particular members of his or her social group; learning is required with regard to these aspects of the social environment. The second example concerns development of circuits for binocular vision. Grobstein and Chow (1976) suggest that the precise binocular register of cortical cells requires adjustment during individual development because the two eyes have somewhat independent developmental histories; their optics, positions, and shapes develop independently and are affected by a variety of internal and environmental factors that are essentially unpredictable. Let us consider one further example, this one involving still other aspects of the environment: The world that an animal confronts upon emerging from hibernation may contain unpredictable features. For example, a new plant or a new species of animal may have come into the environment. Do they represent a threat or a source of nourishment? The "bait-shyness" response (Garcia & Ervin, 1968; Wilcoxin, Dragoin, & Kral, 1969) represents a special kind of learning that helps to adapt to such new circumstances.

The second hypothesis predicts that, other things being equal, a species that has evolved in a varied and unpredictable environment will show more cerebral plasticity in response to environmental demands than will a similar species from a less varied and more predictable environment. Too few species have yet been examined with regard to neural responsiveness to allow even a preliminary evaluation of this hypothesis. Dr. Bennett and I hope soon to begin some initial tests of the hypothesis, in collaboration with Dr. Paul Sherman, an expert in animal behavior and evolutionary theory. Some projected tests will involve different species of ground squirrels—social species, species in which the individuals are solitary, and also species that live in rather changeable environments versus other species that live in rather stable environments. Animals from such species will be tested for responsiveness of the brain both to varied laboratory environments (adaptations of the EC, SC, and IC situations) and also to natural environments; we predict that larger central effects of differential experience will be found in the social than in the solitary species, and in those from changeable as compared with those from stable environments.

The third hypothesis is that, in view of the metabolic cost of a large brain, there is survival value in holding down brain size at times in the individual's life when a low level of demand is placed upon it, but in leaving the brain large enough to meet some sudden demands and plastic enough to increase its capacity when a higher level of demand occurs. The metabolic cost of the central nervous system is substantial. While the human brain represents only about 2% of the weight of the body, it accounts for about 20% of the energy expenditure of the body at rest. Unlike muscle cells, which have a low resting metabolic rate and can store energy against future needs, the cells of the central nervous system must operate at a high metabolic rate simply to maintain their functional integrity, and they cannot store energy. Thus another type of compromise is required between the benefits conferred by a large complex brain and the metabolic costs entailed in maintaining it.

One test of this hypothesis would be to measure brain size of animals that hibernate, or that go through other phases of life during which little demand for behavioral adjustment occurs and during which energy is at a premium. The hypothesis would predict some reduction in brain weight during hibernation, and a rapid increase when the animal emerges to face new demands of both the social and the inanimate environment. We plan also to undertake some tests of this hypothesis formulated to account for structural plasticity of the nervous system.

Acknowledgments

I would like to thank the many collaborators who have shared in the various phases of the research reported in this chapter, especially Edward L. Bennett, Marie Alberti, Hiromi Morimoto, and Ken Chin.

References

Bennett, E. L. Cerebral effects of differential experience and training. In M. R. Rosenzweig & E. L. Bennett (Eds.), *Neural mechanisms of learning and memory.* Cambridge, Mass.: MIT Press, 1976. Pp. 279–287.

Bennett, E. L., Rosenzweig, M. R., Morimoto, H., & Herbert, M. Maze training alters brain weights and cortical RNA/DNA ratios. *Behavioral and Neural Biology*, 1979, *26*, 1–22.

Bonnet, C. *Oeuvres d'histoire naturelle et de philosophie.* Neuchatel: S. Fauche, 1779–1783.

Bischoff, T. L. W. *Das Hirngewicht des Menschen.* Bonn: Neusser, 1880.

Brandt, A. Sur le rapport du poids du cerveau à celui du corps chez differns animaux. *Bulletin de la Société Impériale des Naturalistes de Moscou*, 1867, *40* (Part 2), 525–543.

Bremermann, H. Quantitive aspects of goal-seeking self-organizing systems. *Progress in theoretical biology*, 1967, *1*, 59–77.

Cajal, R. S. La fine structure des centres nerveux. *Proceedings Royal Society of London*, 1894, *55*, 444–468.

Coleman, W. R. *Georges Cuvier, zoologist.* Cambridge, Mass.: Harvard University Press, 1964.

Cragg, B. G. Changes in visual cortex on first exposure of rats to light: Effect on synaptic dimensions. *Nature*, 1967, *215*, 251–253.

Cummins, R. A., Livesey, P. J., Evans, J. G. M., & Walsh, R. N. A developmental theory of environmental enrichment. *Science*, 1977, *197*, 692–694.

Cuvier, G. *Leçons d'anatomie comparée* Vol. 2. Paris: Baudoin, 1800.

Cuvier, G. *Recherches sur les ossemens fossiles*. Paris: Dufour et d'Ocagne, 1822.

Diamond, M. C. Extensive cortical depth measurements and neuronal size increases in the cortex of environmentally enriched rats. *Journal of Comparative Neurology*, 1967, *131*, 357–364.

Diamond, M. C., Law, F., Rhodes, H., Lindner, B., Rosenzweig, M. R. Krech, D., & Bennett, E. L. Increases in cortical depth and glia number in rats subjected to enriched environment. *Journal of Comparative Neurology*, 1966, *128*, 117–125.

Diamond, M. C., Lindner, B., Johnson, R., Bennett, E. L., & Rosenzweig, M. R. Differences in occipital cortical synapses from environmentally enriched, impoverished, and standard colony rats. *Journal of Neuroscience Research*, 1975, *1*, 109–119.

Ferchmin, P., Bennett, E. L., & Rosenzweig, M. R. Direct contact with enriched environment is required to alter cerebral weight in rats. *Journal of Comparative and Physiological Psychology*, 1975, *88*, 360–367.

Foster, M., & Sherrington, C. S. *A text book of physiology. Part 3. The central nervous system.* New York: Macmillian and Co., 1897.

Garcia, J., & Ervin, F. R. Gustatory-visual and telereceptor-cutaneous conditioning—adaptation in internal and external milieus. *Communications in Behavioral Biology*, 1968, *1*, 389–415.

Globus, A., Rosenzweig, M. R., Bennett, E. L., & Diamond, M. C. Effects of differential experience on dendritic spine counts. *Journal of Comparative and Physiological Psychology*, 1973, *82*, 175–181.

Greenough, W. T. Enduring brain effects of differential experience and training. In M. R. Rosenzweig & E. L. Bennett (Eds.), *Neural mechanisms of learning and memory*. Cambridge, Mass.: MIT Press, 1976. Pp. 255–278.

Grobstein, P., & Chow, K. L. Receptive field organization in the mammalian visual cortex: The role of individual experience in development. In G. Gottlieb (Ed.), *Studies on the development of behavior and the nervous system (Vol. 3), Neural and behavioral specificity.* New York: Academic Press, 1976. Pp. 155–193.

Grouse, L. D., Schrier, B. K., Bennett, E. L., Rosenzweig, M. R., & Nelson, P. G. Sequence diversity studies of rat brain RNA: Effects of environmental complexity on rat brain RNA diversity. *Journal of Neurochemistry*, 1978, *30*, 191–203.

Jerison, H. J. *Evolution of the brain and intelligence*. New York: Academic Press, 1973.

Journal de Physique (Paris), 1793, *43*, 73.

Kandel, E. R. *Cellular basis of behavior*. San Francisco: W. H. Freeman Co., 1976.

Krasne, F. B. Invertebrate systems as a means of gaining insight into the nature of learning and memory. In M. R. Rosenzweig & E. L. Bennett (Eds.), *Neural mechanisms of learning and memory*. Cambridge, Mass.: MIT Press, 1976. Pp. 401–429.

Krech, D., Rosenzweig, M. R., & Bennett, E. L. Effects of environmental complexity and training on brain chemistry. *Journal of Comparative and Physiological Psychology*, 1960, *53*, 509–519.

Kroeber, A. L. *Anthropology*, New York: Harcourt, Brace & World, 1948.

Krompecher, S., & Lipak, J. A simple method for determining cerebralization: Brain weight and intelligence. *Journal of Comparative Neurology*, 1966, *127*, 113–120.

Lugaro, E. I recenti progressi dell'anatomia del sistema nervoso in rapporto alla psicologia ed alla psichiatria. *Rivista di patologia nervosa e mentale*, 1899, *4*, 481–514, 537–547.

Magendie, F. *An elementary compendium of physiology.* (translated by E. Milligan.) Edinburgh: J. Carfrae, 1831.

Miller, G. A. *Psychology: The science of mental life.* New York: Harper & Row, 1962.

Møllgaard, D., Diamond, M. C., Bennett, E. L., Rosenzweig, M. R., & Lindner, B. Quantitative synaptic changes with differential experience in rat brain. *Intern. J. Neuroscience*, 1971, 2, 113–128.

Pearson, K. *The life, letters and labours of Francis Galton* Vol. 2. Cambridge, England: Cambridge University Press, 1924.

Platt, J. R. Strong inference. *Science*, 1964, 146, 347–353.

Riege, W. H., & Morimoto, H. Effects of chronic stress and differential environments upon brain weights and biogenic amine levels in rats. *Journal of Comparative and Physiological Psychology*, 1970, 71, 396–404.

Rosenzweig, M. R., & Bennett, E. L. Effects of differential environments on brain weights and enzyme activities in gerbils, rats, and mice. *Developmental Psychobiology*, 1969, 2, 87–95.

Rosenzweig, M. R., & Bennett, E. L. Cerebral changes in rats exposed individually to an enriched environment. *J. Comp. Physiol. Psych.*, 1972, 80, 304–313.

Rosenzweig, M. R., & Bennett, E. L. Enriched environments: Facts, factors, and fantasies. In L. Petrinovich & J. L. McGaugh (Eds.), *Knowing, thinking and believing*. New York: Plenum Press, 1976. Pp. 179–212.

Rosenzweig, M. R., & Bennett, E. L. Effects of environmental enrichment or impoverishment on learning and on brain values in rodents. In A. Oliverio (Ed.), *Genetics, environment, and intelligence*. Amsterdam: Elsevier–North-Holland, 1977. Pp. 163–195.

Rosenzweig, M. R., & Bennett, E. L. Experimental influences on brain anatomy and brain chemistry in rodents. In G. Gottlieb (Ed.), *Studies on the development of behavior and the nervous system. Vol. 4. Early influences*. New York: Academic Press, 1978. Pp. 289–327.

Rosenzweig, M. R., Bennett, E. L., & Diamond, M. C. Cerebral effects of differential environments occur in hypophysectomized rats. *Journal of Comparative and Physiological Psychology*, 1972, 79, 56–66.

Rosenzweig, M. R., Bennett, E. L., Herbert, M., & Morimoto, H. Social grouping cannot account for cerebral effects of enriched environments. *Brain Research*, 1978, 153, 563–576.

Rosenzweig, M. R., Krech, D., & Bennett, E. L. Heredity, environment, brain biochemistry, and learning. In *Current trends in psychological theory*. Pittsburgh: University of Pittsburgh Press, 1961. Pp. 87–110.

Snell, O. Die Abhängigkeit des Hirngewichtes von dem Körpergewicht und den geistingen Fähigkeiten. *Archiv für Psychiatrie und Nervenkrankheiten*, 1892, 23, 436–446.

Soemmering, S. T. *Von Baue des menschlichen Koerpers*, Vol. 5, Part 1. Frankfurt am Main: Barrentrapp and Wenner, 1791.

Soemmering, S. T. *Ueber die Korperliche Verschiedenheit des Negers von Europaer*. Frankfurt am Mainz, 1785 (Extracts are given as an appendix in C. White, *An account of the regular gradation in man and in different animals and vegetables*. London, 1799).

Szeligo, F., & Leblond, C. P. Response of the three main types of glial cells of cortex and corpus callosum in rats handled during suckling or exposed to enriched, control and impoverished environments following weaning. *Journal of Comparative Neurology*, 1977, 172, 247–264.

Tanzi, E. I fatti e le induzioni nell'odierna isologia del sistema nervoso. *Revista Sperimentale di Freniatria e di Medicina Legale*, 1893, 19, 419–472.

Van Valen, L. Brain size and intelligence in man. *American Journal of Physical Anthropology*, 1974, 40, 417–424.

Walsh, R. N., & Cummins, R. A. Mechanisms mediating the production of environmentally induced brain changes. *Psychological Bulletin*, 1975, 82, 986–1000.

West, R. W., & Greenough, W. T. Effect of environmental complexity on cortical synapses of rats: Preliminary results. *Behavioral Biology,* 1972, *7,* 279–284.

White, C. *An account of the regular gradation in man and in different animals and vegetables.* London: C. Dilly, 1799.

Wilcoxin, H., Dragoin, W., & Kral, P. Illness-induced aversions in rat and quail: Relative salience of visual and gustatory cues. *Science,* 1971, *171,* 826–828.

Williams, G. C. *Adaptation and natural selection.* Princeton, N.J.: Princeton University Press, 1966.

Chapter XV

Experience-Induced Changes in Brain Fine Structure: Their Behavioral Implications[1]

WILLIAM T. GREENOUGH
JANICE M. JURASKA

The other chapters in this volume have summarized views of the relationships between evolution, genetics, brain size, and behavior. Possible relationships between *genetically dependent* brain size and behavior, especially intelligent behavior, have been investigated from several perspectives. Jerison (1973; also see Jerison's chapter in this volume) has argued that the size of the brain can be viewed as an index of intelligence of various species across evolutionary time. In another paradigm, strains of mice have been selectively bred for high brain weight. They are superior to mice selectively bred for low brain weight and controls in some discrimination tasks (e.g., Elias, 1969; Wimer & Prater, 1966). Unfortunately, high brain weight mice are not superior in all learning tasks (Ahroon & Fuller, 1976; also see Fuller and Jensen's chapters in this volume); these brain size differences cannot easily be related to the development of behavior (Fuller & Geils, 1973).

In the preceding chapter, Rosenzweig has discussed historical and modern research approaches to *experience-induced* changes in brain size. This research provides information of potential use to those who wish to understand the relationship between brain size and behavior. In this

[1]Work described here and not otherwise reported has been supported by NSF Grants BMS 75 08596 and BNS 77 23660, NIH Grant MH 28529, and the James McKeen Cattell Foundation. Dr. Juraska was supported by NIMH postdoctoral award MH 07286 during preparation of this chapter.

295

DEVELOPMENT AND EVOLUTION
OF BRAIN SIZE

chapter, we will examine the evidence that supports the following major points:

1. Genetic differences in overall brain size, or regional brain size, usually correspond to differences in *neuron* (and associated glial) *numbers*. Differences in the size of equivalent cells from brains of widely different size, such as those of rat and man, are remarkably small. In contrast, differences induced by *experience* typically do not involve differences in the number of neurons, although glial cell numbers may change. Rather, such differences appear to be associated with changes in the number or properties of *synaptic connections* between neurons.
2. The synaptic effects following experience often correspond regionally to gross differences in brain size (cortical thickness, etc.).
3. Brain changes induced by differential sensory input are predictable in that effects occur in regions of the brain corresponding to the processing centers for that input.
4. Behavioral output corresponds to some degree to the region in which brain size differences are induced. The types of behavior affected by lesions of a region also appear to be affected when the anatomy of the region is altered by differential experience.

Experience-Induced Changes at the Neuron Level

A number of correlates of experience-induced changes in the size of brain structures have been described at the level of the individual cell, as Rosenzweig's chapter has noted. Since, with the exception of a few regions, neuronal proliferation is largely complete prior to the time that differential experience manipulations occur, the effects of such manipulations appear in the properties of already existing neurons. While these effects are reflected in relatively gross differences in cell size and in supportive tissue, changes in the synaptic connections between neurons indicate that the functional organization of the brain is altered by experience. The changes fall into two basic classes: changes in the *number* of synapses and changes in the *properties* of synapses. The bulk of the data have come from manipulations of two types: sensory deprivation and differential environmental housing.

Visual Deprivation Effects on Brain Anatomy

Sensory deprivation is an extreme form of experience and would be expected to influence sensory areas of the brain and behavior. Visual deprivation is the most thoroughly studied form of deprivation since it is relatively easy to accomplish. It can take several forms. Eye enucleation will not be reviewed here because it involves degeneration of some central pathways and, obviously, results in a blind animal, making brain–behavior relationships meaningless. Dark rearing and lid suture are the most common noninvasive types of visual deprivation. Both are readily reversible. Lid suturing can be performed binocularly or monocularly. The latter has the added advantage of depriving only part of the animal's visual system so that there is a within subject control. However, it also has a disadvantage in that for some species it may result in competition between inputs from the two eyes to the brain.

GROSS STRUCTURE AND CELL SIZE

The size of specific visual areas of the brain is reduced by visual deprivation. Using monocular lid suturing (from the time of eye opening) in rats, Fifková and Hassler (1969) found a decrease in the volume of the brain on the side contralateral to the deprived eye. (The vast majority of optic fibers in the rat cross to the opposite side of the brain.) Both the dorsal lateral geniculate nucleus (LGN) and the visual cortex contralateral to the deprived eye showed a significant decrease in volume. Also, Gyllensten, Malmfors, and Norrlin (1965) found that the visual cortex decreased in thickness after dark rearing mice from birth to 2–4 months.

Such gross measures of regional brain size changes indicate finer changes, many of which have been described. In the deprived LGN of the rat, Fifková and Hassler (1969) found a decrease in the number of neurons after monocular suturing. Using the same paradigm in kittens, Wiesel and Hubel (1963) found atrophy of the layers of the LGN receiving input from the deprived eye. They also observed a large decrease in cell size (25–40%) in these layers, as well as decreases in intercellular space. Similar but less severe changes have been reported after monocular suturing of rabbits' eyes (Chow & Spear, 1974). After dark rearing, Gyllensten et al. (1965) found extranuclear material decreases in the LGN of mice.

Thus the lateral geniculate, a relay nucleus in the visual system, exhibits plastic changes with visual deprivation. However, of seemingly greater relevance to our discussion of brain–behavior relationships are the changes that occur in the visual cortex. After monocular deprivation of rats, Fifková (1970c) reported that layers III and IV of the contralateral visual cortex showed increases in cell density, which are indicative of decreases in intercellular material. Gyllensten (1959) also found in layers II–IV a reduction of internuclear material and a decrease in size of cell nuclei in the visual cortex of dark reared mice.

CHANGES AT THE SYNAPTIC LEVEL

Since dendrites and axons are found in what is termed the intercellular material, it seems likely that these elements decrease after visual deprivation. Such data would indicate changes in the number or location of synapses. Valverde (1976) has presented preliminary evidence that the lengths of intracortical axons are shortened following visual deprivation in mice. Coleman and Riesen (1968) found that stellate neurons in the cat visual cortex tended to have fewer and shorter higher order (farther out from the cell body) dendritic branches after dark rearing. Orientation of dendritic branches has also been reported to change after dark rearing in rats (Borges & Berry, 1976). Valverde (1967) found large decreases in numbers of dendritic spines, representing postsynaptic sites, on the apical shafts of layer V pyramidal neurons in dark reared mouse cortex. Similarly, Fifková (1970c) showed a decrease in spine density in the same layer after monocular suturing in rats. In rabbits, on the other hand, no changes in dendritic branching or spine density were found after dark rearing (Globus & Schiebel, 1967). However, some spine deformations were observed. Undoubtedly many of these changes vary across species.

A few studies have indicated that changes in the properties of synapses, as well as the number of synapses, may occur following manipulations of visual experience. Using electron microscopy, Cragg (1969) found a decrease in the diameter of LGN axon terminals, but an increase in axon terminal density when rats had been dark reared and subsequently exposed to light. In the superficial visual cortex, exposure of dark reared rats to light increased the size of synaptic contacts; in the deeper cortical layers, contacts were smaller but more frequent per unit tissue volume (Cragg, 1967). Cragg suggested that superficial synapses grew larger, while new synapses formed in deeper layers. The latter region corresponds roughly to the area in which Valverde (1971) reported increased dendritic spine frequency following light exposure. Using monocular closure, Fifková (1970a) found a relative decrease in axodendritic synaptic frequency, coupled with an increase in average synaptic contact size in the hemisphere receiving input from the closed eye. Axosomatic synaptic contacts decreased in size in the deprived cortex (Fifková, 1970b). Together these studies suggest that the size of synapses, as well as the numbers, may be altered by experience.

In addition, there is preliminary evidence that visual manipulations may alter the number of vesicles in synaptic terminals. Garey and Pettigrew (1974) using cats, reported that relative to visually deprived hemispheres, synapses of hemispheres receiving visual input had more vesicles. Similarly, Vrensen and DeGroot (1974, 1975) described sizable decreases in synaptic vesicle numbers following monocular closure or dark rearing in rabbits. Moreover, the reduction in vesicle numbers persisted in the dark reared rabbits for at least a year following exposure to normal light. Vrensen and DeGroot suggested that dark rearing may diminish the ability of synapses to synthesize or to store neurotransmitters.

Thus far this review has only included studies of deprivation that started at or before the time of eye opening. There have been attempts at visually depriving older animals, but the results have been mixed. Gyllensten et al. (1965) observed decreases in internuclear material in the LGN and the visual cortex of adult mice placed in darkness. Fifková (1970c) found that changes in volume of both the LGN and cortex could be induced in adult rats that were monocularly sutured, whereas after monocular deprivation of adult cats, Wiesel and Hubel (1963) found no changes in LGN cell size. The species of animal used, the type of deprivation, and the measures taken all may influence whether deprivation effects can be found in adults.

The degree to which the system can recover from deprivation once exposed to light is also of interest. Fifková (1970c) reported virtually no recovery in the size of the LGN and visual cortex after monocular deprivation in rats. This is consistent with the lack of electrophysiological recovery after monocular deprivation in cats (Wiesel & Hubel, 1965). On the other hand, Valverde (1971) found in mice that dendritic spine density showed some recovery, but not to the level of light reared controls. While more work on recovery from deprivation is needed, the current evidence is that deprivation effects are not as pronounced in adults, and that recovery from developmental deprivation is less than complete. This leads to the conclusion that there is a sensitive period for the effects of visual deprivation during development.

Thus we know that with visual deprivation the cortex and lateral geniculate change in structure, both in size and at a finer level. The overall significance of these changes for the organism and its behavior are not fully known. However, they do correlate with both physiological and behavioral measures of function. It has been suggested regularly that these light-dependent differences in the number and properties of synapses underlie light-dependent maturation or maintenance of visual ability.

Differential Postweaning Experience

Visual deprivation is more severe than the extremes an animal generally experiences in its natural environment. More subtle manipulations are possible, and again these can alter both brain and behavior. Rosenzweig described a commonly used paradigm in the preceding chapter. Briefly, animals are housed singly in standard laboratory cages (isolated condition or IC), in social conditions (SC) with other animals, or in a condition enriched or complex (EC) relative to standard laboratory conditions. In EC, other animals and various toy objects are available to the subject. Frequently, littermates across conditions are compared to minimize preexperimental variance. Although the enriched experience has principally involved rodents, there is some work with other species that examines the behavior of isolate and socially reared animals. Clearly there are differences in the levels of stimulation that animals in these groups receive. Such paradigms may help to elucidate the sorts of experiences and anatomical changes that accompany more complex behavior.

Rosenzweig has summarized some anatomical consequences of enriched rearing in his chapter. Gross brain weight and size increases are found with enriched rearing. These effects are mainly cortical, especially in the occipital or visual cortex. Again the effects indicate differences in both the number and characteristics of synapses.

Indications of differential numbers of synapses have come primarily from studies employing Golgi stains. These stains impregnate entire neurons such that the dendritic (and axonal in certain rapid Golgi procedures) processes can be followed. A small percentage of cells stain, so that the stained cells are easy to visualize in good preparations. Their processes can be recorded in their entirety within a thick tissue section (100 microns). We have done so either with a camera lucida, a microscope tracing device, or more recently with a computer drawing system in which sequential points along neuronal processes are recorded in three dimensions. Estimates of the total amount of dendritic material can be obtained from either the relative numbers of intersections between dendrites and an overlay of concentric rings (or spheres, in a three dimensional analysis), or from direct measures of the length of dendrites. In addition, we quantify the number of dendrites at each order away from the cell body, indicating where differences occur within the dendritic tree. These measures are shown in Figure XV.1.

The occipital cortex showed the greatest effects in the studies described by Rosenzweig (preceding chapter). Following preliminary work by Holloway (1966), we examined this region and found clear differences in the extent of the dendritic tree in several types of neurons. EC rats had the most extensive branching, SC rats were intermediate, and IC rats had the least extensive dendritic tree. As seen in Figure XV.2, the differences appeared in the outer regions of the dendritic tree, and were

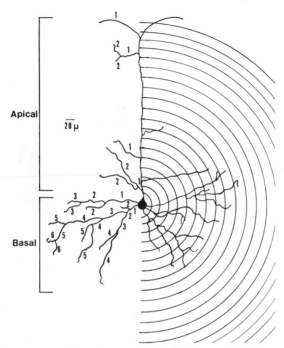

FIGURE XV.1. The amount of dendritic material for both apical and basilar branches of cortical neurons is analyzed in two ways: 1. The intersections between dendrites and a series of concentric rings are counted (right); 2. The number and length of dendrites at each order (defined by bifurcations) from the cell body or apical shaft are measured (left). [From Greenough, 1975.]

evident in all three measures (Greenough & Volkmar, 1973; Volkmar & Greenough, 1972). We have replicated these studies, and while the magnitude of the differences may vary across replications, the results are consistent in animals placed in differential environments for 30 days following weaning.

These differences indicate the presence of more dendritic surface for synapses and imply that more synapses are present on each neuron. However, it is possible that synapses are merely further apart on these longer dendrites, such that no net difference exists. This possibility is contradicted by the Globus, Rosenzweig, Bennett, and Diamond (1973) findings, which are described in Rosenzweig's chapter. Globus *et al.* found that the frequency of spines along occipital neuronal dendrites in EC rats is greater or equal to IC rats, depending on dendritic location.

Indications that characteristics of synapses at the ultrastructural level

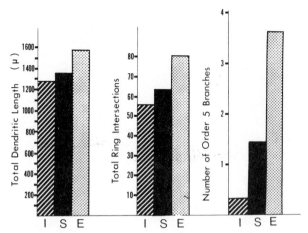

FIGURE XV.2. A comparison of measures of the extent of dendritic processes in stellate neurons of cortical layer IV in rats reared in isolation (I), social (S), and complex (E) environments. [From Greenough, Volkmar, & Fleischmann 1976.]

may be altered by differential rearing have arisen from electron microscopic studies. The size of axodendritic synapses, reflected in the length of the postsynaptic thickening, is greater on the average in EC than in IC rats for some cortical layers (Diamond, Lindner, Johnson, Bennett, & Rosenzweig, 1975; Møllgaard, Diamond, Bennett, Rosenzweig, & Lindner, 1971; West & Greenough, 1972). In addition, we have recently found that the relative frequency of perforations in the postsynaptic thickening (subsynaptic plate perforations, or SSPPs) is affected by rearing conditions. These SSPPs, which are seen as discontinuities in the two dimensional section through the postsynaptic thickening, appear as perforations in a postsynaptic plate in serial reconstructions (Peters & Kaiserman-Abramof, 1969), as shown in Figure XV.3. Greenough, West, and DeVoogd (1978) found that the frequency with which these holes appeared in axodendritic synapses was higher in EC rats than in IC rats, while SCs were intermediate. We have also seen changes in the frequency of these perforations with other experience manipulations and with age. While the size changes could be interpreted as an indication of increased synaptic efficacy, the possible role of SSPPs in synaptic function is less obvious.

Thus after differential rearing, there appear to be both more synapses and synapses with different characteristics in the groups exposed to greater environmental complexity. These differences are correlated with enhanced behavioral ability discussed later in this chapter.

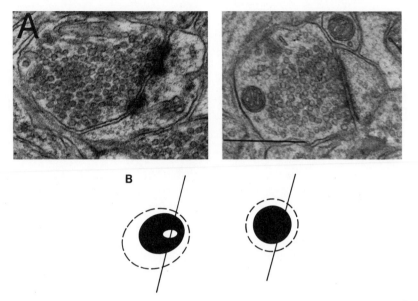

FIGURE XV.3. (a) Electron micrographs shown of round vesicle, axodendritic synapses. The synapse at the right does not contain an SSPP while the one at the left does, Bar = .5. (b) Possible configurations of the above synapses viewed perpendicular to the plane of section. Lines indicate possible plane of section. [This form of illustration is adapted from Peters & Kaiserman-Abramof, 1969.]

Relations between Gross and Fine Structure Changes

We have previously noted that the gross structural effects of visual deprivation on visual centers are paralleled by fine structural changes in those regions. A degree of correspondence is also evident in a comparison of studies of gross and fine measures in nonvisual brain regions after visual deprivation. Gyllensten, Malmfors, and Norrlin (1965, 1966) described both relative shrinkage of visual cortex and relative growth of auditory cortex in mice kept in the dark for long periods. The auditory growth may possibly occur to compensate for loss of visual orienting ability. In a Golgi study, Ryugo, Ryugo, Globus, and Killackey (1975) similarly reported that mice whose eyes were removed at birth had both reduced spine frequency on deep pyramidal cells of visual cortex and increased numbers of spines on corresponding cells in the auditory cortex.

A similar correspondence between regional effects on gross and fine structure has appeared in environmental complexity research. We have already noted that the changes in occipital cortex depth reported by Rosenzweig are paralleled by a variety of finer structural changes. Also in temporal cortex, Greenough, Volkmar, and Juraska (1973) found that dendritic branching differences mirrored the cortical thickening differences described by Diamond, Rosenzweig, Bennett, Lindner, and Lyon (1972). We also failed to find dendritic changes in the frontolateral cortex (Greenough, Volkmar, & Juraska, 1973), a region that Diamond *et al.* (1972) reported not to differ in thickness. While these studies suggest a close relationship between regional size and neuron level changes, the relationship may not hold in all cases. Diamond *et al.* (1972) have found cortical depth differences in occipital cortex, regardless of the age at which subjects enter the differential environments (see also Riege, 1971). While our preliminary data do not rule out small effects, we have not been able to find the full dendritic effect in adults that we have seen when the rats were placed in the environments at weaning.

These studies and others discussed previously also indicate that sensory deprivation effects occur in the brain regions associated with the deprived modality and generally not elsewhere (excluding compensatory hypertrophy). Similarly, specific regional patterns of brain change, including areas unaffected by the treatments, are seen in environmental complexity research. In contrast, if general effects on brain arousal, metabolism, or hormonal state were the cause of changes following complex rearing, they would be more evenly distributed throughout the brain.

In summary, the gross regional size changes that accompany differences in experience are associated with changes at the neuronal level in the number, pattern, and qualities of synaptic connections. This indicates that the organization of selected regions has been modified by experience. Clearly this has implications for behavior.

Relationships to Behavior

Visual Deprivation

A number of deficits in visual behavior have been reported following visual deprivation. Immediately after binocular deprivation, dark rearing, or monocular deprivation, animals (cats are generally used) appear functionally blind. They bump into obstacles, fail to blink at approaching objects, do not reach for objects or visually place, that is, extend, their paws when brought toward a surface (reviewed in Ganz, 1975). Recovery from this apparent blindness occurs, although it is quite slow in the monocularly sutured eye. Part of the original deficit relates to the lack of visual-motor experience that accompanies visual deprivation, and this can readily be reversed (Held & Hein, 1963). However, there are permanent losses in visual behavior.

Monocular suturing results in the most persistent deficits in cats, particularly when imposed during an early critical period (Dews & Wiesel, 1970). Animals recover from their initial blindness (bumping into objects, etc.) much more slowly and incompletely after monocular deprivation than after binocular deprivation (Ganz & Fitch, 1968). The monocularly deprived also exhibit more severe deficits on visual discrimination problems (Dews & Wiesel, 1970; Ganz, Hirsch, & Tieman, 1972). Suturing of the nondeprived eye appears to aid in some recovery of the deprived eye (Dews & Wiesel, 1970), and removing the nondeprived eye rapidly produces pronounced recovery (Smith & Loop, 1978).

Dark reared rats have been found to perform as well as light reared rats on a visual cliff, although with long periods in darkness more time in light is required for normal performance (Nealy & Riley, 1963). However, in most visual cliff testing very deep sides are used. When a more shallow cliff is employed, dark reared animals show deficits in depth perception that are not readily reversed (Walk & Walters, 1973). Tees (1974) showed that such subtle tests of depth perception on a visual cliff improve with age in light reared rats. Dark reared rats also show some increments in depth perception with age, but with a longer time in darkness there is deterioration. Thus experience in light seems necessary to maintain as well as to increment some perceptual abilities. Most of the anatomical studies of light deprivation have not been done longitudinally. Therefore, it is not known whether visual experience has a maintenance as well as an inductive effect on such factors as neuron growth and synaptogenesis.

In addition to depth perception, dark reared animals show deficiencies in various visual discriminations. Cats that have been reared in the dark or diffuse light are slower to discriminate between complex stimuli such as an X versus an N (Riesen, 1965) or a cross versus a circle (Meyers & McCleary, 1964).

Some of the most elegant studies of the visual deficiencies found in dark reared hooded rats have been performed by Tees. He demonstrated that dark reared rats learned simple pattern discriminations as well as light reared rats. However, it took more trials for the dark reared to learn the more difficult X versus N discrimination (Tees, 1968b). Task difficulty alone is not the sole determinant of poorer performance for the dark reared rats. They could learn very difficult light intensity discriminations as well as the controls, even though these tasks took the controls more trials than the X versus N discrimination (Tees, 1968a). It may be that the X versus N discrimination requires a degree of spatial integration that visually inexperienced rats find difficult (Tees, 1976). Further experiments revealed that while both groups were using luminous flux cues in solving the intensity discrimination, the light reared controls were using luminance cues more than the dark reared (Tees, 1971). Thus, even when there are no differences in trials to criterion in a task, the strategy used may differ with visual experience.

Paralleling the selectivity of anatomical effects on the visual system, Tees and Cartwright (1972) also have shown that the deficits after dark rearing are specific to visual information and not due to some overall learning deficiency. Using a sensory preconditioning paradigm, they found no deficit in the dark reared group when associating two auditory stimuli, but did find less learning than the light reared when visual and auditory stimuli were paried. This demonstrates a difference in readiness to attend to particular types of stimuli without a difference in learning ability per se.

Thus the behavioral deficits accompanying visual deprivation may sometimes be subtle. Specific relationships between anatomical and behavioral effects of visual manipulations have yet to be established, in part because anatomical and behavioral studies have rarely been coordinated with regard to procedures. It seems quite likely that the deficits in anatomically detectable organization of visual brain regions underlie the behavioral deficits, at least to some degree.

Differential Postweaning Experience

While the effects of visual deprivation are seen primarily in visually related behavior, the behavioral changes following complex, social, and isolation rearing are broader and more difficult to classify. Likewise, the behavioral effects are harder to relate to the various regional brain changes that have been described.

Because animals reared in complex environments exhibit regional increases in numbers and sizes of synapses, as well as gross size, it has been predicted that they should be superior in information processing and better able to perform complex behavioral tasks. Evidence that this is true, in fact, predates the brain findings. Hebb (1949) reported that rats raised as pets at home were superior to laboratory rats in a Hebb-Williams maze and other tasks.

A variety of investigators since have similarly found that rats reared in a more complex environment are superior to isolated or socially housed rats in various types of mazes (e.g., Brown, 1968; Forgays &

Forgays, 1952; Greenough, Madden, & Fleischmann, 1972; Hymovitch, 1952), reversal learning (Krech, Rosenzweig & Bennett, 1962; Morgan, 1973), and alternation (Nyman, 1967). All of these tasks could be considered to be relatively complex for a rat. On simple tasks the results are more mixed. Although Greenough, Yuwiler, and Dollinger (1973) reported that EC rats were superior to ICs in a brightness discrimination, others have reported no differences in visual discrimination learning (Bingham & Griffiths, 1952; Krech et al., 1962). Also Freeman and Ray (1972) found that enriched rats performed more poorly than controls in a passive-avoidance situation, while Greenough, Fulcher, Yuwiler, and Geller (1970) found them to be superior. Some of the variability in results could stem from differences in the type and degree of enriched experience given. Age is also an important variable which will be discussed later. In general, the most pronounced behavioral differences occur when the differential environments are instituted at weaning.

Are there general behavioral qualities that lead to the superior performance of rats reared in complex environments? Since the visual cortex is the most affected cortical area, superior visual ability could underlie behavioral differences. However, blinded rats reared in complex environments also showed cortical depth changes (Krech, Rosenzweig, & Bennett, 1963) and behavioral superiority on mazes when compared to blinded isolated rats (Hymovitch, 1952; Lash & Goldstein, 1965). Visual experience undoubtedly does play a role, but it is not the only type of experience that is occurring. It has been proposed that isolated animals perform poorly on tasks such as mazes because they have an increased exploratory drive and thus make more errors (Myers & Fox, 1963; Woods, Fiske, Ruckelshaus, 1961; Zimbardo & Montgomery, 1957). However, the results from activity in an open field are mixed. Isolated animals have been found to be more active (Morgan, 1973; Zimbardo & Montgomery, 1957), less active (Gardner, Boitano, Mancino, D'Amico, & Gardner, 1975), and not different (Brown, 1968; Freeman & Ray, 1972) relative to EC animals in an open field situation. Smith (1972) did find isolated rats to be more active in the open field but did not find a correlation for individual animals between open field scores and errors in a Hebb-Williams maze. Greater emotionality of isolated animals could also contribute to performance differences. However, Greenough, Madden, and Fleishmann (1972) found differences on a Lashley III maze even after isolated animals had been calmed by daily handling. The hypothesis that isolated animals are poorer performers due to motor deficits has also not been supported (Morgan, 1973). Greenough, Wood, and Madden (1972) presented data consistent with the idea that the information processing capacity of mice in a complex environment is greater. They found that with spaced trials, mice that were reared in either EC or SC learned a Lashley III maze faster than IC mice. However, with massed trials the EC mice were superior to the other groups. EC mice appeared to be the only group capable of keeping pace with massed trials.

There is also evidence that after the enriched experience, animals sample more or at least different cues. Several investigators have found that enriched rats made fewer errors than isolated rats in a Hebb-Williams maze but fell to the isolated level when the maze was rotated (Brown, 1968; Forgays & Forgays, 1952; Hymovitch, 1952). This indicates that the enriched animals were using extra-maze cues. However, Ravizza and Herschberger (1966) ran their Hebb-Williams maze with a curtain around it and still found that enriched rats were superior. Thus the use of different cues is not the only difference between the enriched and the isolated; given the opportunity, the enriched may use different or a wider variety of cues to solve a problem.

There does not seem to be any single explanation for why EC animals are superior in some behavioral tasks. Perhaps the experience changes the organism on a number of dimensions. Two hypotheses that have received some support are differences in the use of cues and differences in information-processing speed or capacity, although differences in other aspects of behavioral ability seem likely.

Differential Rearing and the Hippocampus

One instance in which behavioral and brain effects appear mutually predictable involves the hippocampus. Behavioral effects of hippocampal lesions and of IC, relative to EC, rearing appear remarkably similar in several instances. Both hippocampectomized and IC animals are inferior maze learners (Bender, Hostetter & Thomas, 1968; Greenough, Wood & Madden, 1972; Kimble, 1963; Rosenzweig, 1971); both are inferior on discrimination reversal learning (Rosenzweig, 1971; Teitelbaum, 1964), alternation tasks (Dalland, 1970; Nyman, 1967), and passive avoidance (Greenough et al., 1970; Isaacson & Wicklegren, 1962). In hippocampal lesion studies, these findings have been interpreted to reflect deficits in perceptual or behavioral inhibition (Altman, Brunner, & Bayer, 1973; Douglas, 1967; Kimble, 1968) or spatial ability (Nadel, O'Keefe, & Black, 1975; Olton, 1977). Further evidence comes from work on social and isolated rats in which isolated rats were slower to habituate to objects in an open field and exhibited greater response perseveration after reinforcement contingencies changed than socially reared rats

(Einon & Morgan, 1977; Morgan, Einon, & Morris, 1977; Morgan, Einon, & Nicholas, 1975). Thus there appear to be similar deficits in hippocampectomized and isolation reared animals. This leads to the prediction that the hippocampus may be affected by differential rearing.

Until recently the evidence was mixed as to whether there are hippocampal changes after differential rearing. Walsh, Budtz-Olsen, Penny, and Cummins (1969) found that the medial hippocampus was thicker in EC rats than in ICs. On the other hand, Diamond, Ingham, Johnson, Bennett, and Rosenzweig (1976) could not find consistent hippocampal changes. In our laboratory, Fleischmann (1972) found that certain hippocampal synapses were larger in enriched rats.

Fiala, Joyce,and Greenough (1978) have found dendritic branching differences in hippocampal granule cells after enriched and isolated rearing that began at weaning. The hippocampus of some animals was Golgi-Cox stained and in others Golgi-Kopsch stained. Granule cells were traced (without knowledge of groups) from 13 littermate male pairs of rats. Dendritic trees of neurons were analyzed for width and height as well as with a Sholl concentric ring analysis (see Figure XV.4). Dendrites were also analyzed for length and number at each order. The EC rats had significantly wider, but not taller, granule cell dendritic fields than the isolates. They also had more first and second order dendritic branches (i.e., those closest to the cell body) and more dendritic inter-

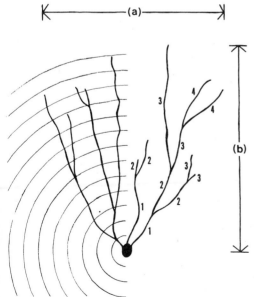

FIGURE XV. 4. The analysis is of the hippocampal granule cells. The dendritic field was measured with a concentric ring analysis (left) and through a tabulation of length and number of dendritic branches at each order from the cell body (right). Also the width (a) and height (b) of the dendritic field was measured. [From Fiala, Joyce, & Greenough, 1978.]

sections with the innermost Sholl rings (Figures XV.5 and XV.6). This contrasts with the cortical effect found in previous work (Greenough, Volkmar, & Juraska, 1973; Volkmar & Greenough, 1972). In all populations of cortical neurons examined, the effects of the enriched rearing experience were found in the higher order dendritic branches and outer Sholl rings, further from the cell body.

Thus the hippocampus provides an example of reasonably strong predictive relationships between behavioral and anatomical measures of the effects of differential rearing. Moreover, the parallel holds across age differences, to some degree. The behavioral literature indicates that there may be critical, or at least more sensitive, periods for differential environmental effects on behavior. Differential experience immediately after weaning has been found to be the most effective time for the behavioral differences seen in some mazes (Forgays & Read, 1962; Hymovitch, 1952), in habituation of object contact in an open field (Einon & Morgan, 1977), and in visual discrimination reversals (Rosenzweig, 1971). In fact, Rosenzweig (1971) reported that the inferiority of isolated rats on the discrimination reversal task only occurred when the environments were imposed at 25 days of age (as opposed to 60 or 90 days). In contrast, superior performance was found for enriched rats on the Lashley III maze, regardless of age at the time of the experience. However, the greatest differences were seen when the environments were instituted immediately postweaning. Thus the impact of postweaning versus adult experience is in part dependent on the task.

This leads to the prediction that some brain effects may be sensitive to the timing of the experience. We have found that the dendritic

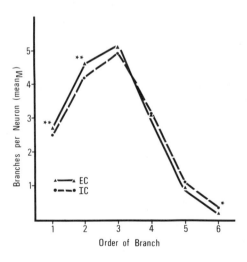

FIGURE XV.5. Number of branches shown at each order of hippocampal granule cells in EC and IC rats. ** is a significant difference at $p < .05$; * indicates a difference of $.10 > p > .05$. [From Fiala, Joyce, & Greenough, 1978.]

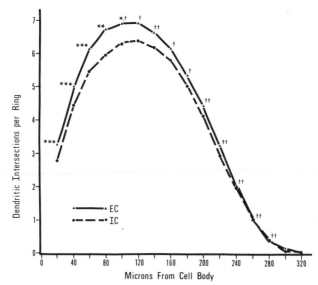

FIGURE XV.6. The results of the concentric ring analysis, with rings at 20 micron intervals, of hippocampal granule cells in EC and IC rats. Significant treatment (EC versus IC) differences are indicated by *** at the .01 level, ** at the .05 level, and * at the .10. Significant litter differences are shown by †† at the .01 level and † at the .05 level.

changes in hippocampal granule cells found after postweaning differential experience were not demonstrable when the experience was started in adulthood (145 days) (Fiala *et al.*, 1978). Thus the hippocampal effect is age dependent. It would be of interest to determine the extent of the parallel between isolation-rearing and hippocampectomy across further behavioral tasks.

Environmental Influence on Primate Cerebellum

Except for a few visual deprivation studies and the hippocampus work cited above, virtually all studies of experiential effects on gross and fine structure of the brain have involved the cerebral cortex. Since we know little about effects elsewhere within the brain, generating behavioral predictions from comparison with brain lesion data (the reverse of the reasoning in the previous section) is not generally possible. Likewise, except for the visual deprivation data, predictions about experience-induced changes in brain of the type in the preceding section have rarely emanated from behavioral analyses. One that has is Prescott's (1971) suggestion that the primate isolation syndrome (Harlow, Dodsworth, &

Harlow, 1965; Mason, 1968) involves somatosensory deprivation and consequent cerebellar-limbic-somatosensory cortex developmental retardation. Prescott proposes that abnormal development of these regions—particularly the cerebellum—underlies the abnormalities in social, self-directed and motor behaviors that comprise the isolation syndrome. To date, there has been little evidence to test this prediction.

Aside from the 1791 Malacarne report described in Rosenzweig's chapter, there is essentially no evidence to indicate experience-produced changes in cerebellar anatomy. While a number of models of cerebellar function seem to require some form of plasticity (e.g., Marr, 1969), only work by Essman (e.g., 1971) suggests that the cerebellum is modified by experience. He has reported that cerebellar DNA, an indication of cell number, was strikingly reduced after isolation rearing in mice.

Recently, in our laboratory, in conjunction with G. P. Sackett of the Washington Primate Research Center, Mary Kay Floeter has obtained preliminary results indicating that fine structural changes do occur in the paraflocculus of the cerebellum in differentially reared monkeys. *Macaca fascicularis* monkeys were reared from 1–2 weeks to 6 months of age in either a sound attenuating chamber with minimal sensory and no social input, in individual cages where they could see other monkeys and had 4 hours of social contact with a peer daily, or in a group of adults and peers in a large room with some play objects. The cerebella were Golgi-Cox stained, and spiny branchlets of Purkinje cells and dendritic fields of granule cells were traced with the aid of a computerized recording system, without knowledge of groups (Figure XV.7). A concentric ring analysis similar to that already described, expanded to three

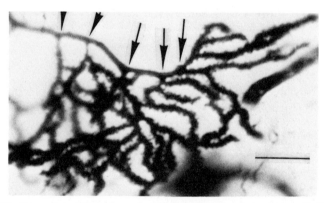

FIGURE XV.7. Examples of Purkinje cell spiny branchlets seen in the cerebellum of the monkey. Arrows show where the individual spiny branchlet units start. Bar = 20 μ. [Courtesy of M. K. Floeter.]

dimensions, was performed. Although no differences were found for the granule cells, the concentric sphere analysis revealed more total sphere intersections for the spiny branchlets in the group housed monkeys than in the partial social and isolated groups (Figure XV.8). The cell body size of Purkinje cells in the uvula was also found to be significantly greater in the group housed animals as opposed to the other two groups (Figure XV.9). Thus group housed monkeys (a condition somewhat comparable to the EC environment for rats) have larger cell bodies and more dendrites in their cerebellar output neurons—the Purkinje cells.

These results fail to confirm the Prescott (1971) predictions, since the intermediate socially experienced group, which did not show a significant behavioral isolation syndrome (Greenough, Floeter, Sackett, Jencius, & Kraff, in preparation), are clearly not more well developed (in terms of cell size and branching) than the isolated animals in these cerebellar regions. However, the data do suggest that the more demanding sensorimotor environment of the large group cage enhanced cerebellar neuronal growth.

The results extend the anatomical effects of differential rearing to monkeys as well as to the cerebellum, a structure that has been largely ignored in such investigations. The cerebellum, unlike the neocortex

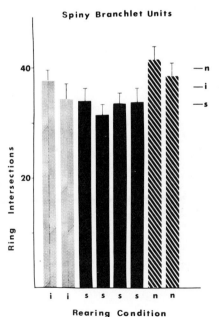

FIGURE XV.8. The results of the concentric ring analysis of Purkinje cell spiny branchlet units for individual monkeys in isolated (i), social (s), and group-housed (n) conditions. The means for each group are indicated on the right.

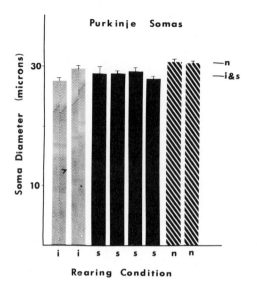

FIGURE XV.9. The average size of Purkinje cell bodies in the cerebellum of individual monkeys in insolated (i), social (s), and group-housed (n) conditions. The group means are indicated on the right.

and hippocampus, is involved in the motor output side of behavior and thus is unique among the areas usually considered to be affected by the rearing environment. This finding lends support to the possibility that areas that do not show gross size changes may also be involved in the anatomical response to the stimulation of the environment.

Conclusions

The new results reported here extend findings of experientially-induced changes in brain structure beyond those previously described in the cerebral cortex and subcortical visual structures. Thus they begin to suggest that anatomically detectable plasticity, at least in fine structure, may be the rule rather than the exception for the higher mammalian brain. Whether plasticity of this sort represents a qualitative difference in mammalian brains is not certain. Most attempts to demonstrate developmental effects of experience manipulations in simpler vertebrates have met with limited success (e.g., Coghill, 1929; Jacobson & Hirsch, 1973), although a recent report of anatomical effects of experience in fish suggests that plasticity may exist at that phyletic level (Coss & Globus, 1978). Clearly, more work along these lines will be necessary to demonstrate the types of plasticity in lower vertebrates that have been amply demonstrated in laboratory mammals.

These indications of widespread anatomical effects of experience suggest caution in attributing behavioral consequences of altered experience to demonstrated correlates in brain anatomy, at least until a more thorough brain and behavioral picture has been obtained. Such an attribution might be strengthened by demonstrating that differential abilities attributed to structural differences no longer exist when those structures have been removed by lesions from the differentially experienced groups. A related approach is to employ different experiences with different brain structure consequences and to compare the effects upon behavior, as has been done in selective visual experience studies.

An alternative approach, which has met with mixed success in the studies described here, is to work from behavioral assessment to predictions regarding structural differences in brain. We have confirmed behaviorally based predictions for hippocampus but not for cerebellum. There is an indication that this approach may be applied to genetically based brain differences as well. Coleman (1972) has examined the hippocampus in the Tryon S_1 ("maze bright") and S_3 ("maze dull") rat strains used by Rosenzweig and his collaborators. Behaviorally, S_1 rats tend to adopt visual "hypotheses" in maze learning, while the S_3 strain is predisposed toward spatial cues (Krechevsky, 1933). Given recent suggestions that the hippocampus plays a role in spatial orientation (Nadel et al., 1975; Olton, 1977), it is perhaps not surprising that Coleman found rats of the S_3 strain to have greater dendritic branching in hippocampal cells.

Clearly, we are not yet able to understand the functional meaning of differences in brain size and fine structure, whether brought about through genetic manipulation or through experiential manipulation. While there is no necessary reason for gross size changes resulting from differential experience and differential genetics to have similar behavioral consequences, there is no evidence or theoretical reason to expect that they do not. Perhaps the best suggestion for progress in both areas is to broaden the anatomical and the behavioral bases of the search for correlates.

Acknowledgments

We thank Raymond L. Jackson for comments on the manuscript, as well as symposium participants. We gratefully acknowledge the assistance of Kathy Wrege, Frederick Snow, and Carol Fahrhenbruch.

References

Ahroon, J. K., & Fuller, J. L. Performance characteristics of maze learning in mice selected for high and low brain weight. *Journal of Comparative and Physiological Psychology*, 1976, *90*, 1184–1190.

Altman, J., Brunner, R. L., & Bayer, S. A. The hippocampus and behavioral maturation. *Behavioral Biology*, 1973, *8*, 557–596.

Bender, R. M., Hostetter, G., & Thomas, G. J. Effects of lesions in hippocampus–entorhinal cortex on maze performance and activity in rats. *Psychonomic Science*, 1968, *10*, 13–14.

Bingham, W. E., & Griffiths, W. J., Jr. The effect of different environments during infancy on adult behavior in the rat. *Journal of Comparative and Physiological Psychology*, 1952, *45*, 307–312.

Borges, S., & Berry, M. Preferential orientation of stellate cell dendrites in the visual cortex of the dark-reared rat. *Brain Research*, 1976, *112*, 141–147.

Brown, R. T. Early experience and problem solving ability. *Journal of Comparative and Physiological Psychology*, 1968, *65*, 433–440.

Chow, K. L., & Spear, P. D. Morphological and functional effects of visual deprivation on the rabbit visual system. *Experimental Neurology*, 1974, *42*, 429–447.

Coghill, G. E. *Anatomy and the problem of behavior*. Cambridge, England: Cambridge University Press, 1929.

Coleman, P. D. Invited discussion. In C. D. Clemente, D. P. Purpura, & F. E. Mayer (Eds.), *Sleep and the maturing nervous system*. New York: Academic Press, 1972.

Coleman, P. D., & Riesen, A. H. Environmental effects on cortical dendritic fields. I. Rearing in the dark. *Journal of Anatomy*, 1968, *102*, 363–374.

Coss, R. G., & Globus, A. Spine stems on tectal interneurons in jewel fish are shortened by social stimulation. *Science*, 1978, *200*, 787–790.

Cragg, B. G. Changes in visual cortex on first exposure of rats to light. *Nature*, 1967, *215*, 251–253.

Cragg, B. G. The effects of vision and dark-rearing on the size and the density of synapses in the lateral geniculate nucleus measured by electron microscopy. *Brain Research*, 1969, *13*, 53–67.

Dalland, T. Response and stimulus perseveration in rats with septal and dorsal hippocampal lesions. *Journal of Comparative and Physiological Psychology*, 1970, *71*, 114–118.

Dews, P. B., & Wiesel, T. N. Consequences of monocular deprivation on visual behavior in kittens. *Journal of Physiology*, 1970, *206*, 437–455.

Diamond, M. C., Ingham, C. A. Johnson, R. E., Bennett, E. L., & Rosenzweig, M. R. Effects of environment on morphology of rat cerebral cortex and hippocampus. *Journal of Neurobiology*, 1976, *7*, 75–85.

Diamond, M. C., Lindner, B. Johnson, R. Bennett, E. L., & Rosenzweig, M. R. Differences in occipital cortical synapses from environmentally enriched, impoverished, and standard colony rats. *Journal of Neuroscience Research*, 1975, *1*, 109–119.

Diamond, M. C., Rosenzweig, M. R., Bennett, E. L., Lindner, B., & Lyon, L. Effects of environmental enrichment and impoverishment on rat cerebral cortex. *Journal of Neurobiology*, 1972, *3*, 47–64.

Douglas, R. J. The hippocampus and behavior. *Psychological Bulletin*, 1967, *67*, 416–422.

Einon, D. F., & Morgan M. J. A critical period for social isolation in the rat. *Developmental Psychobiology*, 1977, *10*, 123–132.

Elias, M. F. Differences in spatial discrimination reversal learning for mice selected for high brain weight and unselected controls. *Perceptual and Motor Skills*, 1969, *28*, 707–712.

Essman, W. B. Isolation-induced behavioral modification: some neurochemical correlates. In M. B. Sterman, D. J. McGinty, & A. M. Adinolfi (Eds.), *Brain development and behavior.* New York: Academic Press, 1971, Pp. 265–276.

Fiala, B. A., Joyce, J. N., & Greenough, W. T. Environmental complexity modulates growth of granule cell dendrites in developing but not adult hippocampus of rats. *Experimental Neurology,* 1978, *59,* 372–383.

Fifková, E. Changes of axosomatic synapses in the visual cortex of monocularly deprived rats. *Journal of Neurobiology,* 1970, *2,* 61–71. (a)

Fifková, E. The effect of monocular deprivation on the synaptic contacts of the visual cortex. *Journal of Neurobiology,* 1970, *1,* 285–294. (b)

Fifková, E. The effect of unilateral deprivation on visual centers in rats. *Journal of Comparative Neurology,* 1970, *140,* 431–438 (c)

Fifková, E., and Hassler, R. Quantitative morphological changes in visual centers of rats after unilateral deprivation. *Journal of Comparative Neurology,* 1969, *135,* 167–178.

Fleischmann, T. B. Effects of differential rearing complexity on synapses of the rat hippocampus (Regio superior-CA1). Unpublished Masters thesis, University of Illinois, Champaign, 1972.

Forgays, D. G., & Forgays, J. W. The nature of the effect of free-environmental experience in the rat. *Journal of Comparative and Physiological Psychology,* 1952, *45,* 322–328.

Forgays, D. G., & Read, J. M. Crucial periods for free-environmental experience in the rat. *Journal of Comparative and Physiological Psychology,* 1962, *55,* 816–818.

Freeman, B. J., & Ray, O. S. Strain, sex and environment effects on appetitively and aversively motivated learning tasks. *Developmental Psychobiology,* 1972, *5,* 101–109.

Fuller, J. L. & Geils, H. D. Behavioral development in mice selected for differences in brain weight. *Developmental Psychobiology,* 1973, *6,* 469–474.

Ganz, L. Orientation in visual space by neonates and its modification by visual deprivation. In A. H. Riesen (Ed.), *The developmental neuropsychology of sensory deprivation.* New York: Academic Press, 1975. Pp. 196–210.

Ganz, L., & Fitch, M. The effect of visual deprivation on perceptual behavior. *Experimental Neurology,* 1968, *22,* 638–660.

Ganz, L., Hirsch, H. V. B., & Tieman, S. B. The nature of perceptual deficits in visually deprived cats. *Brain Research,* 1972, *44,,* 547–560.

Gardner, E. B., Boitano, J. J., Mancino, N. S., D'Amico, D. P., & Gardner, E. L. Environmental enrichment and deprivation: Effects on learning, memory and exploration. *Physiology and Behavior,* 1975, *14,* 321–327.

Garey, L. J., & Pettigrew, J. D. Ultrastructural changes in kitten visual cortex after environmental modification. *Brain Research,* 1974, *66,* 165–172.

Globus, A., Rosenzweig, M. R., Bennett, E. L., & Diamond, M. C. Effects of differential experience on dendritic spine counts in rat cerebral cortex. *Journal of Comparative and Physiological Psychology,* 1973, *82,* 175–181.

Globus, A., & Scheibel, A. B. The effect of visual deprivation on cortical neurons: A Golgi study. *Experimental Neurology,* 1967, *19,* 331–345.

Greenough, W. T. Experiential modification of the developing brain. *American Scientist,* 1975, *63,* 37–46.

Greenough, W. T., Floeter, M. K. Sackett, G. P., Jencius, M. W., & Kraff, C. Experience and monkey brain development: Relationship to primate isolation syndrome. In J. W. Prescott (Ed)., *Consequences of social isolation upon primate brain development and behavior.* New York: Academic Press, in preparation.

Greenough, W. T., Fulcher, J. K., Yuwiler, A., & Geller, E. Enriched rearing and chronic electroshock: effects on brain and behavior in mice. *Physiology and Behavior,* 1970, *5,* 371–373.

Greenough, W. T., Madden, T. C., & Fleischman, T. B. Effects of isolation, daily handling and enriched rearing on maze learning. *Psychonomic Science*, 1972, *27*, 279–280.

Greenough, W. T., West, R. W., & DeVoogd, T. J. Post-synaptic plate perforations: Changes with age and experience in the rat. *Science*, 1978, *202*, 1096–1098.

Greenough, W. T., Wood, W. E., & Madden, T. C. Possible memory storage differences among mice reared in environments varying in complexity. *Behavioral Biology*, 1972, *7*, 717–722.

Greenough, W. T., & Volkmar, F. R. Pattern of dendritic branching in occipital cortex of rats reared in complex environments. *Experimental Neurology*, 1973, *40*, 491–504.

Greenough, W. T., Volkmar, F. R., & Fleischmann, T. B. Environmental effects on brain connectivity and behavior. In D. I. Mostofsky (Ed.), *Behavior control and modification of physiological activity*. Englewood Cliffs, N.J.: Prentice-Hall, 1976. Pp. 220–245.

Greenough, W. T., Volkmar, F. R., & Juraska, J. M. Effects of rearing complexity on dendritic branching in frontolateral and temporal cortex of the rat. *Experimental Neurology*, 1973, *41*, 371–378.

Greenough, W. T., Yuwiler, A., & Dollinger, M. Effects of posttrial eserine administration on learning in "enriched"- and "impoverished"- reared rats. *Behavioral Biology*, 1973, *8*, 261–272.

Gyllensten, L. Postnatal development of the visual cortex in darkness (mice). *Acta Morphologica Neerlando-Scandinavica*, 1959, *2*, 331–345.

Gyllensten, L., Malmfors, T., & Norrlin, M. Effect of visual deprivation on the optic centers of growing and adult mice. *Journal of Comparative Neurology*, 1965, *124*, 149–160.

Gyllensten, L., Malmfors, T., & Norrlin, M. L. Growth alteration in the auditory cortex of visually deprived mice. *Journal of Comparative Neurology*, 1966, *126*, 463–470.

Harlow, H. F., Dodsworth, R. O., & Harlow, M. K. Total isolation in monkeys. *Proceedings of the National Academy of Sciences*, 1965, *54*, 90–97.

Hebb, D. O. *The organization of behavior*, New York: John Wiley & Sons, 1949.

Held, R., & Hein, A. Movement- produced stimulation in the development of visually guided behavior. *Journal of Comparative and Physiological Psychology*, 1963, *56*, 872–876.

Holloway, R. L. Dendritic branching: Some preliminary results of training and complexity in rat visual cortex. *Brain Research*, 1966, *2*, 393–396.

Hymovitch, B. The effects of experimental variations on problem solving in the rat. *Journal of Comparative and Physiological Psychology*, 1952, *45*, 313–321.

Isaacson, R. L., & Wickelgren, W. D. Hippocampal ablation and passive avoidance. *Science*, 1962, *138*, 1104–1106.

Jacobson, M., & Hirsch, H. V. B. Development and maintenance of connectivity in the visual system of the frog. I. The effects of eye rotation and visual deprivation. *Brain Research*, 1973, *49*, 47–65.

Jerison, H. J. *Evolution of the brain and intelligence*. New York: Academic Press, 1973.

Kimble, D. P. The effects of bilateral hippocampal lesions in rats. *Journal of Comparative and Physiological Psychology*, 1963, *56*, 273–283.

Kimble, D. P. Hippocampus and internal inhibition. *Psychological Bulletin*, 1968, *70*, 285–295.

Krech, D., Rosenzweig, M. R., & Bennett, E. L. Relations between brain chemistry and problem solving in rats raised in enriched and impoverished environments. *Journal of Comparative and Physiological Psychology*, 1962, *55*, 801–807.

Krech, D., Rosenzweig, M. R., & Bennett, E. L. Effects of complex environments and blindness on rat brain. *Archives of Neurology*, 1963, *8*, 403–412.

Krechevsky, I. Hereditary nature of "hypotheses". *Journal of Comparative Psychology*, 1933, *16*, 99–116.

Lash, L., & Goldstein, A. G. The effects of pre-puberal environment and post-puberal blindness on maze learning. *Psychonomic Science*, 1965, 2, 5–6.

Marr, D., A theory of cerebellar cortex. *Journal of Physiology*, 1969, 202, 437–470.

Mason, W. A. Early social deprivation in the nonhuman primates: Implications for human behavior. In D. C. Glass, (Ed.), *Environmental influences*. New York: Rockefeller University Press, 1968. Pp. 70–101.

Meyers, B., & McCleary, R. A. Interocular transfer of a pattern discrimination in pattern deprived cats. *Journal of Comparative and Physiological Psychology*, 1964, 57, 16–21.

Møllgaard, K., Diamond, M. C. Bennett, E. L. Rosenzweig, M. R., & Lindner, B. Qualitative synaptic changes with differential experience in rat brain. *International Journal of Neuroscience*, 1971, 2, 113–128.

Morgan, M. J. Effects of post-weaning environment on learning in the rat. *Animal Behavior*, 1973, 21, 429–442.

Morgan, M. J., Einon, D., & Morris, R. G. M. Inhibition and isolation rearing in the rat: Extinction and satiation. *Physiology and Behavior*, 1977, 18, 1–5.

Morgan, M. J., Einon, D. F., & Nicholas, D. The effects of isolation rearing on behavioral inhibition in the rat. *Quarterly Journal of Experimental Psychology*, 1975, 27, 615–634.

Myers, R. D., & Fox, J. Differences in maze performance of group *vs.* isolation reared rats. *Psychological Reports.* 1963, 12, 199–202.

Nadel, L., O'Keefe, J., & Black A. Slam on the brakes: A critique of Altman, Brunner, and Bayer's response-inhibition model of hippocampal function. *Behavioral Biology*, 1975, 14, 151–162.

Nealy, S. M., & Riley, D. A. Loss and recovery of discrimination of visual depth in dark reared rat. *American Journal of Psychology*, 1963, 76, 329–333.

Nyman, A. J. Problem solving in rats as a function of experience at different ages. *Journal of Genetic Psychology*, 1967, 110, 31–39.

Olton, D. S. Spatial memory. *Scientific American*, 1977, 236 (6), 82–98.

Peters, A., & Kaiserman-Abramof, I. R. The small pyramidal neuron of the rat cerebral cortex. The synapses upon dendritic spines. *Zeitschrift für Zellforschung und Mikroskopische Anatomie*, 1969, 100, 487–506.

Prescott, J. Early somatosensory deprivation as an ontogenetic process in the abnormal development of the brain and behavior. In E. Goldsmith & J. Morr-Jankowski (Eds.), *Medical primatology, 1970*. Basel, Switzerland: Karger, 1971. Pp. 356–375.

Ravizza, R. J., & Herschberger, A. C. The effect of prolonged motor restriction upon later behavior of the rat. *Psychological Record*, 1966, 16, 73–80.

Riege, W. H. Environmental influences on brain and behavior of year-old rats. *Developmental Psychobiology*, 1971, 4, 151–167.

Riesen, A. H. Effects of visual deprivation on perceptual function and the neural substrate. In J. DeAjuriaguerra (Ed.), *Symposium bel air II, desafferentation experimentale et Clinique*. Geneva: George & Cie, 1965, Pp. 47–66.

Rosenzweig, M. R. Effects of environment on development of brain and of behavior. In E. Tobach, L. R. Aronson, & E. Shaw (Eds.), *The biopsychology of development*. New York: Academic Press, 1971. Pp. 303–342.

Ryugo, D. K., Ryugo, R., Globus, A., & Killackey, H. P. Increased spine density in auditory cortex following visual or somatic deafferentation. *Brain Research*, 1975, 90, 143–146.

Smith, D. C., & Loop, M. S. Rapid restoration of visual abilities in the monocularly deprived adult cat. *Investigative Opthalmology and Visual Science Supplement*, 1978, 17, 294.

Smith, H. V. Effects of environmental enrichment on open field activity and Hebb-Williams problem solving in rats. *Journal of Comparative and Physiological Psychology,* 1972, *80,* 163–168.

Tees, R. C. Effect of early visual restriction on later visual intensity discrimination in rats. *Journal of Comparative and Physiological Psychology,* 1968, *66,* 224–227. (a)

Tees, R. C. Effect of early restriction on later form discrimination in the rat. *Canadian Journal of Psychology,* 1968, *22,* 294–298. (b)

Tees, R. C. Luminance and luminous flux discrimination in rats after early visual deprivation. *Journal of Comparative and Physiological Psychology,* 1971, *74,* 292–297.

Tees, R. C. Effect of visual deprivation on development of depth perception in the rat. *Journal of Comparative and Physiological Psychology,* 1974, *86,* 300–308.

Tees, R. C. Perceptual development in mammals. In G. Gottlieb (Ed.), *Neural and behavioral specificity.* New York: Academic Press, 1976, Pp. 281–326.

Tees, R. C., & Cartwright, J. Sensory preconditioning in rats following early visual deprivation. *Journal of Comparative and Physiological Psychology,* 1972, *81,* 12–20.

Teitelbaum, H. A comparison of effects of orbitofrontal and hippocampal lesions upon discrimination learning and reversal in the cat. *Experimental Neurology,* 1964, *9,* 452–462.

Valverde, F. Apical dendritic spines of the visual cortex and light deprivation in the mouse. *Experimental Brain Research,* 1967, *3,* 337–352.

Valverde, F. Rate and extent of recovery from dark rearing in the visual cortex of the mouse. *Brain Research,* 1971, *35,* 1–11.

Valverde, F. Aspects of cortical organization related to neurons with intracortical axons. *Journal of Neurocytology,* 1976, *5,* 509–529.

Volkmar, F. R., & Greenough, W. T. Rearing complexity affects branching of dendrites in the visual cortex of the rat. *Science,* 1972, *176,* 1445–1447.

Vrensen, G., & DeGroot, D. The effect of dark rearing and its recovery on synaptic terminals in the visual cortex of rabbits: a quantitative electron microscopic study. *Brain Research,* 1974, *78,* 263–278.

Vrensen, G., & DeGroot, D. The effect of monocular deprivation on synaptic terminals in the visual cortex of rabbits. A quantitative electron microscopic study. *Brain Research,* 1975, *93,* 15–24.

Walk, R. D., & Walters, C. P. Effect of visual deprivation on depth discrimination of hooded rats. *Journal of Comparative and Physiological Psychology,* 1973, *85,* 559–563.

Walsh, R. N., Budtz-Olsen, O. E., Penny, J. E., & Cummins, R. A. The effects of environmental complexity on the histology of the rat hippocampus. *Journal of Comparative Neurology,* 1969, *137,* 361–366.

West, R. W., & Greenough, W. T. Effect of environmental complexity on cortical synapses of rats: Preliminary results. *Behavioral Biology,* 1972, *7,* 279–284.

Wiesel, T. N., & Hubel, D. H. Effects of visual deprivation on morphology and physiology of cells in the cat's lateral geniculate body. *Journal of Neurophysiology,* 1963, *26,* 978–993.

Wiesel, T. N., & Hubel, D. H. Extent of recovery from the effects of visual deprivation in kittens. *Journal of Neurophysiology,* 1965, *28,* 1060–1072.

Wimer, C. C., & Prater, L. Behavioral differences in mice genetically selected for high and low brain weight. *Psychological Reports,* 1966, *19,* 675–681.

Woods, P. J., Fiske, A. S., & Rukelshaus, S. I. The effects of drives conflicting with exploration on the problem-solving behavior of rats reared in free and restricted environments. *Journal of Comparative and Physiological Psychology,* 1961, *54,* 167–169.

Zimbardo, P. G., & Montgomery, K. D. Effects of "free environment" rearing upon exploratory behavior. *Psychological Reports,* 1957, *3,* 589–594.

Chapter XVI

Effects of Early Undernutrition on Brain and Behavior of Developing Mice[1]

Z. MICHAEL NAGY

General Approaches to the Study of Brain Size— Behavior Relationships

A variety of approaches have been used by researchers in their attempts to better understand the relationships between brain size and behavior; these approaches are well represented in the present volume. One approach might be considered a normative one, in which organisms are studied in their natural states, with little attempt to influence experimentally the course of brain or behavioral development. Included in this approach would be the study through various periods of evolution of between-species variations of brain size and intelligence (see Chapters by Holloway and by Jerison, in this volume), the within-species correlations of brain and behaviors during the normal course of maturation (Epstein, this volume), and the cross-species comparisons of brain size and behavioral abilities on a variety of tasks (Riddell, this volume).

A second approach has been to determine the correlations between brain and behavior for a number of inbred animal strains, and for their resulting hybrids established through cross-breeding selective strains (Henderson). Or investigators manipulate brain size genetically through

[1]The research reported in this chapter was supported by National Institute of Child Health and Human Development Grant HD-09145.

321

selective breeding, and determine the effects of this selection procedure on the behaviors, brain sizes, and biochemistries of the resulting lines (see chapters by Dudek & Berman; Fuller; Hahn; and Jensen, this volume).

A third approach has attempted to induce changes in brain size through differential postnatal experiences, and then to examine the resulting correlations between changes in brain and behavior (chapters by Greenough & Juraska, and by Rosenzweig, this volume).

In this chapter, I shall review several studies from our laboratory that have been conducted to better understand the relationships between brain maturation and learning–memory processes. In general, our approach incorporates several features of those already described. First, we have chosen to examine young organisms' emerging capabilities to learn and to remember responses during the early postnatal period of rapid brain growth. On the assumption that the increasing learning and memory capabilities are reflecting the maturation of underlying brain processes, we next attempted to determine whether alterations of the rate of brain maturation have corresponding effects on the emergence of those abilities. It should be noted at this point that the primary interest in our research was not simply in the relationship between brain size and behavior *per se*, but rather in the manner that increasing brain size during early development might reflect the state of functional maturation of a variety of brain areas and processes, and consequential effects upon behavior.

Developmental Approach to Brain–Behavior Relationships

POSTNATAL BRAIN GROWTH

It is now well known that a number of organisms, particularly altricial mammals such as man, dogs, cats, rats, and mice, are born with relatively immature central nervous systems (CNS) and undergo dramatic changes in brain size, structure, organization, and function during the postnatal periods. Many changes continue even into adulthood in some species. It is further known that the maturation of neural CNS·function does not occur at the same rate in all areas, but rather shows the earliest maturation of structure and function at the lower levels of the spinal cord, and the latest development in the forebrain, following a caudal to rostral pattern. In addition, the development of various structures and biochemical processes within particular levels of the CNS occurs at somewhat different rates (as space does not permit a detailed review of postnatal brain maturation, the interested reader should refer to the following: Himwich, 1970, 1973, 1976; Lanier, Dunn, & Van Hartesveldt, 1976; Paoletti & Davison, 1971; Sterman, McGinty, & Adinolfi, 1971; Tobach, Aronson, & Shaw, 1971; Vernadakis & Weiner, 1974).

Behaviorally, these developmental changes in brain structure and function are accompanied by increasing response repertoires that indicate specific periods of a species' development (e.g., Altman & Bulut, 1976; Bolles & Woods, 1964; Fox, 1965; Gottlieb, 1971). It would seem likely, then, that there would be some relationship between these increasing behavioral capacities and the maturing brain. The developmental approach involves identifying those brain structures or processes that may underlie the emerging behavioral patterns during ontogeny.

POSTNATAL CHANGES IN LEARNING AND MEMORY ABILITIES

A large body of literature has now been accumulated, at least for the rat, which traces the learning and memory capabilities from weaning to adulthood in a variety of learning situations. The results are quite consistent (for detailed reviews, see: Campbell, 1967; Campbell & Coulter, 1976; Campbell, Riccio, & Rohrbaugh, 1971; Campbell & Spear, 1972; Spear, 1973; Spear & Campbell, in press). In general, when a learning task requires a response to be made, young rats learn as well as adults. When age-related differences have been noted, they have usually been poorer performance in the younger animals whose perceptual–motor development had not yet achieved adult levels.

On tasks that required a response to be withheld, however, young rats have consistently performed more poorly, and learned more slowly than adults (e.g., Feigley & Spear, 1970; Riccio, Rohrbaugh, & Hodges, 1968; Schulenburg, Riccio, & Stikes, 1971). These task- and age-related learning differences are consistent with evidence that inhibitory control develops slowly, only after the development of excitatory control in the rat. Many investigators have concluded that the poorer learning by younger subjects is due to the relative lack of inhibitory ability at the early ages (see Campbell et al., 1971, for a review of this concept).

When age-related memory functions are examined, younger rats demonstrate markedly poorer memories, particularly at longer retention intervals, than adult animals for learned responses in both kinds of tasks. The hypothesis that these long term memory deficits are due primarily to the neurological immaturity of brain processes underlying memory at the time of original learning has gained considerable support (Campbell & Coulter, 1976).

POSTNATAL CHANGES IN LEARNING AND MEMORY DURING BRAIN
"GROWTH SPURT"

Whereas the majority of studies dealing with age-related learning and memory abilities in rats have typically employed 20–25-day-old weanlings as the youngest age group tested, in our research program we have directed our attention to learning and memory abilities at much earlier ages. More specifically, we have attempted to determine whether young rats and mice first become capable of demonstrating certain kinds of learning and memory capabilities during the periods of most rapid CNS development, or the brain "growth spurt," when the major maturational changes in physiological and biochemical brain growth are taking place (Davison & Dobbing, 1968). For rats and mice, the brain "growth spurt" occurs around 5–20 days after birth.

In a series of papers, Epstein (1974a; 1974b; this volume), following an extensive review of the human developmental literature, has suggested that there appear to be at least four stages of human postnatal development when especially large increases in brain weight are poorly correlated with corresponding increases of general body growth. Epstein further suggests that these periods of brain "growth spurts" are correlated highly with marked increases in intellectual functioning. Thus, it appears that the physical growth of the brain may be correlated with the functional growth of the mind.

At the level of the mouse, Epstein (Epstein & Miller, 1977) has suggested that Dobbing's brain "growth spurt" may actually be comprised of three separate bursts, occurring at approximately 0–6, 9–13, and 17–23 days after birth. If a similar relationship between growth and intellectual growth exists for the mouse as it appears to for the human, one would then expect to find marked increases in learning or memory capabilities in mice during these ages.

Learning and Memory for Simple Escape Training As much of our previous research investigating the development of learning and memory in the mouse and rat has recently been reviewed in detail (Nagy, in press), I shall provide only a brief summary of our major findings at this point. In one set of studies, we examined the ability of mice and rats to learn and remember a simple shock-escape response in a straight alley. The results indicated that both rats and mice are capable of showing improvement as young as 5-days-old within a training session, and can remember this response for at least 1 hr.; however, they do not appear able to remember such training over a 24 hr period until they are 9 days of age (Misanin, Nagy, Keiser, & Bowen, 1971; Nagy, Misanin, Newman, Olsen, & Hinderliter, 1972). Even when the number of original training trials is markedly increased, 7-day-old mice fail to show evidence of 24 hr. memory of prior training, whereas 9-day-old mice demonstrate retention functions that vary directly with the amount of original training (Nagy & Mueller, 1973). These data suggested to us that the physiological and biological processes related to memory for this type of learning had reached functional maturity between 8 to 9 days of age.

Learning and Memory for Discriminated Escape Training In a second series of experiments, we examined the development of learning and memory in mice on a slightly more complex task, the T-maze. On this task, mice between 7 to 13 days of age were trained to escape to the goal arm opposite their initial preference and were then retested 24 hrs later. Over a training session of 25 trials, mice younger than 9 days of age failed to show any improvement in choosing the correct goal arm (Nagy & Murphy, 1974). By 9 days of age, however, the mice were capable of increasing the number of times that the correct arm was chosen, but failed to show 24 hr memory for that training (Nagy & Murphy, 1974; Nagy and Sandmann, 1973). By 11 days of age, the mice showed both learning and 24 hr memory of T-maze training, suggesting that memory mechanisms involved with this type of training had reached functional maturity by 11 days of age. Additional studies that varied the number of training trials (Nagy, Pagano, & Gable, 1976), or the shock intensity (Nagy, 1975), provided further support for this conclusion.

The results of these experiments clearly indicate that marked increases in the learning and memory abilities of young mice occur during the brain "growth spurt" reported to occur in mice between 9 to 13 days of age (Epstein & Miller, 1977). Furthermore, these findings are consistent with the hypothesis that the behavioral emergence of adult-like learning and memory capacities, albeit in immature form, reflects the functional maturity or integration of physiological and biochemical processes underlying adult processes for these tasks. While it would be intriguing to propose a cause-and-effect relationship between brain maturation and the increasing learning and memory abilities of the developing mice, such a proposal is clearly premature. Several important questions must first be answered.

Are Learning and Memory Processes the Same for Infant and Adult? The first question concerns whether the learning and memory processes used by the young mice are indeed the same as those used by adults on these tasks. It is possible that although the behavioral responses are similar for young and adult mice, the processes underlying the behavior may be different; there may be learning and memory processes unique to the early ages that are replaced by different, more complex systems with further maturation.

Although we cannot directly answer this question, we have shown certain manipulations that interfere with adult memory also disrupt memory in the young. For example, we have shown that posttraining hypothermia markedly interferes with 24 hr memory of escape training in the straight alley in 9-day-old mice (Nagy, Anderson, & Mazzaferri, 1976) and rats (Misanin *et al.*, 1971) in much the same manner as has been reported for adults of these species (e.g., Beitel & Porter, 1968; Riccio, Hodges, & Randall, 1968). In another study, we have demonstrated that when T-maze training occurs under conditions of marked inhibition of cerebral protein synthesis, 13-day-old mice show evidence of amnesia for original training when retested 24 hr later (Nagelberg & Nagy, 1977). Numerous studies with adult subjects have reported similar retention deficits (Barraco & Stettner, 1976). While this type of evidence is indirect, it is consistent with the suggestion that the learning and memory processes used by both young and adult mice are the same.

Are Learning and Memory Processes Dependent on Brain Maturation? The second important question that must be answered is whether the maturing brain, or components therein, is in fact responsible for the emerging behavioral capabilities, rather than simply being correlated with their ontogenetic appearance. For example, it may be that a certain amount of environmental experience or stimulation is required before certain kinds of learning and memory abilities become evident behaviorally in the young animal. Brain maturation may simply be occurring at the same time the young mouse is gaining the prerequisite stimulation from its environment.

If brain maturation underlies behavioral capacities, one would then expect manipulations that alter the rate of CNS maturation would also have corresponding effects upon the age at which learning and memory abilities become behaviorally functional. In two experiments, we have provided data consistent with this expectation. When mice are injected with thyroxine over the first several days of postnatal life, a procedure reported to advance the early stages of brain (e.g., Balazs & Richter, 1973; Schapiro, 1971) and behavioral (e.g., Davenport & Gonzalez, 1973; Schapiro, 1971) development, the ability to remember T-maze training occurs at around 9 days of age, as compared to 11 days of age in saline-injected controls (Murphy & Nagy, 1976a). On the other hand, when mice are subjected to postnatal undernutrition, a procedure resulting in the retardation of both brain growth and the emergence of behavioral abilities (e.g., Altman, Sudarshan, Das, McCormick, & Barnes, 1971; Smart & Dobbing, 1971), the capacity to remember prior T-maze training for a 24 hr period does not occur until 13 days of age, 2 days later than for normally nourished mice (Nagy, Porada, & Anderson, 1977). In the case of both experimental manipulations, the effects appeared specific to memory systems, since original training scores at each age for treated mice did not differ from their respective controls.

In summary, the results of these experiments suggest that the memory system involved with a form of instrumental conditioning, in this case T-maze shock-escape, develops at around 9–11 days of age in the mouse, a stage of ontogeny coincident with a purported brain "growth spurt." Furthermore, the behavioral emergence of this memory system appears to be dependent on the functional maturation of underlying brain processes, and these processes appear to be similar to those used by adult mice on similar tasks.

Undernutrition and Development of Inhibitory Capacities

General Ontogenetic Correlation between Inhibitory Behaviors and Neurotransmitters

As noted in a preceding section of this chapter, one of the most consistent age-related differences in learning abilities of altricial animals occurs in those tasks that require a response to be withheld, with young animals typically performing much more poorly than older subjects (Campbell, Riccio, & Rohrbaugh, 1971). For example, when rats between 15–120 days of age are trained on a passive avoidance task, the rate of acquisition improves markedly with increasing age (e.g., Riccio, Rohrbaugh, & Hodges, 1968; Schulenburg et al., 1971). Because rats of comparable ages do not exhibit age-related differences in the acquisition of active avoidance learning, it has been generally concluded that young rats are less able to inhibit responding than are older rats.

There is a striking parallel between these age- and task-related learning differences and postnatal maturation. Supporting the notion that brain maturation follows a pattern of sequential caudal to rostral development of excitatory and inhibitory centers, there is a great deal of pharmacological data demonstrating that maturing rats are responsive to drugs affecting excitatory systems (Campbell & Mabry, 1973) earlier in ontogeny, than the rats are to agents affecting inhibitory systems, such as the cholinergic (Campbell, Lytle, & Fibiger, 1969; Carlton, 1963;

Fibiger, Lytle, & Campbell, 1970) and serotonergic (Mabry & Campbell, 1974) transmitter systems. As these inhibitory neurotransmitter systems appear to become functional at about the same stage of development at which rats begin to show improvement in passive avoidance learning, the third postnatal week, the implication is strong that these systems underlie inhibitory responding.

Rationale and Purpose of Present Research Program

Based upon these findings, the series of experiments to be described in the remaining portion of the chapter were conducted in order to determine the effects of postnatal undernutrition on the ability of the developing mouse to learn and remember a task requiring response inhibition. In addition, we also attempted to determine whether early undernutrition would affect the chronological ages at which mice first responded to anticholinergic and antiserotonergic agents, antagonists of systems implicated with response inhibition. Earlier studies with undernourished animals have demonstrated marked effects upon brain development (see Nowak & Munro, 1977), including decreased cell number (Bass, 1971; Fish & Winick, 1969), axonal proliferation in the forebrain (Cragg, 1972), and the retardation of cholinergic (Adlard & Dobbing, 1971; Eckhert, Barnes, & Levitsky, 1976) and serotonergic (Ramanamurthy, 1977) functioning; we expected our undernourished mice to exhibit several learning deficits on a passive avoidance task. In a previous paper, we reported that undernutrition appeared to delay the ontogenetic appearance of several unlearned behaviors requiring inhibitory control, but had little effect on the age-related ability to learn a task requiring an active response (Nagy *et al.*, 1977).

General Method of Undernutrition

In all of the following experiments, a state of undernutrition was imposed on our experimental subjects by increasing the litter size to 16 pups on the day following birth. Other litters, serving as normally nourished controls, were altered in size to contain either 6 or 8 pups. When the litter sizes were composed, every effort was made to assign randomly pups to mothers that were not their own and to maintain an equal number of each sex within each recomposed litter. Except during the testing sessions, the mothers remained with the pups, and ad-libitum food and water were available to the mothers. No attempt was made to prevent the pups from eating or drinking the available nutrients when they became old enough to do so.

Although this technique for inducing undernutrition has been widely employed, it has come under some criticism, primarily because of the increased variability in maturational growth and behavior that results (Galler & Turkewitz, 1975). However, since alternative methods of undernutrition also introduce confounding variables (Crnic, 1976; Plaut, 1970), we chose to use the litter-size technique. We attempted to control the variability by using only litters and subjects that did not deviate markedly from the average weight at particular ages found in our prior research.

Effects of Litter Size on Brain and Body Growth

Before proceeding with the behavioral studies, we first attempted to determine the effects of our litter size rearing conditions upon the brain and body growth of the pups during postnatal ontogeny. In this study, mouse pups were assigned to litter sizes of 6 or 16 on the day following birth. Beginning at 3 days of age, and continuing every other day through 27 days of age, one male and one female pup were randomly selected from each litter, sacrificed by CO_2 asphyxiation, and weighed to the nearest .1 gm. The brain was then removed by separation from the spinal cord with a cut 1 mm posterior to the posterior tip of the fourth ventricle, and weighed to the nearest milligram. A total of 5 males and 5 females were sampled from each litter size at each age. In addition, 10 males and 10 females were sampled at 60 and 90 days of age. In all instances when pups were removed from the litter, they were replaced by pups of the same age and sex from similar litter sizes. Mice tested at 60 and 90 days of age were weaned at 27 days of age, kept in cages with four age mates of the same sex, from the same litter size, and received ad-libitum food and water until sacrifice.

Rearing pups in litters of 16 resulted in significantly lighter brains as compared to 6 litter mice (see Figure XVI.1, left panel), beginning at 5 days of age. Significant differences in brain size persisted through 90 days of age, despite the fact that pups reared in large litters had free access to food and water from 27 through 90 days of age. Body weight was affected even earlier, with reliable differences being found by 3 days of age (see Figure XVI.1, right panel). However, by 90 days of age, the body weight differences were no longer reliable.

The mean brain–body weight ratios (see Figure XVI.2) also show marked and early differences as a function of litter size. However, in this case, the brain–body weight ratios are higher for mice reared in large litters than are those for mice reared in small litters. While it has been suggested that this kind of finding reflects a brain sparing phenomenon from similar data obtained with the rat, Dobbing (1971) has

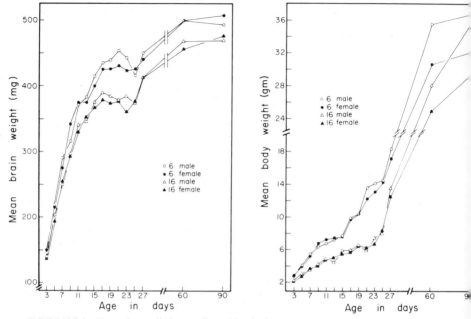

FIGURE XVI.1. Mean brain (left panel) and body (right panel) weights of mice reared in litter sizes of 6 and 16 presented as a function of age.

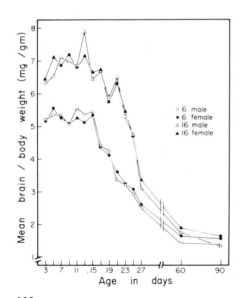

FIGURE XVI.2. Mean brain/body weight ratios of mice reared in litter sizes of 6 and 16 presented as a function of age.

argued that this difference simply reflects the fact that brain weight increases with age before the major increase in body weight. A simple growth retardation produced by undernutrition must, therefore, lead to higher values of the brain–body weight ratios for those mice reared in large litters. As the rate of body growth begins to accelerate in comparison to brain growth rate, the resulting body–weight ratios must, therefore, decrease with increasing age. For the present data, the brain–body weight ratios begin to show marked decreases beginning at 15 days of age for mice reared in small litters, and 21 days of age for mice reared in large litters.

The brain and body weights found in the present study are crude indexes of development and cannot reflect the differential effects of undernutrition on more specific brain areas and processes (e.g., Mc-Khann, Coyle, & Benjamins, 1973; Nowak & Munro, 1977; Winick & Rosso, 1975). However, they are consistent with previous reports on the rat, and suggest that our litter size manipulation affects the general maturational rate of the brain.

Acquisition and Retention of a Passive–Avoidance Response

In one experiment, Ray and Nagy (1978) have shown that mice are capable of learning a passive avoidance response at ages much younger than previously believed possible. When mice between 7 days of age and adulthood were all trained to avoid a shock by withholding a step down response, clear age-related differences in rates of acquisition occurred. When comparisons between mice 15 days of age and older were made, the age-related function previously reported for rats (e.g., Riccio, Rohrbaugh, & Hodges, 1968; Schulenburg et al., 1971) was closely replicated, with learning ability markedly improving with increasing age. However, 7 and 11-day-old mice also learned the task much more rapidly than 15-day-olds, with 7-day-olds learning about as rapidly as adults. In addition to these acquisition data, Ray and Nagy (1978) also reported that mice of all ages demonstrated reliable retention of prior training, compared to control groups, when retested 1 hr later. When retested 24 hr following training, mice 15 days of age and younger performed as poorly as controls without training, while mice 19 days of age and older were significantly better than controls. These results indicate that mice of all ages tested were capable of learning a passive avoidance task and remembering it for at least 1 hr, while further maturation of brain processes necessary for 24 hr retention occurred between 15 to 19 days of age.

In the present experiment, separate groups of mice from litter sizes of 6 and 16 were trained to a common criterion on a step off, passive avoidance apparatus between 7 and 19 days of age, and were retrained to the same criterion following a 1 hr interval. Similarly, groups between 15 to 21 days of age from each litter size were trained to criterion and retrained following a 24 hr interval. Basically, the training procedure consisted of shocking the mouse pup if it stepped off a small elevated platform onto a grid floor within 120 sec (see Nagy, Porada, & Monsour, in press; Ray & Nagy, 1978, for details). Training continued until each mouse withheld stepping off the platform for two consecutive 120 sec trials. Yoked control (YC) mice received similar experience, except were prevented from stepping off the platform by enclosing it with a cardboard cylinder. During retention tests, the cardboard cylinder was not used, and each YC mouse was permitted to step off the platform and receive a brief shock.

During the original training (see Figure XVI.3, left panels), the mean number of trials required to achieve criterion for the trained mice of each litter size formed an inverted U-shaped function, with the maximum number of training trials being required at 15 days of age for the 6 litter mice, and at 17 days of age for the 16 litter mice. Although the age-related differences in rates of acquisition were highly significant within each litter size, the only age at which reliable differences were found between litter sizes was at 15 days of age, where the 16 litter mice acquired the criterion significantly faster than did 6 litter mice.

During the 1 hr retention test, all 6 litter trained mice reachieved criterion reliably faster than did their YC littermates (see Figure XVI.3, center panels), indicating that all ages had acquired the inhibitory response and were capable of remembering it for at least 1 hr. In contrast, the 16 litter mice did not reacquire the task faster than their YC controls until 15 days of age. At 7 and 11 days of age, the YC mice reached criterion as quickly as did those littermates with prior training.

Following a 24 hr retention interval (see Figure XVI.3, right panels), 6 litter mice took significantly fewer trials to reach criterion than controls at 17 days of age and older. For the 16 litter mice, although all trained mice achieved criterion somewhat faster than their YC littermates, the differences were not statistically reliable until 21 days of age.

The results of this experiment indicate that although early undernutrition had some effect upon acquisition of the passive avoidance response across ages, the within-age differences between normally nourished and undernourished mice were quite small. However, undernutrition appeared to have a more profound effect upon the developing memory systems for this type of training. The data suggest that

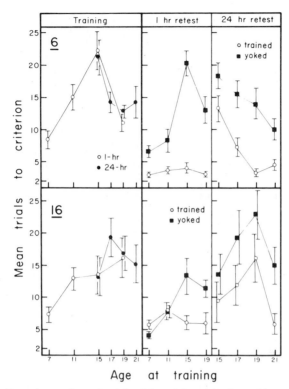

FIGURE XVI.3. Mean (± s.e.) number of training trials required to achieve criterion during original training (left panels) and subsequent 1 hr (center panels) and 24 hr (right panels) retention tests as a function of litter size, age at training, and training condition. [From Nagy, Porada, & Monsour, 1979.]

both short- and long-term memory capabilities were retarded in development for the undernourished mice.

In light of the implicit relationship between age-related learning ability for this type of task and the development of inhibitory neurotransmitter systems, the acquisition results were indeed surprising. If anything, this hypothesized relationship would predict that learning should be poorer with decreasing age. Yet, the younger ages of both nutritional groups learned as quickly as the oldest group studied. While this finding appears to damage the notion that inhibitory neurotransmitter systems are necessary for learning a passive avoidance response, at least two possibilities could account for these findings. First, it is possible that inhibitory neurotransmitter systems other than the cholinergic and serotonergic systems are involved with response inhibition at the very early ages. For example, there are data suggesting that the GABAergic system becomes functional in the inhibitory control of spontaneous activity at an earlier chronological age than does the cholinergic system (Murphy, Meeker, Porada, & Nagy, in press).

A second possibility is that the cholinergic and serotonergic systems are involved in passive avoidance learning at the early ages, but their relative effectiveness in inhibiting responses at different ages varies as a function of the corresponding maturation of the excitatory systems. It is known (e.g., Lanier *et al.*, 1976) that cholinergic and serotonergic neurotransmitters are evident at birth in the rat, although their levels are low compared to older rats. If the levels of catecholamines are also low at the early ages, it would necessarily follow that the level of inhibitory transmitters may be sufficiently high to counteract the excitatory transmitters and allow relatively easy acquisition of a passive avoidance response, as demonstrated by our 7-day-old mice. With increasing maturation, the excitatory systems appear to develop more rapidly than inhibitory systems, and this would result in acquisition becoming more difficult for the young animal. When the inhibitory systems begin their maturational spurt, perhaps beginning around 15 days of age in the mouse, it should then become increasingly easy for the developing mouse to acquire the passive avoidance response.

Ontogenetic Patterns of Spontaneous Activity

In normally nourished mice, spontaneous activity levels measured from the first postnatal week through adulthood characteristically form an inverted U-shaped function, with peak levels occurring at about 13–14 days of age (Nagy, Murphy, & Ray, 1975; Nagy & Ritter, 1976). Primarily on the basis of pharmacological data, it has been suggested that the decline in activity following peak levels represents a functional emergence of brain biochemical systems, such as the forebrain cholinergic and serotonergic systems, sufficient to modulate the earlier developing adrenergic arousal systems (Campbell *et al.*, 1969; Nagy *et al.*, 1975). For example, whereas agents acting on adrenergic arousal systems produce activity increases in rats as young as 10 days of age (Campbell *et al.*, 1969), manipulation of cholinergic or serotonergic transmission does not alter activity levels until after the ontogenetic peak in either rats (Mabry & Campbell, 1973; Campbell *et al.*, 1969) or mice (Murphy & Nagy, 1976b; Porada & Nagy, 1978).

It should be noted that the ontogenetic pattern may not represent a general developmental phenomenon but, rather, an age-related response to fear or stress induced by conditions such as isolation from conspecifics, or removal from familiar environments (Campbell & Raskin, 1978; Randall & Campbell, 1976). Regardless, the notable developmental parallel between the declining activity levels and the initial response to cholinergic and serotonergic manipulations during the third postnatal week suggests that these systems are important in the mediation of inhibitory capacities for activity.

In a paper (Nagy *et al.*, 1977), we reported striking alterations of the age-related activity function for mice undernourished during the suckling period. Although both normally nourished and undernourished pups displayed an inverted U-shaped activity function across days of age, mice reared in large litters exhibited a 3–4 day delay in attainment of peak activity levels, as well as marked hyperactivity during the third postnatal week. These results suggested that one of the more severe effects of postnatal undernutrition may be to retard the functional emergence of neurochemical systems that control the inhibition of spontaneous locomotor activity.

Effects of Inhibitory Blocking Agents on Activity in Undernourished Mice

In order to test the possibility that undernutrition affects developing inhibitory systems, the following series of studies was conducted. We compared the age-related activity responses of small and large litter reared mice to the cholinergic and serotonergic postsynaptic blocking agents, scopolamine and methysergide, respectively. Our intention in conducting this research was not simply to demonstrate a generally retarded activity response to these agents in undernourished mice, but rather to determine whether nutritional deprivation might produce a selective retardation of one or the other of these neurotransmitter systems which would closely correspond with the delayed emergence of inhibitory control evidenced in the passive avoidance experiment.

EFFECTS OF SCOPOLAMINE ON ACTIVITY

In the first study, groups of 6 and 16 litter mice received daily activity testing sessions from 11 through 21 days of age. Activity scores at 11 and 12 days of age served as a basis for equating groups for subsequent drug administration. Beginning at 13 days of age, one-half of the mice from each litter size were injected with scopolamine (1 mg/kg, intraperitoneal [i.p.]), while the remaining half received the saline injection. Immediately following injection, all mice received a 2 hr session in small photocell activity monitoring cages (see Nagy, *et al.*, 1975, for a description of the apparatus).

The results of this experiment (see Figure XVI.4) provided some evi-

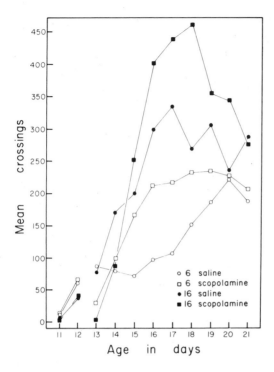

FIGURE XVI.4. Mean number of cage crossings made over a 2 hr session in response to saline or scopolamine injections from 13–21 days of age by mice reared in small and large litters. No injections were administered at 11 and 12 days of age.

dence for a delayed emergence of a cholinergic inhibitory function for large litter mice, although the full extent of the retardation is not clear from these data. For 6 litter mice, scopolamine injections reliably elevated activity, compared to saline controls, from 15 through 18 days of age. In contrast, increases that were statistically significant occurred only at 18 days of age for the 16 litter mice, 3 days later than for the small litter mice. However, the failure to obtain reliable differences may be at least partially attributed to the increased variability displayed by the 16 litter mice (Galler & Turkewitz, 1975); the mean differences between the scopolamine and saline injected 16 litter mice were roughly comparable to those displayed by the 6 litter groups. Thus, it appears that early undernutrition results in a delay of at least 1 day, and possibly 3 days, in the initial developmental activity response to the anticholinergic agent, scopolamine.

EFFECTS OF METHYSERGIDE ON ACTIVITY

In this study, separate groups of 8 and 16 litter mice were tested for activity levels at 11, 13, 15, and 17 days of age. Additional groups of 16 litter mice were also tested at 19 days of age. At each age, all mice received a 30 min adaptation period in the activity cages that served as a basis for equating drug groups. Mice from each litter size and age group were then assigned to one of four drug groups: 0 (saline), 1.0, 2.0, or 3.0 mg/kg methysergide (i.p.). Fifteen minutes later, the mice were returned to the activity cages for a 5 hr session. The longer activity session was employed for the methysergide groups in comparison to the scopolamine groups due to differences in the time courses of the two drugs.

The results (see Figure XVI.5) indicate a clear developmental pattern of sensitivity to methysergide for both litter sizes. For the 8 litter groups, little increase in activity was observed at 11 days of age; at 13 days of age, only the lowest dose (1 mg/kg) produced a reliable increase in activity. At 15 days of age, however, a clear dose–response relationship was observed, with higher doses yielding additional activity increments. By 17 days of age, none of the dose levels resulted in increases in activity. Since subsequent pilot research has shown that mice at this age respond to higher doses of methysergide, the failure to obtain activity differences at 17 days of age among the doses suggests that the behavioral thresholds for this drug increase between 15 and 17 days of age.

For the 16 litter groups, there were minimal drug effects at 11 and 13 days of age, followed at 15 days of age by maximal activity increase with

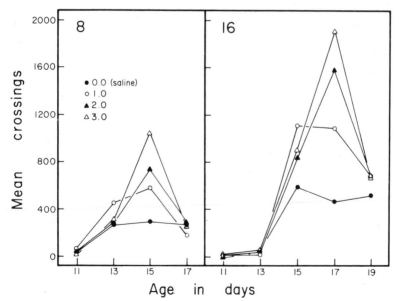

FIGURE XVI.5. Mean number of cage crossing made over a 5 hr session in response to methysergide injections as a function of dose, age, and litter size.

1.0 mg/kg, and a clear dose–response relationship at 17 days of age. By 19 days of age, there was no increase in activity due to methysergide injections. Thus, the developmental emergence of the activity response to methysergide appeared to be delayed by about 2 days for mice undernourished during early development.

IS THE DELAYED RESPONSE TO METHYSERGIDE DUE TO RETARDATION
OF SEROTONERGIC DEVELOPMENT?

Although the preceding results suggest a retarded development of the serotonergic system in undernourished mice, it is possible that the altered activity response to methysergide reflects a dietary deficit of the essential serotonin precursor, L-tryptophan, at the time of testing, rather than a delayed development of this system. Plasma and brain levels of L-tryptophan have been suggested to play a central role in the regulation of brain serotonin levels (Wurtman & Fernstrom, 1976), and reduced amounts of the precursor have been found in the brains of undernourished young rats (Kalyanasundaram, 1976).

To test this possibility, separate groups of 8 and 16 litter mice, aged 11, 13, 15, 17, and 19 days, were assigned to each of four drug treatment conditions: saline-saline, methysergide-saline, saline-L-tryptophan, and methysergide-L-tryptophan. The dosages for L-tryptophan and methysergide were 100 and 1mg/kg, respectively, and the initial injection (saline or methysergide) preceded the second by 30 min. Due to differences in the time courses of these agents, injection of the precursor L-tryptophan followed that of the serotonergic antagonist, methysergide. Immediately following the second injection, the subjects were tested for a 4 hr activity session. If the altered developmental response to methysergide obtained for large litter mice merely reflected a dietary tryptophan deficiency, then the administration of the precursor should produce an activity response to the serotonin antagonist similar to that observed for normally nourished mice.

The results of this experiment (see Figure XVI.6), however, clearly indicate that L-tryptophan administration did not alter the developmental pattern of response to methysergide for either litter size. Therefore, it appears that early undernutrition results in retarded maturation of the serotonergic system.

Conclusions

Overall, the data reviewed in this chapter indicate that dramatic changes in the abilities to acquire and remember certain kinds of in-

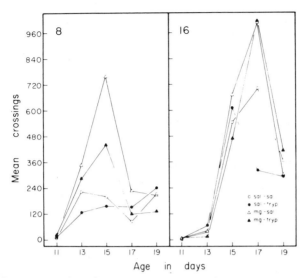

FIGURE XVI.6. Mean number of cage crossings over a 4 hr session in response to saline or methysergide injections in mice receiving either the precursor, L-tryptophan or vehicle, presented as a function of age and litter size.

strumental responses occur during the brain "growth spurt" period. The data are consistent with the hypothesis that physiological and bio-chemical processes underlying these behavioral changes achieve a functional level of maturity, or integration, during this period of brain development.

The strongest support for this hypothesis comes from changes in memory abilities that occur during the brain "growth spurt." For the normally nourished mouse, 24 hr memory of prior escape training appears to emerge between 9–11 days of age, while a similar memory capacity for passive avoidance training becomes evident around 17 days of age. The development of these 24 hr memory capabilities well match the second and third brain "growth spurt" periods reported by Epstein and Miller (1977). Until further data are collected on the development of memory capacities for different tasks, however, it is not yet possible to determine whether major increases in memory capacities can occur at stages of brain development other than the "growth spurt" periods.

With regard to the relationship between brain maturation and learning abilities, only the T-maze data suggest the development of a learning capacity during the brain "growth spurt" period. For the T-maze, we found that learning to go to a particular goal arm develops around 9 days of age in the mouse. On the straight alley, mice were capable of improved escape responses as early as 5 days of age, while on the passive avoidance task, mice between 7 and 21 days of age were capable of learning to a common criterion. This latter finding basically replicated our early report (Ray & Nagy, 1978) that learning of an inhibitory nature was indeed possible at very early ages. The age-related differences, which we found during acquisition of this task, appear to reflect the differential maturation rates and relative balance of developing excitatory and inhibitory systems, and are, therefore, interpreted as indicating differences in performance rather than in learning abilities. The finding that the 1 hr retention scores for normally nourished mice were equivalent across ages would tend to support this interpretation.

The fact that undernutrition appeared to delay the development of memory abilities for passive avoidance training is consistent with earlier results (Nagy *et al.*, 1977), which demonstrated a similar delay of 24 hr memory for T-maze training. Taken together, these results provide further indirect evidence that the ontogenetic increases in memory capacities reflect the functional maturation of brain mechanisms underlying memory processes. We did not expect that undernutrition would have little effect on learning both the T-maze escape and the passive avoidance tasks. If undernutrition caused a general, overall retardation of brain maturation, it would be expected that these learning abilities would have been similarly retarded. The fact that they were not suggests that this undernutrition procedure, or some aspect of it, result in the selective retardation of memory functions, and has relatively little effect upon mechanisms involved with learning at these early ages. If further research confirms these findings, the undernutrition procedure may prove extremely useful in separating the underlying mechanisms involved with memory from those involved with acquisition.

The results of our experiments, which were designed to determine whether undernutrition had selective effects on the developing neurotransmitter systems involved with spontaneous activity, suggest that the serotonergic system was somewhat more affected by early nutritional deprivation than was the cholinergic system. Whether the deficiency in serotonergic functioning is involved directly with undernourished mice having poorer memories of passive avoidance training cannot be determined at this time.

While the results of these experiments are consistent with the hypothesis that the ontogenetic appearance of behavioral capacities reflects the maturation of brain mechanisms involved with these capacities, the determination of clear cause-and-effect relationships between specific brain processes and behaviors is extremely difficult. Both researchers and readers of this area of investigation must constantly be cognizant of the correlative nature of most findings. Even when highly significant correlations are established between changes in behavior and in brain structure or biochemistry, they may reflect coincidental rather than causal relationships. As stated by Dobbing and Smart (1973), "Neurobiologists have only measured parameters which are comparatively easy to measure. No one knows what to measure as a physical index of important aspects of higher mental function. Certainly cell number, brain size, degree of myelination and so forth are no more than tangible examples of structural characteristics, which, by analogy, may react in a similar fashion to whatever structures actually do matter [p. 19]."

Another problem of concern is the attempt to identify individual brain areas or systems as the underlying basis for specific kinds of behavioral change. Although the brain has been conveniently divided by researchers into areas, levels, and systems according to certain structural or behavioral characteristics, the study of such subsystems in isolation may provide data that are totally unrelated to what is going on in the highly integrated brain. Similarly, it may be extremely misleading to study isolated brain processes, or even the integrated brain, while neglecting the interactions of brain and external environment. The results reported by Greenough and Juraska (this volume) and Rosenzweig (this volume) clearly demonstrate that external stimulation can have dramatic effects upon brain growth. When additional manipulations, such as undernutrition, are introduced, these may well affect the manner in which the developing organism interacts with its mother, siblings, and external environment (Crnic, 1976), resulting in different amounts of stimulation, which in turn may affect brain development. For example, biochemical changes associated with prior malnutrition, with correlated changes in behavior, have been reversed by environmental stimuli (Barnes, 1976).

Notwithstanding these kinds of problems, the developmental approach appears viable in furthering our understanding of the relationships between brain and behavior, particularly with regard to learning the memory functions. Clearly a full understanding of these relationships will not result from any single approach, but will require the integration of the various approaches used by the contributors to this volume.

Acknowledgments

While I owe thanks to many undergraduate and graduate students for the long hours which they spent on these experiments, I would like especially to thank Kenneth J. Porada and Ann P. Monsour for their assistance with the experiments reported in the latter part of this chapter.

References

Adlard, B. P. F., & Dobbing, J. Vulnerability of developing brain. III. Development of four enzymes in the brains of normal and undernourished rats. *Brain Research*, 1971, *28*, 97–107.

Altman, J., & Bulut, F. G. Organic maturation and the development of learning capacity. In M. R. Rosenzweig & E. L. Bennett (Eds.), *Neural mechanisms of learning and memory*. Cambridge, Massachusetts: MIT Press, 1976. Pp. 236–240.

Altman, J., Sudarshan, K., Das, G. D., McCormick, N., & Barnes, D. The influence of nutrition on neural and behavioral development. III. Development of some motor, particularly locomotor patterns during infancy. *Developmental Psychobiology*, 1971, *4*, 97–114.

Balazs, R., & Richter, D. Effects of hormones on the biochemical maturation of the brain. In W. Himwich (Ed.), *Biochemistry of the developing brain*. Vol. 1. New York: Marcel Dekker, 1973. Pp. 253–299.

Barnes, R. H. Dual role of environmental deprivation and malnutrition in retarding intellectual development. *The American Journal of Clinical Nutrition*, 1976, *29*, 912–917.

Barraco, R. A., & Stettner, L. J. Antibiotics and memory. *Psychological Bulletin*, 1976, *83*, 242–302.

Bass, N. H. Influence of neonatal undernutrition on the development of rat cerebral cortex: A microchemical study. In R. Paoletti & A. N. Davison (Eds.), *Chemistry and brain development*. New York: Plenum, 1971. Pp. 413–424.

Beitel, R. E., & Porter, P. B. Deficits in retention and impairments in learning induced by severe hypothermia in mice. *Journal of Comparative and Physiological Psychology*, 1968, *66*, 53–59.

Bolles, R. C., & Woods, P. J. The ontogeny of behaviour in the albino rat. *Animal Behaviour*, 1964, *12*, 427–441.

Campbell, B. A. Developmental studies of learning and motivation in infra-primate mammals. In H. W. Stevenson, E. H. Hess, & H. L. Rheingold (Eds.), *Early behavior: Comparative and developmental approaches*. New York: Wiley, 1967. Pp. 43–71.

Campbell, B. A., & Coulter, X. The ontogenesis of learning and memory. In M. R. Rosenzweig, & E. L. Bennett (Eds.), *Neural mechanisms of learning and memory*. Cambridge, Massachusetts: MIT Press, 1976. Pp. 209–235.

Campbell, B. A., Lytle, L. D., & Fibiger, H. C. Ontogeny of adrenergic arousal and cholinergic inhibitory mechanisms in the rat. *Science*, 1969, *166*, 637–638.

Campbell, B. A., & Mabry, P. D. The role of catecholamines in behavioral arousal during ontogenesis. *Psychopharmacologia*, 1973, *31*, 253–264.

Campbell, B. A., & Raskin, L. A. Ontogeny of behavioral arousal: The role of environmental stimuli. *Journal of Comparative and Physiological Psychology*, 1978, *92*, 176–184.

Campbell, B. A., Riccio, D. C., & Rohrbaugh, M. Ontogenesis of learning and memory: Research and theory. In M. Meyer (Ed.), *Second Western Washington Symposium on Learning: Early Learning*. Bellingham: W. Washington College Press, 1971. Pp. 76–109.

Campbell, B. A., & Spear, N. E. Ontogeny of memory. *Psychological Review*, 1972, *79*, 215–236.

Carlton, P. L. Cholinergic mechanisms in the control of behavior by the brain. *Psychological Review*, 1963, *70*, 19–39.

Cragg, B. G. The development of cortical synapses during starvation in the rat. *Brain*, 1972, *95*, 143–150.

Crnic, L. S. Effects of infantile undernutrition on adult learning in rats: Methodological and design problems. *Psychological Bulletin*, 1976, *83*, 715–728.

Davenport, J. W., & Gonzalez, L. M. Neonatal thyroxine stimulation in rats: Accelerated behavioral maturation and subsequent learning deficit. *Journal of Comparative and Physiological Psychology*, 1973, *85*, 397–408.

Davison, A. N., & Dobbing, J. The developing brain. In A. N. Davison, & J. Dobbing (Eds.), *Applied neurochemistry*. Philadelphia: Davis, 1968. Pp. 253–286.

Dobbing, J. Undernutrition and the developing brain. In W. A. Himwich (Ed.), *Developmental neurobiology*. Springfield, Illinois: Thomas, 1970. Pp. 241–261.

Dobbing, J. Undernutrition and the developing brain: The use of animal models to elucidate the human problem. In R. Paoletti & A. N. Davison (Eds.), *Chemistry and brain development*. New York: Plenum, 1971. Pp. 399–412.

Dobbing, J., & Smart, J. L. Early undernutrition, brain development and behavior. In S. A. Barnett (Ed.), *Ethology and development*. London: William Heinemann Medical Books Ltd., 1973. Pp. 16–36.

Eckhert, C. D., Barnes, R. H., & Levitsky, D. A. Regional changes in rat brain choline acetyltransferase and acetycholinesterase activity resulting from undernutrition imposed during different periods of development. *Journal of Neurochemistry*, 1976, *27*, 277–283.

Epstein, H. T. Phrenoblysis: Special brain and mind growth periods. I. Human brain and skull development. *Developmental Psychobiology*, 1974, *7*, 207–216. (a)

Epstein, H. T. Phrenoblysis: Special brain and mind growth periods. II. Human mental development. *Developmental Psychobiology*, 1974, *7*, 217–224. (b)

Epstein, H. T., & Miller, S. A. The developing brain: A suggestion for making more critical interspecies extrapolation. *Nutrition Reports International*, 1977, *16*, 363–366.

Feigley, D. A., & Spear, N. E. Effect of age and punishment condition on long-term retention by the rat of active- and passive-avoidance learning. *Journal of Comparative and Physiological Psychology*, 1970, *73*, 515–526.

Fibiger, H. C., Lytle, L. D., & Campbell, B. A. Cholinergic modulation of adrenergic arousal in the developing rat. *Journal of Comparative and Physiological Psychology*, 1970, *72*, 384–389.

Fish, I., & Winick, M. Effect of malnutrition on regional growth of the developing rat brain. *Experimental Neurology*, 1969, *25*, 534–540.

Fox, M. W. Reflex-ontogeny and behavioural development of the mouse. *Animal Behaviour*, 1965, *13*, 234–241.

Galler, J. R., & Turkewitz, G. Variability of the effects of rearing in a large litter on the development of the rat. *Developmental Psychobiology*, 1975, *8*, 325–331.

Gottlieb, G. Ontogenesis of sensory function in birds and mammals. In E. Tobach, L. R. Aronson, & E. Shaw (Eds.), *The biopsychology of development*. New York: Academic Press, 1971. Pp. 67–128.

Himwich, W. A. (Ed.) *Developmental neurobiology*. Springfield, Illinois: Thomas, 1970.

Himwich, W. A. (Ed.) *Biochemistry of the developing brain*. Vol. 1. New York: Marcel Dekker, 1973.

Himwich, W. A. Developmental neurobiology. In R. G. Grenell, & S. Galay (Eds.), *Biological foundations of psychiatry*. New York: Raven Press, 1976. Pp. 591–632.

Kalyanasundaram, S. Effect of dietary protein and calorie deficiency on tryptophan levels in the developing rat brain. *Journal of Neurochemistry*, 1976, *27*, 1245–1247.

Lanier, L. P., Dunn, A. J., & Van Hartesveldt, C. Development of neurotransmitters and their function in brain. In S. Ehrenpreis, & I. J. Kopin (Eds.), *Reviews of neuroscience*. Vol. 1. New York: Raven Press, 1976. Pp. 195–256.

Mabry, P. D., & Campbell, B. A. Ontogeny of serotonergic inhibition of behavioral arousal in the rat. *Journal of Comparative and Physiological Psychology*, 1974, *86*, 193–201.

McKhann, G. M., Coyle, P. K., & Benjamins, J. A. Nutrition and brain development. In J. I. Nurnberger (Ed.), *Biological and environmental determinants of early development*. Baltimore: Williams & Wilkins, 1973. Pp. 10–22.

Misanin, J. R., Nagy, Z. M., Keiser, E. F., & Bowen, W. Emergence of long-term memory in the neonatal rat. *Journal of Comparative and Physiological Psychology*, 1971, *77*, 188–199.

Murphy, J. M., Meeker, R. B., Porada, K. J., & Nagy, Z. M. GABA-mediated behavioral inhibition during ontogeny in the mouse. *Psychopharmacology*, in press.

Murphy, J. M., & Nagy, Z. M. Neonatal thyroxine stimulation accelerates the maturation of both locomotor and memory processes in mice. *Journal of Comparative and Physiological Psychology*, 1976, *90*, 1082–1091. (a)

Murphy, J. M., & Nagy, Z. M. Development of cholinergic inhibitory capacities in the hyperthyroid mouse. *Pharmacology Biochemistry & Behavior*, 1976, *5*, 449–456. (b)

Nagelberg, D. B., & Nagy, Z. M. Cycloheximide produces adult-like retention deficits of prior learning in infant mice. *Pharmacology Biochemistry & Behavior*, 1977, *7*, 435–441.

Nagy, Z. M. Effect of drive level upon age of onset of 24-hr retention of discriminated escape learning in infant mice. *Bulletin of the Psychonomic Society*, 1975, *6*, 22–24.

Nagy, Z. M. Development of learning and memory processes in infant mice. In N. E. Spear, & B. A. Campbell (Eds.), *Ontogeny of learning and memory*. Hillsadale, New Jersey: Lawrence Erlbaum, in press.

Nagy, Z. M., Anderson, J. A., & Mazzaferri, T. A. Hypothermia causes adult-like retention deficits of prior learning in infant mice. *Development Psychobiology*, 1976, *9*, 447–458.

Nagy, Z. M., Misanin, J. R., Newman, J. A., Olsen, P. L., & Hinderliter, C. F. Ontogeny of memory in the neonatal mouse. *Journal of Comparative and Physiological Psychology*, 1972, *81*, 380–393.

Nagy, Z. M., & Mueller, P. W. Effect of amount of original training upon onset of 24-hour memory capacity in neonatal mice. *Journal of Comparative and Physiological Psychology*, 1973, *85*, 151–159.

Nagy, Z. M., & Murphy, J. M. Learning and retention of a discriminated escape response in infant mice. *Developmental Psychobiology*, 1974, *7*, 185–192.

Nagy, Z. M., Murphy, J. M., & Ray, D. Development of behavioral arousal and inhibition in the Swiss-Webster mouse. *Bulletin of the Psychonomic Society*, 1975, *6*, 146–148.

Nagy, Z. M., Pagano, M. R., & Gable, D. Differential development of 24-hr retention capacities for two components of T-maze escape learning by infant mice. *Animal Learning and Behavior*, 1976, *4*, 25–29.

Nagy, Z. M., Porada, K. J., & Anderson, J. A. Undernutrition by rearing in large litters delays the development of reflexive, locomotor and memory processes in mice. *Journal of Comparative and Physiological Psychology*, 1977, *91*, 682–696.

Nagy, Z. M., Porada, K. J., & Monsour, A. P. Ontogeny of short- and long-term memory capacities for passive avoidance training in undernourished mice. *Developmental Psychobiology*, in press.

Nagy, Z. M., & Ritter, M. Ontogeny of behavioral arousal in the mouse: Effect of prior testing upon age of peak activity. *Bulletin of the Psychonomic Society*, 1976, *7*, 285–288.

Nagy, Z. M., & Sandmann, M. Development of learning and memory of T-maze training in neonatal mice. *Journal of Comparative and Physiological Psychology*, 1973, *83*, 19–26.

Nowak, T. S., & Munro, H. N. Effects of protein-calorie malnutrition on biochemical aspects of brain development. In R. J. Wurtman & J. J. Wurtman (Eds.), *Nutrition and the brain*. Vol. 2. New York: Raven Press, 1977. Pp. 193–260.

Paoletti, R., & Davison, A. N. (Eds.) *Chemistry and brain development*. New York: Plenum, 1971.

Plaut, S. M. Studies of undernutrition in the young rat: Methodological considerations. *Developmental Psychobiology*, 1970, *3*, 157–167.

Porada, K. J., & Nagy, Z. M. Development of serotonergic inhibitory capacities in undernourished mice. Paper presented at the Midwestern Psychological Association Meetings, 1978.

Ramanamurthy, P. S. V. Maternal and early postnatal malnutrition and transmitter amines in rat brain. *Journal of Neurochemistry*, 1977, *28*, 253–254.

Randall, P. K., & Campbell, B. A. Ontogeny of behavioral arousal in rats: Effects of maternal and sibling presence. *Journal of Comparative and Physiological Psychology*, 1976, *90*, 453–459.

Ray, D., & Nagy, Z. M. Emerging cholinergic mechanisms and the ontogeny of response inhibition in the mouse. *Journal of Comparative and Physiological Psychology*, 1978, *92*, 335–349.

Riccio, D. C., Hodges, L. A., & Randall, P. K. Retrograde amnesia produced by hypothermia in rats. *Journal of Comparative and Physiological Psychology*, 1968, *66*, 618–622.

Riccio, D. C., Rohrbaugh, M., & Hodges, L. A. Developmental aspects of passive and active avoidance learning in rats. *Developmental Psychobiology*, 1968, *1*, 108–111.

Schapiro, S. Hormonal and environmental influences on rat brain development and behavior. In M. B. Sterman, D. J. McGinty, & A. M. Adinolfi (Eds.), *Brain development and behavior*. New York: Academic Press, 1971, Pp. 307–334.

Schulenburg, C. J., Riccio, D. C., & Stikes, E. R. Acquisition and retention of a passive-avoidance response as a function of age in rats. *Journal of Comparative and Physiological Psychology*, 1971, *74*, 75–83.

Smart, J. L., & Dobbing, J. Vulnerability of developing brain. II. Effects of early nutritional deprivation on reflex ontogeny and development of behavior in the rat. *Brain Research*, 1971, *28*, 85–95.

Spear, N. E. Retrieval of memory in animals. *Psychological Review*, 1973, *80*, 163–194.

Spear, N. E., & Campbell, B. A. (Eds.), *Ontogeny of learning and memory*. Hillsdale, New Jersey: Lawrence Erlbaum, in press.

Sterman, M. B., McGinty, D. J., & Adinolfi, A. M. (Eds.) *Brain development and behavior*. New York: Academic Press, 1971.

Tobach, E., Aronson, L. R., & Shaw, E. (Eds.), *The biopsychology of development*. New York: Academic Press, 1971.

Vernadakis, A., & Weiner, N. (Eds.), *Advances in behavioral biology*. Vol. 8. *Drugs and the developing brain*. New York: Plenum, 1974.

Winick, M., & Rosso, P. Malnutrition and central nervous system development. In J. W. Prescott, M. S. Read, & D. B. Coursin (Eds.), *Brain function and malnutrition: Neuropsychological methods of assessment*. New York: Wiley, 1975. Pp. 41–51.

Wurtman, R. J., & Fernstrom, J. D. Control of brain neurotransmitter synthesis by precursor availability and nutritional state. *Biochemical Pharmacology*, 1976, *25*, 1691–1696.

Chapter XVII

Genetic Correlations between Brain Size and Some Behaviors of Housemice[1]

NORMAN D. HENDERSON

The relationship of brain characteristics to experience, evolution, and behavior is one of those issues in science that has had a long and cyclical history. As Professor Rosenzweig has already pointed out in this volume, many of the basic issues concerning species differences in brain size and cognitive functioning, the effects of mental exercise on the brain, the relationship of brain and body size, and the relationship of brain characteristics to behavior within species were addressed during the latter half of the eighteenth century. About a century later, interest in these issues was renewed with a focus on neural connections and organization of the brain; scientists asked how neural organization differed as a function of species, development, and experience. The influence of Ramon y Cajal (1894) and Foster and Sherrington (1897) was pronounced on the course of research on relationships between brain and behavior. The work of Lashley (1930) was followed by an explosion of research concerned with neural pathways and their role in integrating behavior.

Although much of this research focused on specific neural structures and their influence on narrow classes of behavior, some investigators continued to pursue the broad questions concerning the relationship of overall brain size and adaptive behavior. The remarkable plasticity of

[1]Research supported by National Science Foundation Grant BNS 71-00821

347

the brain, both in terms of changes in absolute size and in neural structure resulting from environmental experience, has now been well documented (e.g., Greenough, 1975; Rosenzweig & Bennet, 1976). In addition, Jerison (1973) has marshalled considerable evidence demonstrating that brain size indexes that properly correct for body size show a clear evolutionary pattern toward larger brains. He has also demonstrated that, across species, gross brain size provides an accurate estimate of a number of other parameters, such as the volumes of general cortical, subcortical structures, and neuronal connectivity indexes. Thus, nearly 200 years after most of the major questions were asked, and 100 years after several specific hypotheses were made, we are beginning to answer the two broad questions concerning the adaptive significance of brain size on a broad evolutionary scale, and the effects of experiential and nutritional influences on the brain.

On a third broad question—what is the relationship of various brain capacity measures to behavior within species—we have been less successful in providing clear answers, as attested to by several papers presented in this volume. The lack of progress in this area is somewhat surprising, particularly for species like the laboratory mouse, where genetic influences on both behavioral and neural characters are often substantial (e.g., Fuller & Wimer, 1966). Some data on within-species relationships between brain and behavior are beginning to emerge, as reported in chapters by Drs. Epstein, Nagy, and Jensen. I hope to extend these beginnings by describing the correlational results of a behavior genetics research program with *mus musculus*, which included brain size as a variable. In doing so, I will point out some of the methodological and practical constraints involved in trying to find genetic correlations between brain and behavior within a species.

Strategies for Studying Genetic Correlations in Laboratory Animals

Most of the research methods developed for the genetic study of physiological, chemical, and morphological characters in plants and animals have been successfully applied to behavioral variables. Many studies using drosophila, mice, rats, and other species can now be found that have used single gene mutants, artificial selection, inbred strain comparisons, or crossing experiments to answer questions concerning genetic influences on behavior. All of these techniques can be used when studying more than one dependent variable to estimate genetic correlations between variables; but, as one moves from the study of variance of a single measure to covariance between measures, the relative advantages and disadvantages of these genetic strategies become amplified. Each of the methods and their use in animal behavior genetics has been described in basic textbooks (e.g., Thiessen, 1972; McClearn & DeFries, 1973; Ehrman & Parsons, 1976). The following comments, therefore, focus on problems encountered when using these methods for computing genetic correlations between dependent variables.

Single-Gene Research

Finding behavioral traits that are controlled by a single gene has great appeal, because single-gene systems are potentially easier to trace from the initial genetic alteration to final behavior than systems involving many genes. Usually the procedure involves comparing normal animals with mutants known to differ at a single genetic locus. The most powerful procedure involves the use of coisogenic strains—obtained when a mutation arises within an inbred strain, and the mutant line is maintained along with the original inbred line. Mutant and nonmutant animals within the strain thus have exactly the same genotype, except for one gene. If these coisogenic strains are found to differ on an interesting behavioral trait, the single gene on which the strains differ is obviously implicated.

The single gene approach works best when one begins with coisogenic or other mutant lines and screens them on a large number of tests, looking for behaviors affected by the gene. Once one or more behavioral traits are found, the process of tracing the pathway from gene to behavior can begin. The problem is somewhat different, however, when one begins with a particular trait of interest, such as brain weight or discrimination learning or locomotor activity, and then attempts to find a single gene responsible for the behavior. The probability of a payoff is considerably less under these circumstances, since the chances are low that any single gene difference examined will strongly influence the trait that interests the investigator. The problem becomes much more severe when one is interested in the genetic correlation between two characters, since the chance that the single gene affects both traits is the product of two already small probabilities. Even if single genes were largely responsible for many behavioral and neurological characters, the chances are small of finding a number of these characters attributable to the same gene.

Selection Studies

Beginning with Rundquist's (1933) work on artificial selection for high- and low-active rats, investigators interested in the genetics of behavior have often used the technique of artificial selection in order to demonstrate the profound influence of genetics on behavior. The procedure can be extended to the study of more than one variable in two ways— measurement during selection, or the comparison of the stabilized selection lines on the character of interest.

MEASUREMENT DURING SELECTION

Behavioral and morphological characters that one might expect to be genetically correlated with a selected phenotype can be measured in succeeding generations during the selection experiment. Those secondary characters that follow the same course as the artificially selected character may be genetically correlated. For example, if a selection program for large and small brain size was begun with a heterogeneous genetic stock, and a certain measure of learning was shown to change over succeeding generations in a similar manner to that found with brain weight changes, one could suspect that the genes involved in brain size are also involved in the measured learning behavior.

One cannot, however, conclude that gene pleiotropy is involved without further experiments. The selection process may, for example, be systematically altering maternal behavior, which in turn is having a potent influence on subsequent learning performance in the offspring. Although such possibilities can be checked easily, two other problems arise when using measures of correlated responses to selection to estimate genotypic correlations. First is a practical issue—the ability of investigators to anticipate correctly which characters will be of most interest to study during the long period of selection. The second point is that natural and artificial selection produce the most rapid changes when the character being selected for had a high proportion of additive genetic variance. Such traits are often only weakly related to Darwinian fitness, or are traits where an intermediate score is associated with fitness. Many characters, however, may already have been subjected to directional natural selection to the point where relatively little additive genetic variation remains. Selection will proceed much more slowly with such characters, and will be frequently asymmetrical in terms of response to selection in high and low directions. Such characters may not show a strong correlated response to brain weight or another selected character.

COMPARISON OF SELECTED LINES

The constraint deriving all measures of interest at the beginning of a selection study has led to an alternative procedure; one can select for high and low expression of a character for a number of generations, until the lines fail to show continued divergence, and use a high, low, and an intermediate nonselected line as genetic material to study new variables of interest. Tryon's famous maze-bright and maze-dull lines (Tryon, 1940), for example, were studied extensively by Searle (1949) on a number of other learning behaviors. Searle's failure to find consistent differences on these other behaviors led to the conclusion that selection had been highly specific to Tryon's testing situation. Today we have many selected lines of mice, rats, and drosophila used in research, including mice derived from artificial selection studies involving brain size. As several chapters in this volume demonstrate, the Roderick lines and the Fuller BWS lines of mice have provided useful genetic material for examining the effects of brain size on behavior. Any new behavior can be examined using mice of large, intermediate, and small brain size produced by the selection studies. As with all studies involving selected lines, additional experiments must be run to assure that behavioral differences are not due to secondary factors, such as maternal nutritional deficiencies, gross differences in body size, or other factors that differ between the selection lines. Furthermore, comparisons of behavior across lines does not reflect all genotypic influences due to nonadditive genetic effects. Nevertheless, uncovering consistent behavioral differences between lines of mice with large and small brains provides a useful starting point studying the genetic correlation between brain and behavior.

Unfortunately, it can only be a starting point, since estimating correlations between characters requires more degrees of freedom than are obtainable with high, intermediate, and low brain weight lines. Large differences in behavior of lines with large and small brains means little in itself, since it has become almost a truism that genetically different lines of mice are likely to behave differently, whether they are randomly chosen inbred strains, or divergent lines artificially selected for any character. It is important, therefore, to go beyond demonstrating significant group differences and to demonstrate further that significant correlations exist between brain weight and various classes of behavior. The single degree of freedom available in correlations computed from measures based on high, intermediate, and low brain weight lines is simply not sufficient for this purpose. More extensive sampling of genotypes with differing brain weights must supplement work on selected lines.

Inbred Strain Comparisons

One method of obtaining a large number of different genotypes with varying brain sizes is to test a large sample of inbred strains that are known to have a wide range of brain sizes. In this way one can obtain sufficient degrees of freedom to allow meaningful significance tests of correlation coefficients across the different lines. Although wider genetic sampling is achieved, the use of inbred strains poses some difficulties for genetic correlation research. Because no heterozygous animals are involved, between-strain variation primarily reflects additive genetic variance and variance mediated by maternal effects. If the latter is large, correlations between characters of interest may not be primarily genetic in nature. As in the case of selection studies, if nonadditive genetic variation is large on some of the characters measured, the correlations obtained may not be accurate representations of true genotypic correlations. Additive genetic variance is usually considerably larger than maternal and nonadditive genetic variance in most characters; thus, differences in additive genetic correlations and genotypic correlations will be small in most cases.

The more serious problems associated with the use of inbred strains for genetic correlation research involve both inbreeding depression and insufficient representation of a normal range of phenotypes. Because inbred strains are homozygous for many deleterious recessive genes, inbreeding depression effects have been found in a large proportion of characters. Many inbred strains have retinal degeneration, leading to severely impaired visual capacity (Fuller & Wimer, 1966). Obviously, a great deal of between-strain variation attributable to *rd* will be present on tasks requiring visual cues, if such strains are included in behavioral studies; yet most investigators would regard this as an atypical source of variation that would confuse correlations between measures. A high proportion of inbred strains are also homozygous for albinism. Although more subtle than the effects of retinal degeneration, there is now considerable evidence that albinos differ from pigmented animals in many situations involving fear responses to light, hesitancy in novel situations, and generally poorer performance in visual discrimination. Obviously, if a large proportion of between-strain variance on one or more behaviors can be attributed to a simple albinism effect, correlations between these characters may in a large part be due to albinism effects. Similarly, the overrepresentation of other, more subtle, recessive gene effects probably works to influence genetic correlations derived from inbred strains.

Inbreeding depression can also lead to a "floor" effect on many measures of interest. Hybrid and wild mice, for example, sometimes show a wide range of variation on performance tasks, while a large proportion of inbred strains score at essentially chance levels on these tasks, resulting in relatively little between-strain variability. For example, in a vertical-horizontal discrimination task to be discussed shortly, we found only two of six inbred parent strains scoring above chance, while all 30 F_1 hybrid crosses did so (Henderson, 1972). In summary, whereas using multiple inbred strains provides the advantage of extensive genetic sampling, this strategy has a number of disadvantages, which are easily overcome by a more extensive breeding design involving hybrid crosses.

Extensive Breeding Designs

Considerable genetic information can be obtained by applying standard analytic procedures to classical breeding designs which involve the the crossing of two parent lines to produce F_1, F_2, and backcross generations. Although this breeding design could be used in conjunction with a large number of dependent variables measured in parents and various crosses, more extensive breeding plans are appropriate when genetic correlations are of primary interest. One such breeding plan, (originally called the method of complete intercrossing and now more commonly the diallel cross technique), is particularly amenable to biometrical genetic analysis in terms of partitioning variance into a number of genetic and environmental components, and in terms of partitioning covariance between traits in a similar manner. Although other, more efficient extensive breeding designs than the diallel cross are now available, these often pose certain constraints on the choice of primary breeder lines, which make them inappropriate for multivariate research.

THE DIALLEL CROSS DESIGN

A schematic representation of a 6 × 6 diallel cross is shown in Figure XVII. 1. The genetic background of each cross is indicated by a two digit number, the first digit representing the number of its maternal strain, and the second digit the number of its paternal strain. A large number of analyses of diallel crosses has been described that allow for many variations in experimental design and in estimating various genetic parameters (e.g., Griffing, 1956; Hayman, 1954a, 1954b; Jinks, 1954; Jinks & Mather, 1955; Wearden, 1964; Yates, 1947). Each of the methods that allow partitioning of variance into genetic and environmental components can be extended to multiple variables; covariance can be partitioned in a similar manner to produce various genetic and environmental correlations, which each contribute to the final phenotypic correlation between two characters. Griffing (1956) presents a worked example of this procedure, partitioning a phenotypic correlation into its genetic and environmental components. The final phenotypic correlation depends not only on the magnitude of each of the individual component correlations, but also on the proportion of variance accounted for by each component.

Although such procedures are elegant extensions to the concept of partitioning variance, correlations derived in this manner have two drawbacks. First, the sampling distributions for such correlation coefficients are unknown, and therefore significance testing is not possible. Second, such procedures are most amenable to situations where all measures are taken on the same subjects. In many cases when one is dealing with a large number of behavioral variables, repeated testing is not desirable because of carryover effects, and occasionally it is impossible because of other experimental constraints. A less elegant procedure can be used to bypass both these difficulties, namely to use cell means as individual units of analysis for correlational purposes. In this way, different groups of animals of the same genotype can be used to measure different groups of dependent variables. Since these parent strains and F_1 crosses can be reproduced at any time in any other laboratory, the same set of "genetic units" can be reproduced indefinitely (assuming only minor genetic drift); investigators can continue adding variables to an ever expanding correlation matrix based on a fixed set of genetic units.

AVAILABLE GENOTYPES FOR GENETIC CORRELATIONS

Exactly how many "genetic units" are actually available to use in a diallel cross for the purposes of computing genetic correlation coefficients? Although 36 cells are represented in the 6 × 6 diallel shown in Figure XVII. 1, the cells above and below the diagonal, (which is composed of inbred strains), represent reciprocal crosses where only the genotype of dam and sire is reversed. Differences in such reciprocals

Female parent strain

	1	2	3	4	5	6
1	11	21	31	41	51	61
2	12	22	32	42	52	62
3	13	23	33	43	53	63
4	14	24	34	44	54	64
5	15	25	35	45	55	65
6	16	26	36	46	56	66

Male   parent   strain

FIGURE XVII.1. Layout of a 6 × 6 diallel cross.

can be attributed to sex-linked effects, maternal effects, or both. Sex-linked effects would be reflected in a statistically significant interaction between the reciprocal differences and the sex of the animals being tested. In the absence of sex × reciprocal interactions, we can assume that the primary source of any reciprocal differences must be attributed to maternal environmental effects. From a genetic standpoint, in the absence of sex-linked effects reciprocal cells above and below the diagonal are essentially genetic replicates of each other. We thus have 15 rather than 30 genetically distinct F_1 crosses in our 6 × 6 diallel, with our best estimate of any phenotype for each F_1 cross the average of the two reciprocals. Note that while working with F_1 reciprocal *averages* will allow us to compute genetic correlations; we could work equally well with F_1 reciprocal *differences* to produce a correlational study of common maternal influences on our dependent variables.

The next question concerns the appropriateness of including the six inbred lines, produced along the diagonal of the diallel matrix, in our correlations. Their use would extend the number of unique genotypes from 15 to 21, in the case of our 6 × 6 diallel. Unfortunately, the inclusion of these inbred parent strains poses some statistical difficulties in cases where nonadditive genetic variation is found in one or both correlated traits. Essentially, the slope of the regression line for two characters will differ for inbred and hybrid animals in the presence of nonadditive genetic variation. An example of this is shown in Figure XVII.2, where I have plotted the log brain and log body weights for the six inbred lines and the 15 F_1 hybrids produced by the diallel cross. Data are shown for

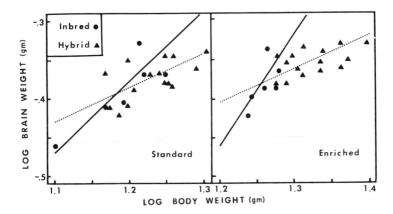

FIGURE XVII.2. The relationship presented between log brain and log body weights for inbred parent strains and their F_1 hybrids reared in standard laboratory cages and enriched environments. In the presence of nonadditive genetic variance, the slopes of the regression lines differ for inbreds and hybrids

animals reared in standard laboratory cages and for animals reared in larger enriched environments, which resulted in somewhat larger animals. The regression lines differ considerably for inbred and hybrids in both cases, as one would expect since both brain and body weights involve significant sources of nonadditive genetic variance. Clearly, indiscriminate pooling of inbred and hybrid groups in these situations would be improper for purposes of computing correlation coefficients. We are, therefore, left with only 15 distinct genetic units derived from our 6 × 6 diallel, providing only 13 degrees of freedom from correlations between measures.

Correlations computed on 15 observational units have large standard errors, even when many observations may be used to determine the mean performance of animals of one of the 15 genotypes. More degrees of freedom (df) can be obtained by using larger diallels, 26 df in an 8 × 8 diallel and 40 df in a 10 × 10 diallel. Although diallels of this size are common in plant research, where dependent variables are quickly and reliably measured, behavioral studies of this magnitude are generally prohibitive, particularly when a large number of dependent variables are to be involved. Unfortunately we must be content with moderate sized breeding designs, which provide relatively little power for detecting significant genetic correlations between brain and behavior. There are several reasons to expect that the magnitude of brain–behavior correlations is unlikely to be high for most behaviors, as we shall discuss later.

The Representative Design Approach to Animal Research

I have previously suggested (Henderson, 1969) that investigators of animal behavior in the laboratory should consider using a *representative design* approach (Brunswick, 1956) in their research, in order to build a stronger case for the external validity of their results. Brunswick's approach stresses the use of multiple variable experiments with extensive sampling of biologically relevant variables. The regular frequency with which interactions between the age, previous experience, genotype, and specific test situations are found in the literature suggests that general statements concerning the effects of any one class of variables may be unwarranted, unless the remaining classes of variables have been sampled at more than one level. A similar situation exists in correlational studies. For example, one might ask how general are the correlation results based on cage reared rats and mice, given the large changes in brain size and some behaviors, which have been found as a result of different rearing conditions. It would be impossible to determine without observation how consistent these behavior correlations are. Similarly, given the low correspondence between different variables supposedly measuring the same construct, such as discrimination learning or locomotor exploration, several measures taken in different test situations should be made for each behavioral domain of interest. It was this research philosophy that led to an extensive developmental genetic study carried out in the Behavior Genetics Laboratory at Oberlin College a number of years ago.

Descriptions of the interaction of genetic and early environmental influences on brain size, discrimination learning, food location ability, and alternation behavior are already available (Henderson, 1970a, 1970b, 1972, 1973). Here I would like to summarize some of the genetic correlations of data that relate brain size to the previous behavioral variables, as well as additional measures of exploratory and locomotor behavior. Since all the genotypes used in that study were derived from crosses of six common inbred laboratory strains of mice, any investigator who wishes to extend this work can simply reproduce these genotypes to examine new variables of interest, and extend my correlation matrices accordingly.

A Study of Gene–Environment Interaction and Genetic Correlations

Environments and Genotypes

Since much of the experimental methodological detail is presented in the preceding references, I will present only a brief description of the general research design and the data collection procedure.

A 6 × 6 diallel matrix was produced by crossing six highly inbred strains (A/J, BALB/cJ, RF/J, C3H/HeJ, C57BL/10J, and DBA/1J) in all possible combinations. Approximately half the mice in each genotype were raised in translucent plastic cages, approximately 14 × 20 × 9 cm, and the remaining half raised in larger cages (55 × 25 × 15 cm) that housed an "enriched" environment. All animals remained in their respective rearing environments until 6 weeks of age, when behavioral testing and brain weight measures were taken. Different groups of animals were assigned to be tested in a visual discrimination swimming maze, a nonvisual T-maze, a battery of measures of exploratory and locomotor behavior, and a food location task. Finally some groups of animals used only for a brief battery of activity measures were sacrificed, and brain and body weights recorded. In all cases care was taken to sample no more than one male and one female from a single litter for any behavioral or brain measure. The design allowed us to carry out a complete biometrical genetic analysis on each of the measures for animals reared in both the enriched and the standard cage environments. The consistency of the genetic architecture across environments, or conversely, the consistency of the enrichment effects across genotypes, could thus be determined.

As indicated above, only the 15 pooled reciprocal F_1 crosses derived from a 6 × 6 diallel are appropriate for the primary genetic correlational research. In some circumstances, correlations between behaviors of the six parent lines may be compared to additive genetic correlations obtained from F_1s, after overall genotypic correlations are explored. The primary analysis therefore consisted of examining the correlations between brain size and a large number of learning and activity measures obtained from 15 distinct genetic groups. Although the correlation matrix of these variables is based on only 13 degrees of freedom, the matrix is replicated under two different environmental conditions, providing additional insight into the stability of the correlations observed.

Behavioral Measures

Animals assigned for testing on the visual discrimination problems were tested for six consecutive days, 12 trials per day, in the two swimming mazes. Half of each genotype received training on the black–white discrimination maze for the first 3 days, followed by testing in the vertical–horizontal maze on Days 4–5. The order was reversed for the remaining animals. Since black–white and vertical–horizontal discrimination tasks were counterbalanced within each genotype, a third measure—improvement on the second discrimination task—was also available for analysis. The original genetic analysis of these data (Henderson, 1972) indicated that this improvement measure showed a higher degree of directional dominance toward positive training transfer than the simple discrimination measures. This finding suggests that the transfer measure may reflect a character that is of greater adaptive significance to the species than one measured by simple black–white or vertical–horizontal discrimination.

Animals tested in the left–right discrimination problems were placed in a T-maze constructed of channel sheet metal, and run under dim red light that minimized visual cues. Shock escape training was continued until an animal made nine consecutive correct responses. After a rest period, the animal was run to the same criterion in the opposite goal arm. Performance during initial acquisition and reversal learning were primary criterion measures. Alternation behavior was also measured in the sheet metal T-maze, and was based on two preliminary exploratory trials in a maze prior to shock escape training. The percentage of animals entering opposite arms on the two test trials was used as an index of alternation behavior for each genotype.

Animals tested in the food location task were deprived of food for 12 hours then placed in a large arena that contained a series of ramps and ladders leading to food located in the upper corner of the test apparatus. Total time to reach the food was used as the primary criterion variable.

Exploratory and ambulatory behavior was measured in a battery of five test boxes. Each animal was tested 5 minutes in each test box on 2 consecutive days. Animals within each genotype received different orders of testing on each of the 2 days. In each box the primary measure consisted of exploratory or locomotor activity recorded automatically by photoelectric cells or contact relays. One test box consisted of a brightly lit open field, the second a series of "rooms" that the animals enter and leave, the third contained two dimly lit mazes separated by a small open area, the fourth consisted of a visual cliff in which activity could be measured over both deep and shallow areas, and the fifth box contained a number of objects wired to contact sensors, as well as vertical and horizontal rods wired to record climbing behavior.

Scores for the various behavioral variables were often transformed to conform with basic biometrical scaling assumptions. For ease in interpreting correlation coefficients, each of the behavioral variables was scaled in such a way that high scores represented "good" learning performance or high activity.

Brain Measures

Although no transformations were necessary for the genetic analysis of brain and body weights, the problem of relative brain size is of obvious concern in a study of brain–behavior relationships. Jerison (1973) has dealt at length with this issue and provides convincing arguments for the use of an *Encephalization Quotient* (*EQ*) as a useful measure of brain size. The *EQ* is the ratio of actual brain size to expected brain size, with expected brain size defined by a power function relating brain and body weights. The power function is most easily obtained from the regressions of log-log plots of brain and body weights, such as those in Figure XVII.2. When measuring across a wide range of species, the relationship $E = kP^{2/3}$ (where E and P are brain and body weights in centimeter-grams-seconds units) fits the data quite well. As one would expect under conditions of considerable range restriction, both the correlation between brain and body weight and the exponent of the power function are considerably smaller for different genotypes within a single species than between species. The brain-body weight relationship for the 15 hybrid groups used in our study was $E = .15P^{.36}$ ($r = .59$) for mice reared in standard cages, and $E = .17P^{.31}$ ($r = .63$) for mice reared in enriched environments. Despite larger brain and body weights for animals reared in enrichment, the brain–body weight relationship was similar for animals reared in both environments. Encephalization quotients were computed for each hybrid cross reared in each environment; actual brain weight is divided by expected brain weight, based on the appropriate preceding equation. Although several additional brain parameters, such as cortical volume, neuron density, neural connectivity, brain size, are associated with improved adaptive capacities, and the number of cortical neurons available beyond those necessary for primitive behavioral functions can also be derived from brain and body weights, absolute brain weight or EQ correlated so highly with each of these derived measures that their inclusion in the present analysis would have been redundant. Eight animals (four male and four female) were used to estimate the average performance of genotypes reared in each environment for the dependent variables in the study.

Results

BRAIN–BEHAVIOR CORRELATIONS WITHIN ENVIRONMENTS

Table XVII.1 summarizes the correlations between brain weight, body weight, and EQ with a number of activity and learning measures. The upper value in each pair is the correlation obtained for animals reared in standard laboratory cages, and the lower value is obtained for animals in the enriched population. Although significant correlations consistent across both enriched and standard cage rearing were observed between body weight and several measures, only two correlations between brain weight or EQ and behavioral measures were significant. Large body weight was associated with higher activity, low defecation, and better performance in a nonvisual left–right T-maze using shock escape. A similar correlation pattern, of much smaller magnitude, existed for brain weight, and probably reflected the overall body size component. When adjusted for body weight, brain size, as reflected by EQ, tended to be slightly negatively correlated with most activity and learning measures.

Table XVII.2 summarizes the orthogonally rotated factor matrices of the genetic correlations among all behaviors shown in Table XVII.1, along with *EQ* and body weight. Despite the small number of observations involved in computing correlations, the factor matrices for animals reared in enriched and in standard cages are quite similar. Factor 1 appears to be a high activity, low defecation factor, which has a positive body weight loading. Factor 2 and Factor 3 reflect visual and nonvisual discrimination learning respectively. Factor 4 results from a single high correlation coefficient in each environment and is not particularly meaningful. The correlations and the subsequent factor analysis of brain and

TABLE XVII. 1

Correlations between Brain Weight, Body Weight, Encephalization Quotient, and Several Behaviors for Animals Reared in Standard Cages (Upper Value) and Enriched Cages (Lower Value)

Measure	Brain weight	Body weight	EQ
Black–white	− .13	.13	− .27
discrimination	− .45	− .27	− .35
Vertical–horizontal	.03	.09	− .02
discrimination	− .42	− .24	− .35
Transfer	− .49	− .11	− .52[a]
task 1–task 2	.17	− .14	.33
T-maze	.21	.55[a]	− .14
initial	.57[a]	.64[a]	.20
T-maze	.44	.29	.33
reversal	.14	.33	− .09
Food	− .33	− .01	− .41
location	− .04	.02	− .07
Alternation	.15	.02	.17
(percentage animals)	− .41	.00	− .53[a]
Open field	.10	.59[a]	− .30
ambulation	.06	.49	− .33
Maze and field	.21	.31	.02
exploration	.24	.33	− .03
Visual cliff	.32	.71[a]	− .13
ambulation	.14	.62[a]	− .34
Visual choice	.08	.52[a]	− .29
exploration	.10	.47	− .27
Number of	.10	.67[a]	− .37
objects touched	.07	.51[a]	− .33
Pole climbing	.10	.54[a]	− .27
activity	− .20	.22	− .43
Open field	− .14	− .36	.08
defecation	.19	− .12	.34

[a] $p < .05$

TABLE XVII.2
Principal Component Factor Matrices Varimax Rotation

Measure	Mice reared in standard cages				Mice reared in enriched cages			
	Factor 1	Factor 2	Factor 3	Factor 4	Factor 1	Factor 2	Factor 3	Factor 4
Black-white discrimination	.30	.79	—	-.27	—	.91	—	—
Vertical–horizontal discrimination	—	.89	—	—	—	.60	—	—
Transfer task 1–task 2	—	.28	—	-.69	—	—	.55	—
T-maze initial	.56	—	.56	—	—	-.55	.66	—
T-maze reversal	—	.52	.49	—	-.45	.25	.36	—
Food location	—	—	-.56	-.26	-.44	.32	-.42	-.44
Alternation	—	—	.81	—	—	—	—	.96
Open field ambulation	.89	.36	—	—	.89	.41	—	—
Maze and field	.42	.68	—	—	.82	—	.54	—
Visual cliff ambulation	.71	.26	—	—	.91	—	—	—
Visual choice exploration	.58	.29	—	—	.82	—	—	—
Objects touched	.89	—	—	-.26	.72	.45	-.37	—
Pole climbing	.76	.26	.29	-.27	.53	.72	-.34	—
EQ (O/E)	—	—	.30	.90	—	-.38	.28	-.47
Body weight	.79	—	—	—	.69	-.36	-.40	—
Open field defacation	-.51	—	—	—	-.31	-.49	—	—

behavior relationships of animals reared in the two environments provide little evidence for consistent brain–behavior relationships.

The lack of statistically significant correlations may be due to the low power of having only 15 genetic units available in a situation where correlation coefficients are not expected to be high. Before considering this possibility, I would like to examine an alternative hypothesis concerning the possible relationship of brain size to long-term adaptations to the environment. Short-term measures of learning or other activity may be less related to absolute brain size than indexes of longer term responses to environmental conditions.

RELATIONSHIP OF BRAIN SIZE TO BEHAVIOR CHANGE RESULTING FROM ENRICHED REARING

In our study, mice were reared in environments that differed considerably in opportunities for perceptual motor stimulation. As a result, several behaviors studied showed a pronounced rearing condition effect. Brain weight, and to a lesser degree body weight, were greater for genotypes reared in the enriched environment. Two discrimination learning measures also showed enrichment effects—improvement on the second swimming visual discrimination task, and reversal learning in the nonvisual shock escape T-maze. Interestingly, both measures are often regarded as measures of flexibility in learning. Animals reared in enrichment showed no better performance on the simple visual and nonvisual discrimination tasks. Among measures reflecting general locomotor exploration and activity, enrichment effects differed depending on the test situations. Food locating ability improved considerably as a result of enrichment, and open field activity, activity in a visual choice situation, and number of objects touched in a test arena all showed increases as results of enriched rearing. Activity level over the deep end of a visual cliff, on the other hand, was less for animals reared in enriched cages. Other measures of ambulation, exploration, and alternation behavior did not show differences as a result of standard or enriched cage rearing. Not surprisingly, animals reared in the large enriched cages also showed less fear in the open field arena, as measured by defecation.

Possibly brain size or changes in brain size are correlated with the degree of behavior change resulting from enrichment. To examine this, correlations were computed on the difference between enriched and standard group scores and brain weight measures, using the 15 F_1 genotypes. The resulting correlation matrix is presented in Table XVII.3. Because EQ values are highly similar for F_1s reared in enriched and standard environments ($r = .82$), an average EQ value for each genotype

TABLE XVII.3
Correlations between Behavior Differences Resulting from Enriched Rearing and Brain–Body Weight Factors

Behavioral measure	Enrichment (effect)	r with EQ (average)	r with EQ (increase)	r with brain weight (increase)	r with body weight (increase)
Black-white discrimination	n.s.	-.28	-.17	.02	.10
Vertical–horizontal discrimination	n.s.	-.41	.11	.20	.14
Transfer task 1–task 2	Improves	.61[a]	-.38	-.45	-.17
T-Maze initial	n.s.	.35	-.01	.26	.43
T-Maze reversal	Improves	-.55[a]	.38	.64[a]	.52[a]
Food location	Improves	.13	-.33	-.38	-.03
Alternation	n.s.	-.36	-.08	-.33	-.45
Open field ambulation	Increases	-.23	.39	.48	.13
Maze and field	n.s.	.30	-.03	.06	.32
Visual cliff ambulation	Decreases	-.41	.17	.32	.39
Visual choice ambulation	Increases	-.14	.19	.33	.32
Objects touched	Increases	-.01	.05	.18	-.01
Pole climbing	n.s.	-.08	.42	.52	-.09
Open field defication	Decreases	.30	.19	.11	-.06

[a] $p < .05$

was computed across rearing conditions. It can be seen that EQ correlates significantly with the two learning measures that showed significant enrichment effects, and correlates marginally with activity on the visual cliff. Enrichment improved transfer of training scores, and genotypes with higher EQs showed the greatest improvement. There was a negative correlation of EQ with positive enrichment effects on T-maze reversal learning, which probably reflects that shock-escape T-maze performance is influenced heavily by body size. EQ must be necessarily correlated negatively with body weight. In both enriched and standard groups, T-maze performance was correlated with body weight, and genotypes showing the greatest improvement in T-maze scores also tended to be genotypes with the greatest body weight increase in enriched environments.

Aside from a tendency for genotypes with high EQ to show a slight decrease in activity from enriched rearing, brain size does not appear to be highly correlated with behavioral changes resulting from long-term exposure to enrichment. Furthermore, relative change in EQ as a result of enrichment also was not correlated with behavior changes. A factor analysis of change scores on all behavioral and brain measures added little insight not already available from the correlations shown in Table XVII.3. EQ loaded on a factor that included improvement in transfer of training in a visual discrimination task, increase in visual cliff activity, and smaller increases in reversal learning performance. EQ was not correlated with the remaining factors, which tended to reflect individual correlation clusters of change scores.

In essence, changes in activity level that result from enrichment do not appear to be related to brain size, and only the two learning measures which showed enrichment effects correlated with brain–body measures. Improvement in training transfer, another result of enrichment, was correlated with relative brain size; improvement in nonvisual reversal learning was correlated with an increase in the general brain–body weight that resulted from enrichment.

It is interesting to pursue further the question of whether genetic correlation between EQ and improvement in training transfer is due primarily to common additive or nonadditive genetic variance. We can get a rough estimate of the additive genetic correlation by pooling all F_1s with a common parent and computing the correlation between the means of the six groupings on the two characters. We can also estimate additive genetic variance by computing the correlation between the two variables, using the mean performance of the six parent strains. Thus, we can calculate two independent estimates of additive genetic correlation, each with some limitations and each with only 4 df. Pooling the two coefficients should produce a reasonable estimate of additive genetic correlation. The Pearson correlation between EQ and enrichment effects on transfer was .80 for pooled F_1 groups, and .51 for inbred parent strains. Averaging these two estimates with Fisher's Z transformation results in an estimate of additive genetic correaltion of .67 with 8 df ($p < .05$). Thus, it appears that the genotypic correlation obtained on the 15 individual F_1 genotypes was due largely to additive genetic variance; this suggests that both EQ and behavioral plasticity (seen in the training transfer scores) can be subject to concurrent selection.

Although the relationship between brain size and the transfer of training measure is an interesting one, it is an exception in an otherwise consistent pattern of nonsignificant brain–behavior correlations. Of the 14 behavioral measures examined, for mice reared in two environments, only two significant correlations with EQ were found, and both were inconsistent across environments. EQ did not load significantly on any of the factors that summarized most of the common variance between behavioral variables. The significant correlations between brain weight and T-maze performance, including improvement in performance as a result of enrichment, appear to be due to general brain and body size increases. It is impossible to tell whether some increase in cognitive capacity due to increased brain size, or some extraneous factor related to body size, is primarily responsible for this relationship. The failure to find genetic correlations between brain size and behavior does not necessarily mean that such correlations do not exist. There are a number of reasons for expecting that if such correlations do exist, they are of a relatively modest magnitude, possibly too small to be detected without considerably larger samples than those used in the present research.

Reasons for Expecting Modest Brain–Behavior Correlations with a Laboratory Species

The extensive work of Selander and Yang (1970), studying isoalelic variation on 10,000 mice collected from over 300 different wild *mus musculus* populations and from a number of inbred laboratory strains, demonstrated conclusively that the gene pool of inbred strains was hardly representative of that found among wild mice. For many polymorphic loci studies, more alleles were represented in wild populations in Texas alone than in all of the inbred strains examined. The genetic variation represented in inbred laboratory strains is apparently only a fraction of the total variation in the species. The degree to which restricted genetic variation of laboratory mice leads to a restriction in phenotypic variation is dependent upon the phenotype being studied. It is likely, however, that restricting genetic variation will often result in narrowing the range of variation in phenotypes. Brain–behavior correlations obtained on laboratory populations are, therefore, often likely to be lower than those that might be found in natural populations, because of the well-known restriction of range effects on correlation.

Another reason one might anticipate low brain–behavior correlations with laboratory animals is that, unlike the situation involving human cognitive abilities, performance on animal learning tasks or other adaptive behaviors do not show consistently high, positive correlations. One can find zero correlations and even negative correlations among various measures of learning, which suggests that a variety of different and sometimes competing mechanisms are involved in these behaviors. We cannot, therefore, expect to find uniformly positive correlations between brain size and different measures of adaptive behaviors. A related issue concerns the relative reliability of cognitive performance measures used for testing humans, and those measures devised to test learning ability of laboratory rodents. Unlike its emphasis in the test and measurements field, measurement reliability is often secondary to other concerns in animal testing procedures. Except for work with extremely heterogeneous stock, the reliability of behavioral variables used in animal research probably ranges from .3 to .6 in most cases, considerably attenuating any brain–behavior correlations that may exist.

Of increasingly important concern to investigators of animal behavior is the meaningfulness of dependent variables with respect to the natural behaviors of the studied species. Laboratory measures of learning probably do tap some behaviors that have adaptive value for a species in its natural ecological niche, but the measures probably also correlate highly with general factors peculiar to laboratory test situations, such as reaction to shock or handling, which have little relation to evolutionary adaptive significance. A single learning measure will also contain variance specific to the individual task, as well as "error" variation; this may account for a rather large proportion of the total between-subject variance found. The single behavioral measure, therefore, consists of many sources of systematic and random variation, only a fraction of which is likely to overlap with brain size. A single measure of animal performance, such as trials to criterion on a specific learning task, is rather similar to a single item on a personality or aptitude test, which will have relatively little discriminating power if used alone. Investigators need a large number of similar items reflecting a common construct in order to obtain a clear picture of the relationship between a given structure and some other measure.

Brain size and more elaborate parameters of brain structure are probably imperfect in many of the ways just described for behavioral variables. Across a wide range of species, whole brain size may correlate highly with a large number of brain parameters, but this may not be the case within a species. The hippocampal region of the forebrain, for example, has been increasingly implicated in learning processes; however, the factor analysis of genetic correlations of brain volumes of inbred mice described by Wimer this volume, suggests that a brain weight-neocortex factor and a separate hippocampal-forebrain factor may exist for *mus musculus*. Furthermore, gross anatomical measures of the hippocampus seem less related to behavior changes than measures of neuronal activity (e.g., O'Keefe & Nadel, 1974). Although whole brain size may be correlated with this neuronal activity of the hippocampus, it is not likely to be a particularly strong relationship within a species. Finally, even when focusing on more specific areas of the brain, the hierarchical organization of brain function may elude even fine anatomical and neurophysiological measures.

Implications for Further Research

The prospects for finding unambiguous genetic relationships between behavioral variables and brain size within a species do not appear to be very promising with the present level of research effort. If we can expect that brain–behavior correlations will be of relatively low magnitude, such as in the .2–.3 range, considerably larger genetic samples will be necessary to detect such effects than have been used thus far. Using the preceding approach, for example, 10 × 10 or larger diallels would be necessary to achieve sufficient power to detect significant but modest correlations. If the data in the preceding study are indicative of the kind of brain–behavior relationships that are most likely to exist, we might have to focus on fairly complex measures of adaption to an environment, and also measure gradual changes in behavioral responses to environmental changes. Change scores involve the differences among scores based on repeated measurements, or on different independent groups of each genotype being studied. As a consequence, error variation is compounded; thus, relatively large samples within each genotype may be necessary to produce resonably reliable data. Although *EQ* appears to be an adequate estimate of several other brain parameters across species, this may not be true within species. Far more detailed measurements of brain components, such as those described by Drs. Wimer and Greenough in this volume, may be essential for detecting brain-behavior relationships.

The task, then, is a formidable one. Large samples of many genotypes, measurements of complex behaviors that change with differing environmental situations, and more detailed measures of brain structure appear to be minimal requirements for investigating the genetic relationship between brain and behavior within a species. It is unlikely many investigators will invest efforts in a project of this magnitude, yet, in the absence of a conceptual breakthrough that would focus investigators' efforts, smaller studies may continue to provide only minimal information on the relationship of brain characteristics to adaptive behavior.

References

Brunswick, E. *Perception and the representative design of psychological experiments* (2nd ed.). Berkeley, California: University of California Press, 1956.

Ehrman, L., & Parsons, P. A. *The genetics of behavior.* Sunderland, Massachusetts: Sinauer Associates, 1976.

Foster, M., & Sherrington, C. S. *A textbook of physiology.* (7th ed.). London: McMillan, 1897.

Fuller, J. L., & Wimer, R. E. Neural, sensory and motor functions. In E. L. Green (Ed.), *Biology of the laboratory mouse.* (2nd ed.). New York: McGraw-Hill, 1966.

Greenough, W. T. Experimental modification of the developing brain. *American Scientist,* 1975, *63,* 37–46.

Griffing, B. Concept of general and specific combining ability in relation to diallel crossing systems. *Australian Journal of Biological Sciences,* 1956, *9,* 463–493.

Hayman, B. I. The analysis of variance of diallel tables. *Biometrics,* 1954, *10* 235–244. (a)

Hayman, B. I. The theory and analysis of diallel crosses. *Genetics,* 1954, *39,* 789–809. (b)

Henderson, N. D. Prior treatment effects on open field emotionality: The need for representative design. *Annals of the New York Academy of Science,* 1969, *159,* 860–868.

Henderson, N. D. Genetic influences on the behavior of mice can be obscured by laboratory rearing. *Journal of Comparative and Physiological Psychology,* 1970, *72,* 505–511. (a)

Henderson, N. D. A genetic analysis of spontaneous alternation in mice. *Behavior Genetics,* 1970, *1,* 125–132. (b)

Henderson, N. D. Relative effects of early rearing environment and genotype on discrimination learning in house mice. *Journal of Comparative and Physiological Psychology,* 1972, *79,* 243–253.

Henderson, N. D. Brain weight changes resulting from enriched rearing conditions: a diallel cross analysis. *Developmental Psychobiology,* 1973, *6,* 367–376.

Jerison, H. J. *Evolution of the brain and intelligence.* New York: Academic Press, 1973.

Jinks, J. L. The analysis of continuous variation in a diallel cross of *Nicotiana rustica* varieties. *Genetics,* 1954, *39,* 767–788.

Jinks, J. L., & Mather, K. Stability in the development of heterozygotes and homozygotes. *Proceedings of the Royal Society,* B. 1955, *143,* 561–578.

Lashley, K. S. Basic neural mechanisms in behavior. *Psychological Review,* 1930, *37,* 1–24.

McClearn, G. E., & DeFries, J. C. *Introduction to behavioral genetics*. San Francisco: Freeman & Co., 1973.

O'Keefe, J. & Nadel, L. *The hippocampus as a cognitive map*. London: Oxford University Press, 1974.

Ramon y Cajal. La fine structure des centres nerveaus. *Proceedings of the Royal Society of London*, 1894, *55*, 444–468.

Rosenzweig, M. R., & Bennet, E. L. Enriched environments: Facts, factors and fantasies. In L. Petrinovich & J. L. McGaugh (Eds.), *Knowing, thinking and believing*. New York: Plenum Press, 1976.

Rundquist, E. A. Inheritance of spontaneous activity in rats. *Journal of Comparative Psychology*, 1933, *16*, 415–438.

Searle, L. V. The organization of hereditary maze-brightness and maze dullness. *Genetic Psychology Monographs*, 1949, *39*, 279–325.

Selander, R. K., & Yang, S. Y. Biochemical genetics and behavior in wild house mouse populations. In G. Lindzey, & D. D. Thiessen (Eds.), *Contributions to behavior genetic analysis: The mouse as a prototype*. New York: Appleton-Century-Crofts, 1970.

Thiessen, D. D. *Gene organization and behavior*. New York: Random House, 1972.

Tryon R. C. Genetic differences in maze learning ability in rats. *Yearbook of National Social Studies Education*, 1940, *39*, 111–119.

Wearden, S. Alternative analysis of the diallel cross. *Heredity*, 1964, *19*, 669–680.

Yates, F. The analysis of data from all possible reciprocal crosses between a set of parental lines. *Heredity*, 1947, *1*, 287–301.

Chapter XVIII

The Role of Development in the Brain–Behavior Relationship

MARTIN E. HAHN
CRAIG JENSEN
BRUCE C. DUDEK

In the symposium that served as the nucleus for this volume, Norm Henderson presented the last paper. As he was beginning, he jokingly pointed out that summarizing the entire symposium would be an easy task as we had, up to that point, only discussed the topics of: genetics of DNA, polygenes, normal probability, log-log plots, factor analysis of endocasts, discriminate analyses of brain parts, Piaget and growth spurts in the brain, the logic of recombinant inbred strains, analyses of residual correlations between brains and behavior, super nutrition and fetal brain development, audiogenic seizure onset, dopamine and norepinephrine levels in the brain, avoidance learning functions, cross-fostering effects on early behavior, infantile mouse learning and memory, correlations between variances in brain weight and absolute brain weights, dendritic spines and pyramidal cells, and a few other things.

We were tempted to refrain from any summary, but as we read all the papers in the volume, certain integrating ideas became overwhelmingly apparent. Before proceeding to our attempts at integration, we will summarize the new information presented by our contributors on the three questions that are central to the volume. The reader will note that in the summary, as compared to the first chapter, it is more difficult to discuss singly any of the central questions. All of the authors in the volume contributed to this happy situation by incorporating the ideas and conclusions of other participants into their own papers. As a prac-

DEVELOPMENT AND EVOLUTION
OF BRAIN SIZE

tical consequence, we modified the second question by excluding discussion of the behavioral results of genetic selection, and discussed that topic instead under the question of the importance of brain size for behavior.

What Is the Importance of Brain Size for Behavior?

On this question, a simple summary statement is possible—brain size is associated powerfully with behavior. Associations were observed within and between species on several tasks, and with variation in brain size introduced by several "treatments," for example, evolution, artificial selection, development, parental effects, and enriched environments.

Riddell described a research project designed to separate intelligence, (a general ability), from species' special abilities. After describing the search for a procedure likely to make that separation, he found that learning set performance was strongly related to N_c (Jerison's concept of extra cortical neurons) across species from rats to man. This demonstration is particularly impressive because of the difficulties of making valid cross-species comparisons.

Jensen had shown previously that lines of mice genetically selected for differential brain size did not exhibit any consistent relationship between brain size and behavior. When he investigated the same problem within heterogeneous stocks of mice, however, he found that brain size was positively correlated with performance on a variety of learning tasks. Jensen further argued that the failure to find a relationship between brain size and behavior in the selected lines demonstrates the appearance of special abilities, (via selection of correlated characters or random fixation of alleles), and therefore does not provide evidence against a brain size–behavior relationship.

In a different approach to the problem of brain size and behavior, Epstein reviewed evidence relating differential brain sizes, resulting from growth during development, and differential brain functioning. Though his chapter was full of interesting ideas, perhaps the most far reaching was that in humans, brain growth spurts are correlated highly with Piagetian stages of cognitive development. He added additional support for this relationship by pointing out that brain growth showed an additional spurt not associated with any Piagetian stage. Epstein then cited recent evidence for an additional cognitive stage that coincides with that predicted from the brain growth data.

The findings of Nagy added further support to the brain growth–behavior change concepts discussed by Epstein. In particular, Nagy found that in mice 24 hour memory of prior escapes, in a shock escape situation, appears between 9 and 11 days of age and is thus in the 9–13 day brain growth spurt for mice reported by Epstein. Thus, this period of rapid brain growth is associated with changes in memo. y capacity.

Hahn examined the effects of brain size on behavior after brain size is altered by selection and fostering. For most measures, brain size was positively correlated with rapid behavioral development. In addition, when cross-fostering resulted in increased or decreased brain size, some behaviors moved in tandem. Some behaviors, however, showed differences due to selection but not fostering. The results, therefore suggest that changes in brain size, resulting from genetic or environmental sources, have behavioral correlates; Hahn's results also indicate that the picture is complex, and that factors in addition to brain size may be operating.

Fuller also found that genetic selection resulted in behavioral change. In his chapter, Fuller noted that temporal patterns in brain growth were present in BWS-H and L mice (Fuller lines selected for high and low brain weight), but those changes were more complex than simple acceleration or retardation. In spite of the complexity, brain size was associated with differential susceptibility to audiogenic seizures. It is possible that the complex results found by Fuller and by Hahn are attributable to the action of correlated characters, or of random fixation, during brain weight selection. Those concepts were used by Jensen to explain similar results in selected lines, and these concepts were discussed thoroughly by Roderick in his chapter.

Though we have outlined evidence for a relationship between brain size and behavior, we have not attempted to describe the nature of that relationship. Though a full description is beyond the scope of this volume, much depends on the way in which the term "brain size" is used. We will pursue the usages and their implications later in this chapter.

What Are the Effects of Genetic Selection on Brain Substructures?

The essential notion embodied in this question is that of functional relationships among different anatomical systems. In an evolutionary sense, Holloway has referred to this as reorganization. The epigenetic viewpoint of the developing brain focuses on the temporal patterns of maturational events, which shape the adult form of nervous systems. By form, we mean both morphological and biochemical structure. Pertinent phenotypes under consideration here include dendritic arborization and the kinetics of neurotransmitter-receptor interaction. If, as Holloway has suggested, brain evolution is based on reorganizational or epigenetic events, then its effects should be observable in the relationships of brain substructures, or biochemical characters. Several chapters address this topic.

Holloway used allometric techniques to examine the predictive power of brain and body weights for defined anatomical structures in several primate species. His analyses showed that brain substructure sizes were predictable from brain and body weights. In addition, the residuals from his regressions contained enough predictive power to classify species in their correct taxa about 80% of the time. These results indicate an evolutionary tendency toward reorganization of the brain, in addition to the tendency toward encephalization shown by Jerison.

Wimer extended and supported Holloway's findings by demonstrating reorganization of substructures within a species. Initially, she performed a factor analysis on several brain and body measures for 11 inbred strains of mice. Her results indicate two factors—a general size factor involving the volumes of hippocampus, and of other forebrain structures. She then performed a factor analysis on measures taken on the Roderick–Wimer selected lines. This analysis indicated that the lines sorted out on both factors, and though there was some suggestion of line × replication differences, the most supported conclusion was that brain weight selection resulted in bigger and smaller brains, and proportional changes in substructures.

Two points in the papers of Holloway and Wimer invite further discussion. First, common to both papers is a separation of a general size factor and a hippocampal factor. It is of interest that the hippocampus achieves much of its development postnatally and seems to be related to cognitive processes. Perhaps genetic control over development of the hippocampus is somewhat separate from control of other areas. The second point deals with the relative importance of encephalization and reorganization. The predictive power of brain and body size for substructures is quite high compared to that for reorganization. Perhaps the portion of variance explained by reorganization is a misleading statistic, however, since evolution toward reorganization or encephalization would seem to have many behavioral implications.

In the chapters by Zamenhof and van Marthens, and by Dudek and Berman, the biochemical correlates of brain weight selection were examined. The results indicate that the gross biochemical characteristics of both the Roderick–Wimer and Fuller BWS lines were similar. DNA, thus cell count, was higher in high brain weight mice than in the low lines. This difference held for both adults and neonates, where DNA presumably reflected only neuron and neuroblast numbers. Thus it is likely that genetic selection for adult brain weight had its most marked effects postnatally, but was probably initiated by differential prenatal neuroblast formation. There were also some differences in the brain chemistry of mice of the two selection programs. The high and low Roderick–Wimer lines did not show difference in cell size (protein/ DNA). In the Fuller lines, the H line animals not only had more brain cells, but those cells were also larger. Thus the differentiation made by Greenough and Juraska, that genes determined cell numbers and environments determine cell size, does seem to hold in this case.

A final point from these studies relates to neurotransmitters as reported by Dudek and Berman. Their findings that neurotransmitter content and concentrations were related to mouse brain size may offer a unique way in which correlations between neural and behavioral development may be studied. Specifically, genetic and environmental influences over development of neurotransmitter systems should be reflected in behavioral development dependent on those systems.

Behavioral Consequences?

Henderson states that there has been a lack of progress in answering the question of whether genetic and environmental manipulations of brain size have similar behavioral consequences. However, the similarities in the behavioral outcomes resulting from those two "treatments" are impressive enough to indicate that an affirmative answer to this question is likely, when further research has been completed.

Greenough and Juraska provide an extensive review and discussion of the environmental side of this question. As they pointed out, enriched animals have larger brains than isolated animals, and learn complex tasks more rapidly. The results were not always consistent with a bigger brain–brighter animal hypothesis, however, since isolated animals performed better than enriched animals on some simple tasks.

Wimer reviewed the behavioral data for animals with differential brain size produced by genetic selection. She pointed out that high brain weight mice were consistently better learners during the early generations of selection in the Roderick–Wimer lines. However, in later generations, the consistent relationship began to break down. In addition, results from the Fuller BWS lines have shown no consistent relationship between brain size and learning ability. As has been discussed previously by Roderick, Jensen, and Hahn, care must be exercised when using the selected lines to test the brain-behavior relationship, especially after selection has proceeded for many generations.

Using mice that differed genetically, but had not undergone genetic selection, Jensen clearly demonstrated a relationship between brain size and learning ability. The heterogeneous population of mice used by Jensen may provide a better tool to evaluate brain–behavior relationships than selected lines.

Henderson examined the joint influences of genes and enrichment on the brain–behavior relationship. Interestingly, he found a relationship between brain size and a transfer of training measure (a task similar to that used to discriminate among species by Riddell). However, the transfer of training measure was only 1 of 14 behavioral measures examined, and in only two cases did learning correlate with brain size (*EQ* in this case). Henderson also found that enrichment improved transfer of training scores, and genotypes with larger brains demonstrated the greatest improvement. Thus, at least for this measure, brain size influenced by genes and brain size influenced by enrichment produced similar performance.

Overall, the chapters in this volume point toward but do not provide a definitive answer on whether environmental and genetic manipulations of brain size have similar behavioral consequences. We suggest that a solid answer to this question will require further work in at least two areas.

1. It has been suggested by Greenough and Juraska that the effects of genetic and environmental manipulations on brain substructures produce differences in numbers of neurons, and differences in numbers or properties of synaptic connections between neurons, respectively. We suggest that more work is required in this area.
2. The consequences of differing brain size by environmental or genetic effects have been examined primarily on learning behavior (some of Henderson's measures and the developing behaviors studied by Hahn are exceptions). We suggest, in agreement with Henderson, that a much greater number of behaviors need to be examined to assess truly the behavioral consequences of differential brain size.

Integrating Theme: The Role of Development in the Evolution of Brain Size

Taken together, the preceding chapters demonstrate that brain size can be manipulated in a variety of ways, and that changes in brain size are associated with a variety of behavioral changes (see Figure XVIII.1). Although a relationship has been demonstrated, the nature of that

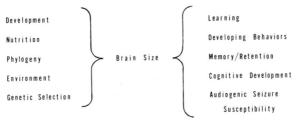

FIGURE XVIII.1. Various manipulations of brain size are associated with various behavioral changes.

relationship has not been made explicit. What is the role of brain size: causative agent, intervening variable, or the sum of the parts? In our opinion, brains size per se is not a causative agent. Rather, brain size estimates features of the brain that are more closely aligned with behavioral changes. Greenough and Juraska's dendritic trees, Dudek and Berman's neurotransmitters, and Zamenhof and van Marthens' cell numbers seem to make for a better understanding of behavioral processes than does brain size. The significance of brain size is the uncanny accuracy with which it estimates other anatomical features (Jerison & Wimer, this volume). Since brain size is an accurate statistic, it becomes a useful bit of shorthand to abbreviate the many changes that occur in the developing, evolving brain. Implicit in this view is that brain size is not a character on which natural selection could have acted directly. If that is the case, we must look to some explanation other than natural selection for the evolution of brain size. We think that the explanation may be found in the concept of development.

If there is a single integrating theme in this volume, it is the role of development. Development, like brain size, is a shorthand phrase. It is a way of referring to a number of events involved in the construction and integration of systems over time. More specifically for our purposes, development of the nervous system refers to the integration of sensory-motor, and association systems, over time. Furthermore, we view development as epigenetic in the same sense that Holloway used the term, that is information about the state of developing structures feeds back to the genetic level. We view development relating to brain size and behavior as summarized in the Figure XVIII. 2. A summary of the events depicted in the figure is as follows:

1. Selection operates on developing behaviors (e.g., the ability to find and attach to a mother's nipple, the use of behavior to regulate body temperature or the ability to give a distress vocalization).
2. Developing behaviors are based in the developing nervous system. By developing nervous system, we mean the growth, differentia-

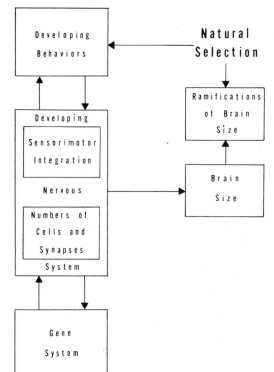

FIGURE XVIII.2. A view of the relationships among natural selection, developing behaviors, and brain size.

tion, and integration of sensory-motor and association systems. The nervous system exhibits a number of properties while developing, for example, rate of development, organization, and plasticity, all of which have potentially powerful influences on behavior. We have delineated two components in the nervous system: (*a*) integration of systems, (primarily an organizational component); and (*b*) numbers of cells, numbers of interconnections (primarily a size component). These two components certainly are related, but would seem to have somewhat separate gene systems underlying them, and also have different impact on brain size. Together, as the nervous system, they determine brain size.

3. The developing nervous system is structured by genotype × environment interaction, with feedback to the genetic level as development takes place.

4. Increases in brain size are not directly selected for, but are the result of brain growth during development, as outlined above. Increased brain size is not directly selected against, but its rami-

fications, e.g., metabolic cost (see Rosenzweig), or size of female birth canal in humans, may be selected against.

In this theory, rapid behavioral development might foster fitness. The developing behaviors are established by a rapidly growing and integrating nervous system. Periods of rapid growth would result in rapid increases in brain size and could result in adult differences, if the growth lasted for varying periods in different individuals. Brain size could not increase in an unlimited fashion, however, because its ramifications would be selected against. Perhaps, as Rosenzweig has hypothesized, brain plasticity in response to environmental demands affords a compromise between costs and benefits of brain size. Furthermore, in this theory, brain size would be positively correlated with cell numbers and other subbrain components, such as sensory-motor integration and behavioral development. It should be emphasized that "our" view is a synthesis of points from all the contributors. In particular, it is similar to portions of Holloway's chapter in which he argues that brain size is not a phenotype—rather the phenotype is the timing of natural events within the central nervous system. Our ideas were also inspired by Cairns' (1976) discussion of the relationship between ontogeny and phylogeny.

Is there any evidence for or against this position? At this writing, we know of no direct evidence testing the theory, but some indirect evidence does exist. As reported in this volume, Fuller's BWS lines and the Roderick-Wimer lines were the product of genetic selection for brain size. While brain size was altered by selection, it has also been shown that behavioral development also changed—a predictable result if developing behaviors and brain size are correlated as in our theory.

Falconer, Gauld, and Roberts (1978) showed that selective breeding for body size resulted in accelerated or decelerated processes of cellular growth—reflected in larger and more numerous cells. This phenomenon was paralleled in the Fuller BWS lines for brain size (see Dudek and Berman) and indicates at least a correlation between overall size of the brain or body and rates of cell growth. Further, our position is consistent with the very interesting results presented by Jerison. He showed that brain size was normally distributed and exhibited constant coefficients of variation across species over evolutionary time. This finding suggests that the shaper of brain size during evolution was an indirect stabilizing selection, rather than a direct and directional selection pressure. Unfortunately, none of the preceding studies directly test our theory.

We suggest that a place to begin in evaluating our theory would be to determine whether developing behaviors and brain size are correlated, as the theory predicts. A correlation study of brain weight and developing behavior in a heterogeneous population, followed by a selection for developing behavior, and examination of brain weight as selection progressed, should provide such information. In addition, it would be valuable to examine the genetic architecture of developing behaviors, using the theoretical framework outlined by Broadhurst and Jinks (1974). Such an analysis would allow statements about the fitness status of developing behaviors. Regardless of the outcome such studies, and many more that could be suggested, are necessary to further delineate the brain–behavior relationship.

Acknowledgments

We thank all of our participants. Without their fine contributions and efforts at integration, no final chapter would have been possible. Of course, errors or misconceptions in the concluding chapter are our own.

References

Broadhurst, P. L., & Jinks, J. L. What genetic architecture can tell us about the natural selection of behavioral traits. In J. H. F. van Abeelen (Ed.), *The genetics of behavior.* Amsterdam: The North-Holland Publishing Co., 1974.

Cairns, R. B. The ontogeny and phylogeny of social interactions. In M. E. Hahn & E. C. Simmel (Eds.), *Communicative behavior and evolution.* New York: Academic Press, 1976. Pp. 115–136.

Falconer, D. S. Gauld, I. K., & Roberts, R. C. Cell number and cell sizes in organs of mice selected for small and large body size. *Genetic Research at Cambridge,* 1978, *31,* 287–301.

Author Index

Numbers in italics refer to the pages on which the complete references are listed.

Subject Index